This is the first volume to look in depth at the way the brain responds to trauma and subsequently integrates and influences behavioural, metabolic, neurohumoral, cardiovascular and immune functions. It is becoming increasingly clear that the brain has an important role in the control and integration of the responses to injury and infection. It is well established that some of these responses, such as fever and neuroendocrine changes, are directly influenced by the central nervous system. These, and other more recent advances, provide new insights into this area and provide a basis for the more effective understanding and clinical management of trauma patients. The authors, all international authorities in their fields, discuss established and recent data from experimental and clinical studies and consider the implications of these findings for the treatment of the trauma patient.

# BRAIN CONTROL OF RESPONSES TO TRAUMA

# BRAIN CONTROL OF RESPONSES TO TRAUMA

*Edited by*

NANCY J. ROTHWELL
*School of Biological Sciences, University of Manchester*

FRANK BERKENBOSCH
*Department of Pharmacology, The Free University, Amsterdam*

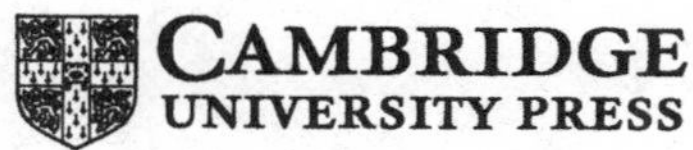

CAMBRIDGE
UNIVERSITY PRESS

CAMBRIDGE UNIVERSITY PRESS
Cambridge, New York, Melbourne, Madrid, Cape Town,
Singapore, São Paulo, Delhi, Tokyo, Mexico City

Cambridge University Press
The Edinburgh Building, Cambridge CB2 8RU, UK

Published in the United States of America by Cambridge University Press, New York

www.cambridge.org
Information on this title: www.cambridge.org/9780521338660



First published 1994
First paperback edition 2011

*A catalogue record for this publication is available from the British Library*

*Library of Congress Cataloguing in Publication data*
Brain control of response to trauma / edited by Nancy J. Rothwell,
Frank Berkenbosch.
p. cm.
Includes index.
ISBN 0 521 41939 5
1. Wounds and injuries. 2. Neuropsychology.
3. Neuroendocrinology. 4. Brain – Pathophysiology. I. Rothwell,
Nancy. II. Berkenbosch, Frank.
[DNLM: 1. Brain – physiology. 2. Wounds and Injuries. WL 102
B8123 1994]
RD93.B68 1994
612.8′2 – dc20 93-47587 CIP
DNLM/DLC
for Library of Congress

ISBN 978-0-521-41939-0 Hardback
ISBN 978-0-521-33866-0 Paperback

# Contents


*Contributors* *page* viii
1 Introduction *Nancy J. Rothwell* 1
2 Responses to injury *Harry B. Stoner* 3
3 Experimental approaches to the central nervous system control of responses to trauma *Roderick A. Little and Nancy J. Rothwell* 22
4 Neurohormonal control of cytokines during injury *Istvan Berczi and Eva Nagy* 32
5 Brain regions involved in modulation of immune responses *Brigitte Deleplanque and Pierre J. Neveu* 108
6 Psychological and neurobiological consequences of trauma *Barbara O. Rothbaum and Charles B. Nemeroff* 123
7 Central nervous system control of sickness behavior *Stephen Kent, Rose-Marie Bluthé, Glyn Goodall, Keith W. Kelley and Robert Dantzer* 152
8 Psychological and behavioural aspects of pain *Holger Ursin, Inger M. Endresen, Anders Lund and Norma Mjellem* 183
9 Central control of cardiovascular responses to injury *Emrys Kirkman and Roderick A. Little* 202
10 Neuroendocrine responses to physical trauma *Frank Berkenbosch* 239
11 Central control of metabolic and thermoregulatory responses to injury *Angela L. Cooper and Nancy J. Rothwell* 260
12 Central control of pain *Robert W. Clarke* 295
13 The final word . . . *Nancy J. Rothwell* 332
*Index* 334

# Contributors

Frank Berkenbosch
*Department of Pharmacology, Medical Faculty, Free University, van der Boechorststraat 7, 1081 BT Amsterdam, The Netherlands*

Istvan Berczi
*Department of Immunology, Faculty of Medicine, University of Manitoba, 795 McDermot Avenue, Winnipeg, Manitoba R3E 0W3, Canada*

Rose-Marie Bluthé
*INSERM-U 176, Rue Camille St Saëns, 33077 Bordeaux Cedex, France*

Robert W. Clarke
*Department of Physiology and Environmental Science, University of Nottingham, Sutton Bonington Campus, Loughborough, Leicester LE12 5RD, UK*

Angela L. Cooper
*Department of Physiological Sciences, Stopford Building, University of Manchester, Oxford Road, Manchester M13 9PT, UK*

Robert Dantzer
*INSERM-U 176, Rue Camille St Saëns, 33077 Bordeaux Cedex, France*

Brigitte Deleplanque
*Psychologie des Comportements Adaptifs, INSERM-U 259, Université de Bordeaux II, Domaine de Carnière 33077, Bordeaux, France*

Inger M. Endresen
*Department of Biological and Medical Psychology, Division of Physiological Psychology, University of Bergen, Arstadveien 21, N-5009 Bergen, Norway*

Glyn Goodall
*INSERM-U 176, Rue Camille St Saëns, 33077 Bordeaux Cedex, France*

Keith W. Kelley
*INSERM-U 176, Rue Camille St Saëns, 33077 Bordeaux Cedex, France*

Stephen Kent
*INSERM-U 176, Rue Camille St Saëns, 33077 Bordeaux Cedex, France*

Emrys Kirkman
*North Western Injury Research Centre, Stopford Building, University of Manchester, Oxford Road, Manchester M13 9PT, UK*

Roderick A. Little
*North Western Injury Research Centre, Stopford Building, University of Manchester, Oxford Road, Manchester M13 9PT, UK*

Anders Lund
*Department of Physiology, University of Bergen, Arstadveien 19, N-5009 Bergen, Norway*

Norma Mjellem
*Department of Physiology, University of Bergen, Aarstadveien 19, N-5009 Bergen, Norway*

Eva Nagy
*Department of Immunology, Faculty of Medicine, University of Manitoba, 795 McDermot Avenue, Winnipeg, Manitoba R3E 0W3, Canada*

Charles B. Nemeroff
*Department of Psychiatry and Behavioral Sciences, Emory University School of Medicine, 1365 Clifton Road, Atlanta, Georgia 30322, USA*

Pierre J. Neveu
*Psychologie des Comportements Adaptifs, INSERM-U 259, Université de Bordeaux II, Rue Camille Saint Saëns, 33077 Bordeaux Cedex, France*

Barbara O. Rothbaum
*Department of Psychiatry and Behavioral Sciences, Emory University School of Medicine, 1365 Clifton Road, Atlanta, Georgia 30322, USA*

Nancy J. Rothwell
*School of Biological Sciences, Stopford Building, University of Manchester, Oxford Road, Manchester M13 9PT, UK*

Harry B. Stoner
*North Western Injury Research Centre, Stopford Building, University of Manchester, Oxford Road, Manchester, M13 9PT, UK*

Holger Ursin
*Department of Biological and Medical Psychology, Division of Physiological Psychology, University of Bergen, Arstadveien 21, N-5009 Bergen, Norway*

# 1
# Introduction

NANCY J. ROTHWELL

It is obvious to most biologists and clinicians that in mammals the central nervous system coordinates and regulates many complex physiological events. In order to do this, it must receive information from the internal and external environment, integrate this information and elicit appropriate efferent signals required to respond to a stimulus and maintain homeostatic function.

The concept of the brain as a regulator of responses to pathogenic insults is somewhat recent and still poses many unanswered questions. This may have resulted in part from a tendency for studies on injury and inflammation to focus on local tissue factors and immune mediators. It has, of course, long been known that certain aspects of the host defence response, such as fever, are under central nervous system control. However, concepts such as the effects of stress on susceptibility to disease, or the sustained psychological responses following trauma, were only poorly understood and were considered by some to be undefined and unsuitable for rigorous scientific analysis. This situation is changing rapidly, not least because of the identification of molecules and mechanisms underlying direct communications between the brain and the immune system, and the realisation that these are not distinct and unrelated biological entities.

The objectives of this book have been to discuss current knowledge about how the brain responds to and influences host responses to trauma, and to consider the mechanisms of these interactions, the clinical relevance and potential for novel therapeutic interventions. In spite of enormous advances in this field over the past decade, it will be clear that for each question that has been answered, a number of others have been raised.

The planning of this book and most of the work in editing was carried out collaboratively with Dr Frank Berkenbosch at the University of

Amsterdam. Frank died tragically at the age of only thirty-nine, shortly before completion of this book. With the agreement of all of the contributors, the book has been dedicated to his memory. I believe that this is a fitting tribute, not simply because of his work on many of the subjects covered in this book, or because of his scientific and social interaction with several of the contributors, but also because the very nature of the subject closely reflects Frank's outstanding contribution to scientific research. His work spanned neuroendocrinology, immunology, fever, responses to stress, injury and infection, and sought to answer basic scientific questions as well as to solve important clinical problems. He contributed novel findings and innovative approaches, collaborated with scientists in different countries with varied backgrounds and interests, and stimulated discussion and enthusiasm in science. Last, but not least, to those who knew him well, Frank Berkenbosch was an extremely likeable and warm individual with a great sense of humour, who will be sadly missed.

# 2

# Responses to injury

HARRY B. STONER

## Historical aspects

Injury is such a frequent occurrence that its effects must have been among the earliest of the biological responses to have been investigated. Indeed, the salient features of the local response, inflammation, have been known from the time of Celsus (quoted by Majno, 1964) in the first century A.D. Realisation that there was a general response by the body to a local injury came later and was probably first described by Paré in 1582. Paré was a military surgeon, and later advances have almost always been linked to warfare. For most of the time injury and its effects can be conveniently ignored by doctor and lay-person alike but in wartime it obtrudes on general consciousness. Hence, our appreciation of these responses was advanced by military surgeons such as Clowes (1591), Hunter (1794), Guthrie (1815) and above all by Larrey (see Dible, 1970), who laid the foundations for the modern treatment of trauma.

Despite numerous conflicts, progress since the work of Larrey has been extremely slow for, although it was realised that injury provoked a response by the body, little attempt was made to understand the coordination of the response.

### *Causation of 'shock'*

Much of the time between the two World Wars was spent in the search for a single cause for what was usually called 'shock'. This term was probably first used in the English literature by Latta (1795) but has never been clearly defined (Grant & Reeve, 1951). Three candidates were considered as possible causes – fluid loss, toxic factors and nervous influences. The last of these had been introduced by Crile (1899), who sought to explain the cardiovascular decline of the injured patient by

Table 2.1. *Phases of response to injury*

| Phase | Activator | Mediator | Response |
|---|---|---|---|
| Pre-injury | Danger | Special senses | *Defence reactions*<br>Loss of thermoregulatory and cardio-vascular homeostasis<br>Diversion of blood supply to brain, heart and muscles |
| Early, 'ebb' | Trauma | Afferent nociceptive stimuli<br>Fluid loss<br>Toxic factors | *Physiological responses*<br>Activation of sympathetic–adrenal medullary system with redistribution of blood and liberation of energy stores<br>Liberation of vasopressin<br>Production of hypothalamic releasing hormones<br>Liberation of ACTH, growth hormone<br>Stimulation of adrenal cortex<br>Impaired homeostasis<br>Thermoregulatory<br>Cardiovascular |
| Late, necrobiosis (shock) | Failure of $O_2$ transport | Hypoxaemia<br>Toxic factors | *Pathological responses*<br>Organ and tissue failure leading to death<br>Rising plasma [lactate] |
| 'Flow' (recovery) | Wound-organ | Lactate, prostaglandins, cytokines, autocoids | Increased cardiac output<br>Increased $O_2$ consumption<br>Negative N balance, fever |

fatigue of the nervous centres involved. This was soon dismissed and interest in the later attempts by O'Shaughnessy & Slome (1934; Slome & O'Shaughnessy, 1938) and by Overman & Wang (1947) to determine the role of the afferent nervous barrage from the injured tissue was short lived. The main argument was between fluid loss and toxic factors and was generally thought to have been decided by Blalock (1931) in favour of fluid loss – either externally as in haemorrhage or internally as in the oedema around damaged tissue. This seemed to bring together haemorrhage and tissue damage under a single umbrella. While it is true that the fluid loss into damaged tissue was often underestimated, real differences between the responses to haemorrhage and tissue damage were ignored. It is only during the last 50 years that the view has slowly developed that the responses to injury form a continuum, from the time of injury (even before in some cases) to eventual recovery or death, in which various factors play major roles at different times.

One reason for slow progress in this subject is scientific compartmentation. Although it has been recognised that the responses to injury involve many functions of the body each investigator seems to have seen them only in terms of his or her discipline – as a cardiovascular phenomenon, as an endocrine response or as a metabolic phenomenon. With overspecialisation few have been able to see the totality of the response. This has delayed the understanding of the order of events after injury. The existence of an order was pointed out by Cuthbertson (1942) and the subsequent development of his 'ebb and flow' idea (Stoner, 1993) indicated that injury was first followed by a period, the 'ebb phase', in which tissue oxygenation was adequate and during which widespread changes occurred. This was followed, either by a failure of $O_2$ transport and decline to death (shock/necrobiosis) or recovery through a 'flow phase'. Each phase has clear markers and a different causation (Table 2.1).

### *Endocrine response*

It might have been thought that the study of the endocrine response to trauma would have led quickly to that of the role of the central nervous system. This was not to be and compartmentation again seems to have been to blame. Physiologists engrossed in the experimental study of 'sham rage' and the defence reaction did not pass on to surgeons the relevance of their findings that showed that changes usually associated with injury could have begun even before it happened, if the danger was appreciated. Similarly, when knowledge of the endocrine response to injuries began to grow from the work of Cannon (1929) on the adrenal medulla and sympathetic nervous system, endocrinologists seemed more concerned with the peripheral effects of the hormones than with the way in which the endocrine response was triggered through the central nervous system.

This was also the case when the importance of the adrenal cortex in the response to injury began to be appreciated in the 1940s. Although the link between the anterior lobe of the pituitary and the adrenal cortex was soon discovered, it was some time before the role of the hypothalamus in stimulating the pituitary–adrenal axis was realised. Before that, other mechanisms such as positive feedback and stimulation of the anterior hypophysis by adrenaline were considered. Positive feedback due to early consumption of adrenocortical hormones was never demonstrated and although adrenaline is a factor in the release of adrenocorticotrophic hormone (ACTH) (Buckingham, 1985) and the circulating levels of adrenaline can be very high after severe injury (Little *et al.*, 1985; Frayn *et al.*, 1985), high enough to penetrate those parts of the brain with a poor blood–brain barrier, it is not the main stimulus. Understanding of this followed the demonstration of the direction of flow in the pituitary portal system and the isolation of the corticotrophin-releasing hormone produced by the parvocellular nuclei of the paraventricular hypothalamus.

Despite this, people seemed able to continue to view the hypothalamus as different, almost separate, from the rest of the brain in spite of its wealth of anatomical connections. Little was done to investigate how the parvocellular nuclei of the paraventricular hypothalamus were stimulated by distant trauma. An exception is the work by Swingle *et al.* (1944), Gibbs (1969*a*, *b*), Greer *et al.* (1970) and Feldman *et al.* (1971). From their work it would seem that, after trauma, nociceptive impulses, not necessarily associated with pain, ascend in the contralateral spinothalamic tracts and stimulate the appropriate hypothalamic neurones, although the precise intracerebral pathways are not known.

Although, since the work of Cannon, there has been a growing appreciation of the importance of the early activation of the sympathetic–adrenal medullary system in diverting blood to the brain, heart and muscles and in liberating energy-yielding substrates from the stores of glycogen and triacylglycerol and, later, of the importance of the hypothalamic–pituitary–adrenal axis, the role of the posterior hypophysis has often been ignored. It was shown by Ginsburg & Heller (1953) that vasopressin was very rapidly released in response to haemorrhage and it is also released in response to accidental trauma (Anderson *et al.*, 1989).

In fact, vasopressin is probably the first of the pituitary hormones to be secreted. Vasopressin will reinforce the effects of the sympathetic–adrenal medullary system, since it is a pressor compound and induces hepatic glycogenolysis (Clark, 1928). Hems & Whitton (1980) have pointed out that the early breakdown of glycogen will have a bonus because it will free the water associated with the glycogen molecule, which can then be used to counteract a volume deficit.

The clinician should realise that the endocrine response to trauma is very rapid and is usually fully developed by the time the patient reaches hospital, say, in an urban area, 20–30 min after the accident.

### *Role of the central nervous system*

Despite the growing appreciation of the importance of the endocrine response to injury, it was still some time before a role in response to injury was allotted to the brain as a whole. By the 1950s it had been shown that there were differences between the response to simple fluid loss, as in haemorrhage, and loss of fluid accompanying tissue damage (Tabor & Rosenthal, 1947). It has also been shown that the effects of fluid loss were aggravated by afferent nerve stimulation (Overman & Wang, 1947). The implications of these findings were widely ignored, particularly by clinicians. An exception was Tibbs (1956), who pointed out that patients could tolerate much greater blood loss if it was not accompanied by tissue damage.

### *Control of body temperature in the 'ebb' phase*

Tabor & Rosenthal (1947) showed that whole body $O_2$ consumption by mice after haemorrhage or bilateral hind-limb ischaemia was less than appropriate at environmental temperatures below thermoneutral. After haemorrhage this was due to failure of $O_2$ transport and could be corrected by administering $O_2$, but this was not the case in the early stage of the response to limb ischaemia. A detailed examination of the reasons for this difference has shown that the animals with bilateral hind-limb ischaemia were unable to thermoregulate properly. This disability is found in other species and after other injuries (e.g. burns; Stoner, 1991). It also occurs earlier than was described by Tabor & Rosenthal (1947), for it commences during the period of limb ischaemia, not just after the tourniquets have been removed (Stoner, 1971). At this early stage after an injury, the reduced response to cold was not due to failure to appreciate the stimulus (Stoner, 1972) or to failure of the peripheral response mechanism. Trauma inhibits both the non-shivering and shivering thermogenic responses to a cold stimulus so that a colder stimulus has to be applied to the exterior of the animal or to the hypothalamus in order to produce a response. However, once the response had been initiated the gain of the response was the same as in the normal state (Stoner, 1969, 1971, 1974).

Further work showed that the alterations in thermoregulatory heat production were due to nociceptive afferent impulses, not necessarily painful ones, carried from the injured areas by non-medullated and fine medullated fibres i.e. C and A$\delta$, with the impulses from the dorsal horns ascending in contralateral spinothalamic tracts. The primary target for these impulses appears to be noradrenergic pools in the hindbrain. When these neurone pools are stimulated, impulses ascend in the ventral bundle to liberate noradrenaline in the region of the dorsomedial nucleus of the hypothalamus and so inhibit shivering (Stoner & Elson, 1971; Stoner *et al.*, 1973; Stoner & Marshall, 1975*a*, *b*, 1977; Stoner & Hunt, 1976; Stoner, 1977; Marshall & Stoner, 1979*a*, *b*). It is not known if the same neurone pools and transmitters are involved in the inhibition of non-shivering thermogenesis, which is apparently more resistant to inhibition than shivering thermogenesis. For instance, in the injury produced in the rat by hindlimb tourniquets, $O_2$ consumption can still be increased to maintain body temperature in response to the postural decrease in insulation during the period of limb ischaemia (Stoner & Marshall, 1971), although shivering is inhibited at that time (Stoner, 1971).

An effect of these changes in the small mammal is a fall in core temperature in environments where it would normally be maintained. However, the acute effects of injury on thermoregulation are not confined to heat production, for the heat loss pathway is also inhibited. In the injured rat more heat has to be applied to the hypothalamus to dilate the arteriovenous anastomoses in the tail than in the normal rat (Stoner, 1972).

The central neural network for thermoregulation is probably similar in all mammals (Bligh, 1979), but the relative importance of the two controlling paths, heat production and heat loss, varies with body weight (Heldmaier, 1971). In a small mammal like the rat, the main variable is heat production, whereas in larger mammals, including adult humans, it is heat loss. A consequence of differences in body weight can be seen in the changes in core temperature after trauma when the environmental temperature is below the thermoneutral zone. In rats and mice under these conditions trauma leads to a rapid fall in core temperature, whereas in humans such falls are seen only after severe injuries, when failure of $O_2$ transport may be a factor (Little & Stoner, 1981). Nevertheless, the same type of central change after injury can be demonstrated in the human as in the rat. For instance, shivering is not seen in injured patients when their body temperature falls below the normal threshold for its onset (Little & Stoner, 1981; L. Martineau, personal communication). On the other hand the threshold for the onset of sweating is raised in the child with burn injury (Childs *et al.*, 1990*b*).

Behavioural thermoregulation is important in all species and this too is affected by injury. In humans there is a very good negative relationship between the preferred temperature for water sprayed on the back of the hand and the core temperature. This relationship is lost in patients with moderately severe injuries (fractures). The injured patients examined all opted for a high water temperature irrespective of core temperature (Little *et al.*, 1986). The desire for a warm environment has been described after burn injury (Wilmore, 1977; Henane *et al.*, 1981).

The overall effect of these changes is to reduce the responses to both heat and cold and widen the 'dead space' (thermoneutral zone) between the onset of thermoregulatory heat production and loss. In the human and the rat the normal bounds of this zone are 28–32 °C. The effect of injury, in the 'ebb' phase, does not represent a change in thermoregulatory set-point, for then the thresholds would have moved in the same, not opposite, direction. This is confirmed in humans, since the change in behavioural thermoregulation after trauma is very different from that seen after a change in set-point (Cabanac & Massonnet, 1974).

### *Cardiovascular homeostasis*

Thermoregulation is not the only homeostatic system to be disrupted by trauma, for the baroreceptor control of the cardiovascular system is also disturbed. Again this is due to nociceptive afferent impulses generated in damaged tissue and reaching the spinal cord via C and A$\delta$ fibres. In this case the primary target in the brain is different and is probably in the periaqueductal grey matter (PAG). From there, impulses go to the hypothalamus and vagal nuclei leading to inhibition of a number of reflex responses. Noradrenaline is not involved as a central transmitter in these effects but is important in another reflex response to damaged tissue, particularly ischaemic muscle, namely the rise in systolic blood pressure in the Alam and Smirk reflex (Alam & Smirk, 1937, 1938*a*, *b*; Stoner & Marshall, 1975*a*). A detailed description of the cardiovascular or homeostatic changes following trauma are given in Chapter 3; they may be summarized here as follows.

In addition to the Alam and Smirk reflex, tissue damage leads to inhibition of those reflexes in which the afferent limb arises from the arterial baroreceptors. Consequently in injured patients and animals there is a reduced reflex response to body tilting, the Valsalva manoeuvre, phenylephrine infusion or direct stimulation of the carotid baroreceptors by neck suction (Little, 1979; Little & Stoner, 1983; Little *et al.*, 1984; Redfern *et al.*, 1984; Anderson *et al.*, 1990). Not only is there a decrease in the sensitivity of the responses but, in the case of the last two, there is also resetting of the responses. The difference between the effects of simple fluid loss and tissue damage is even greater than in the case of thermoregulation, as after haemorrhage the sensitivity of the baroreceptor reflexes can be increased.

These effects of nociceptive afferent stimuli may explain why the outlook after haemorrhage combined with tissue damage is worse than after haemorrhage alone. Nevertheless, it is surprising that an injury should be accompanied by impairment of a homeostatic system on which so much is thought to depend. It is also remarkable that in humans these changes appear after injuries of very moderate severity (injury severity scores 4 and 9) (Baker *et al.*, 1974) that are not life-threatening.

A further action of the nociceptive stimuli on a response to a very severe injury should be mentioned. When haemorrhage is sufficiently severe to reduce cardiac filling to such a degree that it deforms the heart and stimulates cardiac C fibres it leads to vagal bradycardia. This vagal response is also inhibited by nociceptive afferent impulses from damaged tissue so that the blood loss required to produce the bradycardia is increased (Little, 1989).

It would seem from what has been written above that inhibition of homeostasis, both thermoregulatory and cardiovascular, is likely when muscle is damaged either directly by vascular occlusion or indirectly by fractures, which will also interfere to a varying degree with local muscle nutrition. It is likely that the afferent nociceptive impulses that arise from these damaged tissues commence their centripetal journey from polymodal receptors stimulated by such factors as a change in pH (Mense & Stahnke, 1983; Hoheisel & Mense, 1990). The fibres that carry these impulses are themselves resistant to hypoxia (Ochoa *et al.*, 1972).

### *Relation to defence (arousal) reaction*

The changes in homeostasis described above are those that occur after injury. Similar changes, e.g. inhibition of thermoregulation (Stitt, 1976) and of the baroreceptor reflexes (Folkov & Neil, 1971), form part of the defence (arousal) reaction along with active vasodilation of the arterial supply to the musculature. These changes can precede an injury because they are brought into play by the appreciation of danger through the special senses. Although the same midbrain structures (hypothalamus, PAG) are involved, the genesis of these changes implies the cooperation of many more parts of the brain – visual, auditory and olfactory cortices and, it is thought, the amygdala.

These changes form part of Cannon's 'fight or flight' response. If the danger passes without injury then the bodily disturbance will also pass away and conditions return to normal. However, if injury occurs, the impairment of homeostasis will continue into the 'ebb' phase.

### *Duration of response*

When the injury is not preceded by any sense of danger, i.e. there is no defence reaction, the inhibition of homeostasis is established quite quickly. For instance, in ischaemic limb injury in the rat, denervation of the limbs with bupivacaine is effective in preventing inhibition of shivering in response to cold only if it is carried out within 15 min of applying the tourniquets (Stoner & Marshall, 1982). Later denervation is ineffective. The fact that these changes in the function of the central nervous system are inaugurated around the time of the injury has clear clinical implications. It is obviously important to treat the injured patient as soon as possible in order to reduce fear, to reduce the size of the injury and to limit the barrage of nociceptive afferent impulses.

Although we are concerned here with research on accidental trauma, the findings also have implications for elective surgery. Nociceptive afferent impulses arising during operative trauma will have similar effects that will not disappear when the patient recovers from anaesthesia. It is important to realise that surgical patients have difficulty in regaining euthermia after an operation and also in accommodating changes in fluid distribution. These events must be taken into account not only in planning the treatment but also in interpreting the variables such as pulse rate (Little, 1989). Regional anaesthesia could be more widely used in the postoperative management of patients. Inhibition of homeostasis will continue through the 'ebb' phase. This phase may be very short after serious trauma. What happens next depends on $O_2$ transport.

### *Necrobiosis*

If the injury is very serious, or if the early treatment has not been sufficiently vigorous, the transport of $O_2$ to the tissues may fail and then a state of necrobiosis, often called shock, will supervene (Stoner, 1993). In this state, which may end in death, the inhibition of homeostasis will continue and be reinforced by progressive failure of the effector organs and, indeed, of the central mechanisms, through lack of $O_2$. Ensuring that tissues receive satisfactory amounts of $O_2$, which may be more than under normal conditions (Shoemaker, 1986), must be the prime aim in treatment of the injured at all stages.

### *Cerebral perfusion*

This is an appropriate point to indicate that the brain can function only if it receives adequate amounts of $O_2$ and substrate, usually glucose. Of all the organs, the brain is perhaps the most sensitive in this respect. This means that the brain must be adequately perfused with blood and this depends on the blood pressure or more particularly the cerebral perfusion pressure, i.e. the difference between the mean arterial pressure and the cerebrospinal fluid pressure. Cerebral blood flow is autoregulated so that with normovolaemia the flow does not fall until the systolic pressure drops below 40 mmHg (1 mmHg $\approx$ 133 Pa). This system may not function so well in the injured (Yates, 1990). It is of particular interest that in most models of fatal haemorrhage the blood pressure is reduced to about 40 mmHg and held there, often for long periods (Wiggers, 1950). These matters have been discussed elsewhere (Stoner & Cremer, 1985), both in relation to peripheral trauma and to head injury itself. The study of reduced cerebral perfusion is almost a separate subject and there is a large literature on the lesions of the brain it produces. However, the possibility of such effects must always be borne in mind when hypotension occurs. This is especially the case in work on haemorrhagic shock using the Wiggers model, or its variants, where very low blood pressures are produced[1]. Ischaemic brain damage would seem inevitable when these methods are used to produce 'irreversible shock'.

Fortunately for the thesis that the central nervous system is involved in the response to trauma, changes in the homeostasis of thermoregulation, both physiological and behavioural, and the cardiovascular system can be demonstrated at times when hypotension is not a problem.

### *'Flow' phase*

If recovery occurs, the injured patient passes into the 'flow' phase but the impaired homeostasis of the earlier stage does not rapidly disappear. In the rat with a non-lethal scald, for instance, it is 3 days before the rat starts to respond, tentatively, to a cold stimulus (Stoner, 1968). In injured people the changes in behavioural thermoregulation disappear very slowly as do those in the baroreflexes. It may be 2 to 3 weeks before the patient's responses are normal (Little *et al.*, 1986; Anderson *et al.*, 1990). It is remarkable that quite small injuries are so rapidly followed by major changes in reflex behaviour that persist for such a long time.

However, the 'flow' phase is not just a simple return to normal for there are many additional changes, and it is often described as a period of hypermetabolism. This is because $O_2$ consumption is usually increased and there is a net loss of nitrogenous tissue, particularly in the form of muscle. The full explanation of these changes is not yet clear but many of them appear to be due to the presence of the wound and its interaction with the rest of the body (Wilmore & Stoner, 1994). The wound behaves as if it is a separate organ that has been added to the body. Consisting of healing soft tissues and bone, it makes considerable demands of the body. It needs blood to fill and perfuse the new vessels, which will not be under nervous control. Cardiac output may have to be doubled to meet this demand, akin to that of an arteriovenous fistula. The wound requires heat, particularly if it has an exposed granulating surface from which water is evaporating. The energy supplies of the wound are derived from aerobic glycolysis rather than the usual mitochondrial oxidation. This consumes large amounts of glucose and feeds back into the body large amounts of lactate, which are reconverted into glucose in the liver, an oxygen-requiring process. In addition to lactate the wound also feeds back into the body various autocoids and cytokines. The cytokines are produced by the activated macrophages and other cells of the wound. The interleukin family of cytokines is of special interest, since it contains pyrogens, which cause fever by raising the hypothalamic set-point. The action of the interleukins will be considered in Chapter 4.

**Interpretations and questions**

The central nervous system is clearly involved in all stages of the body's response to injury. Does this knowledge help us to treat the injured patient? At the present time the treatment of the injured patient can be very briefly summarised as the arrest of haemorrhage, the maintenance of an airway and tissue oxygenation, early evacuation, the replacement of lost fluid, the early removal of dead tissue, the reduction of fractures and the disposition of the body, for instance by surgical repair and reconstruction, so that healing may occur. Although we now possess a range of drugs capable of influencing nervous function, our knowledge is still insufficient to allow their use in these patients, apart from the control of pain. If we are going to attempt 'central therapy' we must first know the precise nature and mechanism of the central nervous system responses to trauma and our knowledge of these is still incomplete.

We must also be able to interpret these responses. What is their object? What are they intended to achieve? Do they have survival value? This may seem like a teleological approach to the problem but in biology this can often be justified (Krebs, 1954). Without some idea of whether these responses are 'good' or 'bad', whether or not they are helpful to the injured person/animal, whether they have been developed to increase the chances of survival or whether they are just evolutionary remnants that can be altered as we think fit, we shall not be able to proceed. As yet only partial answers can be given to these questions.

The changes in the body during the defence reaction seem useful. Faced with danger there is no point in carefully controlling the blood pressure or temperature. The changes that occur seem well suited to 'fight or flight' and should have survival value.

However, why should the inhibition of homeostasis continue into the 'ebb' phase and beyond? At these times the effects of homeostasis might be considered beneficial – indeed, it is often taught that this is the object of these mechanisms. While these mechanisms play their expected part in the response to simple fluid loss and may have their sensitivity increased for the occasion (Little *et al.*, 1984), they are inhibited when other factors such as damaged tissue are introduced. Strange as it may seem, this is also beneficial, at least for the small mammal.

An example of this benefit in the injured small mammal is the optimum environmental temperature for survival that is below the thermoneutral zone (Tabor & Rosenthal, 1947; Green & Stoner, 1950; Haist, 1960). For the rat this optimum temperature is about 20 °C, so that the core temperature falls moderately but not to such a low level that when the rat starts to recover it cannot restore its body temperature unaided. (If the core temperature falls below 30 °C the injured rat will usually die.) The beneficial effect of a moderate hypothermia in the injured small mammal may be explained by its effect in reducing the consumption of the body's energy stores at a time when foraging may not be possible (Stoner, 1976). The accompanying hyperglycaemia and switch to fat as the main fuel for oxidation will also be beneficial (Stoner, 1987).

If the fall in core temperature is prevented, by increasing the environmental temperature or by pharmacological means, the mortality rate is increased and the survival time shortened (Tabor & Rosenthal, 1947; Green & Stoner, 1950; Stoner, 1958, 1961; Stoner & Little, 1969*a*, *b*). The intraventricular injection of 6-hydroxydopamine 7 days before injury also increased the sensitivity of rats to ischaemic limb injury but it is not certain that this was due to the effect of the drug's action on the central noradrenergic terminals producing the changes in thermoregulation (Stoner & Marshall, 1975*a*). It may reflect an action of 6-hydroxydopamine on central noradrenergic terminals involved with the cardiovascular system, for instance in the Alam and Smirk reflex (Redfern *et al.*, 1984). While it is possible to see benefit in the inhibition of thermoregulatory homeostasis, it is difficult to understand what benefit is derived at this time after injury from inhibition of cardiovascular homeostasis.

Before considering these alterations in reflex activity as they relate to injured humans, it should be pointed out that if they are evolutionary adaptations to meet the ever present threat of trauma they have been made on the basis that the injured animal will not receive treatment. Treatment can change the situation. Tabor and Rosenthal (1947) found that when injured mice were treated with 0.9% (w/v) NaCl the optimum environmental temperature rose from 19 to 25 °C.

For injured humans the questions are the same. How valuable is the inhibition of homeostasis when the patient will soon be treated? The degree of inhibition is related to the size of the injury. Treatment by fluid replacement and surgery will reduce the injury but perhaps not quickly enough to reduce the size of the nervous response. The early effects on homeostasis may persist; do we need them? Again, what are the aims of the changes in homeostasis? Are they ones that we should sustain and assist or can they be disregarded? Our attitude might vary with the time after injury. Chien (1967), discussing the role of sympathetic vasoconstriction in the response to trauma, pointed out that there are times when it would be useful to increase the vasoconstriction whereas at others it would be better to reduce it.

Although the same paths of thermoregulation are inhibited by trauma in the human and the rat, because the main controlling variable is different (heat loss in the human, heat production in the rat) the overall effect on body temperature is different (see above). Hypothermia can be used therapeutically in patients, e.g. in head injury and during carotid endarterectomy, but there is no early fall in core temperature after trauma, indeed it tends to rise after injuries of minor or moderate severity (see Carli *et al.*, 1992; for the effect of elective operation). With the patient's desire for a warm environment it is fortunate that there is no evidence that nursing the patient in a thermoneutral (28–32 °C) environment has the disastrous effect seen in the rat. However, exposure to higher or localised heat (heat cradles) may not be without effect.

Pyrexia often occurs during recovery from an injury in humans, most frequently during the 'flow' phase. The merits, or otherwise, of fever have long been debated. It is doubtful if there is a simple answer to the question. Although in the adult patient pyrexia is usually a 'flow' phase phenomenon, in burned children, where it is common, the maximum temperature is reached about 12 h after the burn (Childs, 1988). The mechanism of this pyrexia is not entirely understood but it may involve pyrogenic interleukins (Childs *et al.*, 1990*a*) and is reduced by cyclooxygenase inhibitors, although their effect is transient (Childs & Little, 1988). Here the best course is probably to treat the patient in a thermoneutral environment. Since the height of the pyrexia is not affected by the ambient temperature, this will reduce the amount of heat that has to be stored to produce this pyrexia. It may also alter the way in which the extra heat is obtained. Morimoto *et al.* (1988) showed, in the rabbit, that the heat required to produce a pyrexia after the injection of a pyrogen in a cool environment was achieved by increasing heat production, whereas in a warm environment the same pyrexia was produced by decreasing heat loss. For a sick patient the latter method is preferable, since it is less of a drain on the body's energy reserves.

Only some aspects of the effect of peripheral injury on the behaviour of the central nervous system have been discussed here. Many other aspects are dealt with in other chapters of this book. It is a large subject that is just beginning to unfurl. None of the changes can yet be completely explained or understood and this limits our use of the wide range of centrally active drugs that are becoming available in increasing number. There is plenty of scope for the further study of this subject and the results should lead to a considerable improvement in our ability to treat the injured patient.

## Note

1. The aim of the Wiggers dog model (Wiggers, 1950) is to produce a fatal haemorrhagic state. The systolic blood pressure of the anaesthetised dog is suddenly reduced to 50 mmHg and kept there by further bleeding for 90 min. The blood pressure is then reduced to 30 mmHg for a further 45 min when all the blood is restored to the circulation. The recovery of the blood pressure is short lived and the dog usually dies (82%, in Wiggers, 1950) within 6 h.

## References


Alam, M. & Smirk, F. H. (1937). Observations in man upon a blood pressure raising reflex arising from the voluntary muscles. *J. Physiol.*, **89**, 372–83.

Alam, M. & Smirk, F. H. (1938*a*). Observations in man upon a pulse accelerating reflex from the voluntary muscles of the legs. *J. Physiol.*, **92**, 167–77.

Alam, M. & Smirk, F. H. (1938*b*). Observations in man concerning the effects of different types of sensory stimulation upon the blood pressure. *Clin. Sci.*, **3**, 253–8.

Anderson, I. D., Forsling, M. L., Little, R. A. & Pyman, J. A. (1989). Acute injury is a potent stimulus for vasopressin release in man. *J. Physiol.*, **416**, 28P.

Anderson, I. D., Little, R. A. & Irving, M. H. (1990). An effect of trauma on human cardiovascular control: baroreflex suppression. *J. Trauma*, **30**, 974–82.

Baker, S. P., O'Neil, B., Haddon, W. & Long, W. B. (1974). The injury severity score; a method for describing patients with multiple injuries and evaluating emergency care. *J. Trauma*, **14**, 187–96.

Blalock, A. (1931). Experimental shock VI-X. *Arch. Surg.*, **22**, 598–648.

Bligh, J. (1979). The central neurology of mammalian thermoregulation. *Neurosci.*, **4**, 1213–36.

Buckingham, J. C. (1985). Hypothalamus–pituitary responses to trauma. *Br. Med. Bull.*, **41**, 203–11.

Cabanac, M. & Massonnet, B. (1974). Temperature regulation during fever; change of set-point or change of gain? A tentative answer from a behavioural study in man. *J. Physiol.*, **238**, 561–8.

Cannon, W. B. (1929). *Bodily Changes in Pain, Hunger, Fear and Rage*, 2nd edn. New York: Appleton.

Carli, F., Webster, J., Nandi, P., Macdonald, I. A., Pearson, J. & Mehta, R. (1992). Thermogenesis after surgery: effect of perioperative heat conservation and epidural anesthesia. *Am. J. Physiol.*, **263**, E441–7.

Chien, S. (1967). Role of the sympathetic nervous system in haemorrhage. *Physiol. Rev.*, **47**, 214–88.

Childs, C. (1988). Fever in burned children. *Burns*, **14**, 1–6.

Childs, C. & Little, R. A. (1988). Paracetamol in the management of burned children with fever. *Burns*, **14**, 343–8

Childs, C., Ratcliffe, R. J., Holt, J., Hopkins, S. J. & Little, R. A. (1990*a*). The relationship between interleukin-1, interleukin-6 and pyrexia in burned children. *Prog. Leucocyte Biol.*, **106**, 295–300.

Childs, C., Stoner, H. B. & Little, R. A. (1990*b*). Evidence for a central inhibition of heat loss during the acute phase of burn injury in children. *Arch. Emerg. Med.*, **7**, 303–4.
Clark, G. A. (1928). The origin of the glucose in the hyperglycaemia induced by pituitrin. *J. Physiol.*, **68**, 324–30.
Clowes, W. (1591). *Proved Practice for Young Chirurgeons. A Profitable and Necessary Book of Observations.* London: Wydow Broome.
Crile, G. W. (1899). *An Experimental Research into Surgical Shock.* Philadelphia: Lippincott.
Cuthbertson, D. P. (1942). Post-shock metabolic response. *Lancet*, **i**, 433–7.
Dible, J. H. (1970). *Napoleon's Surgeon.* London: Heinemann.
Feldman, S., Conforti, N. & Chowers, I. (1971). The role of the medial forebrain bundle in mediating adrenocortical responses to neurogenic stimuli. *J. Endocrinol.*, **51**, 745–9.
Folkov, B. & Neil, E. (1971). *Circulation.* Oxford: Oxford University Press.
Frayn, K. N., Little, R. A., Maycock, P. & Stoner, H. B. (1985). The relationship of plasma catecholamines to acute metabolic and hormonal responses to injury in man. *Circ. Shock*, **16**, 229–40.
Gibbs, F. P. (1969*a*). Central nervous system lesions that block release of ACTH caused by traumatic stress. *Am. J. Physiol.*, **217**, 78–83.
Gibbs, F. P. (1969*b*). Area of pons necessary for traumatic stress-induced ACTH release under pentobarbital anesthesia. *Am. J. Physiol.*, **217**, 84–8.
Ginsburg, M. & Heller, H. (1953). Antidiuretic activity in blood obtained from various parts of the cardiovascular system. *J. Endocrinol.*, **9**, 274–82.
Grant, R. T. & Reeve, E. B. (1951). Observations on the general effects of injury in man. *Spec. Rep. Ser. Med. Res. Counc.* (London), 277.
Green, H. N. & Stoner, H. B. (1950). *Biological Actions of the Adenine Nucleotides.* London: Lewis.
Greer, M. A., Allen, C. F., Gibbs, F. P. & Gullickson, C. (1970). Pathways at the hypothalamic level through which traumatic stress activates ACTH secretion. *Endocrinology*, **86**, 1404–9.
Guthrie, G. J. (1815). *Gunshot Wounds of the Extremities.* London.
Haist, R. E. (1960). Influence of environment on the metabolic response to injury. In *The Biochemical Response to Injury*, ed. H. B. Stoner & C. J. Threlfall, pp. 313–40. Oxford: Blackwell.
Heldmaier, G. (1971). Zitterfreie Wärmebildung und Körpergrösse bei Säugetieran. *Z. vergl. Physiol.*, **73**, 222–48.
Hems, D. A. & Whitton, P. D. (1980). Control of hepatic glycogenolysis. *Physiol. Rev.*, **60**, 1–50.
Henane, R., Bittel, J. & Banssillon, V. (1981). Partitional calorimetry measurement of energy exchanges in severely burned patients. *Burns*, **7**, 180–9.
Hoheisel, V. & Mense, S. (1990). Response behaviour of cat dorsal horn neurones receiving input from skeletal muscle and other deep somatic tissue. *J. Physiol.*, **426**, 265–80.
Hunter, J. (1794). *A Treatise on the Blood, Inflammation and Gunshot Wounds.* London: Nicol.
Krebs, H. A. (1954). Excursion into the borderland of biochemistry and philosophy. *Bull. Johns Hopkins Hosp.*, **95**, 45–51.
Latta, J. (1795). *A Practical System of Surgery*, vol. 2. Edinburgh.
Little, R. A. (1979). Effect of non-haemorrhagic injury on the cardiovascular response to tilting in the rat. *Br. J. Exp. Pathol.*, **60**, 303–13.

Little, R. A. (1989). 1988 Fitts Lecture: Heart rate changes after haemorrhage and injury – a reappraisal. *J. Trauma*, **29**, 903–6.

Little, R. A., Frayn, K. N., Randall, P., Stoner, H. B. & Maycock, P. (1985). Plasma catecholamine concentrations in acute states of stress and trauma. *Arch. Emerg. Med.*, **2**, 46–52.

Little, R. A., Randall, P., Redfern, W. S., Stoner, H. B. & Marshall, H. W. (1984). Components of injury (haemorrhage and tissue ischaemia) affecting cardiovascular reflexes in man and rat. *Q. J. Exp. Physiol.*, **69**, 753–62.

Little, R. A. & Stoner, H. B. (1981). Body temperature after accidental injury. *Br. J. Surg.*, **68**, 221–4.

Little, R. A. & Stoner, H. B. (1983). Effect of injury on the reflex control of pulse rate in man. *Circ. Shock*, **10**, 161–71.

Little, R. A., Stoner, H. B., Randall, P. & Carlson, G. (1986). An effect of injury on thermoregulation in man. *Q. J. Exp. Physiol.*, **71**, 295–306.

Majno, G. (1964). Mechanisms of abnormal vascular permeability in acute inflammation. In *Injury, Inflammation and Immunity*, ed. C. Thomas, J. W. Uhr & L. Grant, pp. 58–93. Baltimore: Williams & Wilkins.

Marshall, H. W. & Stoner, H. B. (1979*a*). The effect of dopamine on shivering in the rat. *J. Physiol.*, **288**, 393–9.

Marshall, H. W. & Stoner, H. B. (1979*b*). Catecholaminergic $\alpha$-receptors and shivering in the rat. *J. Physiol.*, **292**, 27–34.

Mense, S. & Stahnke, M. (1983). Responses in muscle afferent fibres of slow conduction velocity to contractions and ischaemia in the cat. *J. Physiol.*, **342**, 383–97.

Morimoto, A., Murakami, N., Nakamori, T. & Watanabe, T. (1988). Ventromedial hypothalamus is highly sensitive to prostaglandin $E_2$ for producing fever in rabbits. *J. Physiol.*, **397**, 259–68.

Ochoa, J., Fowler, T. J. & Gilliatt, R. W. (1972). Anatomical changes in peripheral nerves compressed by a pneumatic tourniquet. *J. Anat.*, **113**, 433–55.

O'Shaughnessy, L. & Slome, D. (1934). Etiology of traumatic shock. *Br. J. Surg.*, **22**, 589–618.

Overman, R. R. & Wang, S. C. (1947). The contributory role of the afferent nervous factor in experimental shock, sublethal hemorrhage and sciatic nerve stimulation. *Am. J. Physiol.*, **148**, 289–95.

Paré, A. (1582). *Les Oeuvres d'Ambroise Paré*. Paris: Dupuye.

Redfern, W. S., Little, R. A., Stoner, H. B. & Marshall, H. W. (1984). Effect of limb ischaemia on blood pressure and the blood pressure–heart rate reflex in the rat. *Q. J. Exp. Physiol.*, **69**, 763–79.

Shoemaker, W. C. (1986). Hemodynamic and oxygen transport patterns in septic shock: physiologic mechanisms and therapeutic implications. In *Perspectives on Sepsis and Septic Shock*, ed. W. J. Sibbald & C. L. Sprung, pp. 203–34. Fullerton, CA: Society of Critical Care Medicine.

Slome, D. & O'Shaughnessy, L. (1938). The nervous factor in traumatic shock. *Br. J. Surg.*, **25**, 900–9.

Stitt, J. T. (1976). Inhibition of thermoregulatory outflow in conscious rabbits during periods of sustained arousal. *J. Physiol.*, **260**, 31P.

Stoner, H. B. (1958). Studies on the mechanism of shock. The influence of environment on the changes in oxygen consumption, tissue temperature and blood flow produced by limb ischaemia. *Br. J. Exp. Path.*, **39**, 251–77.

Stoner, H. B. (1961). The biochemical response to injury. *Scientific Basis of Medicine Annual Reviews*, pp. 172–99. London: Athlone Press.

Stoner, H. B. (1968). Mechanism of body temperature changes after burns and other injuries. *Ann. NY Acad. Sci.*, **150**, 722–37.
Stoner, H. B. (1969). Studies on the mechanisms of shock. The impairment of thermoregulation by trauma. *Br. J. Exp. Path.*, **50**, 125–38.
Stoner, H. B. (1971). Effect of injury on shivering thermogenesis in the rat. *J. Physiol.*, **214**, 599–615.
Stoner, H. B. (1972). Effect of injury on the responses to thermal stimulation of the hypothalamus. *J. Appl. Physiol.*, **33**, 665–71.
Stoner, H. B. (1974). Inhibition of thermoregulatory non-shivering thermogenesis by trauma in cold-acclimated rats. *J. Physiol.*, **238**, 657–70.
Stoner, H. B. (1976). An integrated neuroendocrine response to injury. In: *Metabolism and the Response to Injury*, ed. A. W. Wilkinson & D. Cuthbertson, pp. 194–201. Tunbridge Wells: Pitman Medical.
Stoner, H. B. (1977). The role of catecholamines in the effects of trauma on thermoregulation studied in rats treated with 6-hydroxydopamine. *Br. J. Exp. Path.*, **58**, 42–9.
Stoner, H. B. (1987). Interpretation of the metabolic effects of trauma and sepsis. *J. Clin. Pathol.*, **40**, 1108–17.
Stoner, H. B. (1991). The burned patient's response to the environment. *J. Burn Care Rehabil.*, **12**, 402–10.
Stoner, H. B. (1993). Responses to trauma. Fifty years of 'ebb' and 'flow'. *Circ. Shock*, **39**, 316–19.
Stoner, H. B. & Cremer, J. E. (1985). Maintenance of metabolic integrity in the brain after trauma. *Br. Med. Bull.*, **41**, 246–50.
Stoner, H. B. & Elson, P. M. (1971). The effect of injury on monoamine concentrations in the rat hypothalamus. *J. Neurochem.*, **18**, 1837–46.
Stoner, H. B., Elson, P. M. & Koltay, E. (1973). The effects of limb ischaemia on the turnover of noradrenaline in the hypothalamus and brain stem of the rat. *J. Neurochem.*, **21**, 223–31.
Stoner, H. B. & Hunt, A. (1976). The effect of trauma on the activity of central noradrenergic neurones. *Brain Res.*, **112**, 337–46.
Stoner, H. B. & Little, R. A. (1969*a*). Studies on the mechanism of shock. The effect of cocaine and theophylline on the temperature response to injury in the cold-acclimated rat. *Br. J. Exp. Pathol.*, **50**, 97–106.
Stoner, H. B. & Little, R. A. (1969*b*). Studies on the mechanism of shock. The effect of catecholamines on the temperature responses to injury in the rat. *Br. J. Exp. Pathol.*, **50**, 107–24.
Stoner, H. B. & Marshall, H. W. (1971). Studies on the mechanism of shock. Thermoregulation during limb ischaemia. *Br. J. Exp. Pathol.*, **52**, 650–5.
Stoner, H. B. & Marshall, H. W. (1975*a*). Studies on the mechanism of shock. The importance of central catecholaminergic neurons in the response to injury. *Br. J. Exp. Pathol.*, **56**, 157–66.
Stoner, H. B. & Marshall, H. W. (1975*b*). Effect of trauma on the formaldehyde-induced fluorescence of noradrenaline in the hypothalamus and brain stem of the rat. *Brain Res.*, **97**, 1–15.
Stoner, H. B. & Marshall, H. W. (1977). Localization of the brain regions concerned in the inhibition of shivering by trauma. *Br. J. Exp. Pathol.*, **58**, 50–6.
Stoner, H. B. & Marshall, H. W. (1982). Neural pathways mediating the inhibition of shivering by non-thermal afferent impulses from ischaemic limbs. *Exp. Neurol.*, **78**, 275–84.
Swingle, W. W., Kleinberg, W., Remington, J. W., Eversole, W. J. & Overman,

R. R. (1944). Experimental analysis of the nervous factor in shock induced by muscle trauma in normal dogs. *Am. J. Physiol.*, **141**, 54–63.

Tabor, H. & Rosenthal, S. M. (1947). Body temperature and oxygen consumption in traumatic shock and hemorrhage in mice. *Am. J. Physiol.*, **149**, 449–64.

Tibbs, D. J. (1956). Blood volumes in gastroduodenal haemorrhage. *Lancet*, **ii**, 266–74.

Wiggers, C. J. (1950). *Physiology of Shock*. New York: The Commonwealth Fund.

Wilmore, D. W. (1977). *The Metabolic Management of the Critically Ill*. New York: Plenum.

Wilmore, D. W. & Stoner, H. B. (1994). The wound organ. In *Scientific Foundations of Trauma*, ed. G. Cooper, H. A. F. Dudley, D. S. Gann, R. A. Little & R. L. Maynard. Oxford: Butterworth–Heinemann, in press.

Yates, D. W. (1990). Changes in the distribution of cardiac output in the rat after trauma with special reference to the cerebral circulation. MD thesis, Cambridge University, Cambridge.

# 3

# Experimental approaches to the central nervous system control of responses to trauma

RODERICK A. LITTLE and NANCY J. ROTHWELL

## Introduction

The 1990s has been proclaimed the 'decade of the brain', reflecting intense and rapidly expanding research into basic neurosciences and neurological disorders. This development has arisen from fundamental scientific advances in understanding the processes within the brain and the interactions and mechanisms by which the central nervous system (CNS) responds to and controls peripheral systems, and from the increasing prevalence of neurological disorders. Of particular relevance to this book have been the important advances made in the field of neuroimmunology, where multiple, bidirectional communications have been observed between the nervous system and the immune system. Increased awareness of the impact of psychological status on responses to disease and injury, and long-term effects of trauma on subsequent behaviour might further contribute to our basic understanding of clinical management of trauma patients. Unravelling the role of the brain in controlling responses to injury and the complex interactions between the CNS and host defence responses is a daunting but exciting challenge, with enormous potential benefits. Specific aspects of this subject are discussed in detail elsewhere in this book. However, in this chapter we attempt to introduce the experimental approaches available for studying CNS control of responses to trauma, and to consider their relative advantages and associated ethical, logistic and scientific drawbacks and limitations.

## Problems of research into trauma

Ideally, scientific research is based on experimental testing of defined hypotheses. However, even in controlled animal or cellular systems this ideal is often difficult to achieve, and studies on normal humans or on patients present more serious and often insurmountable problems. Biological research has moved towards more reductionist approaches where studies on isolated cell systems and molecular mechanisms can provide definitive answers and clearly defined experimental systems. However, for many problems in biological and clinical research, of which the present topic is an excellent example, a more integrated approach is necessary, since numerous cells, organs and physiological systems are involved.

Research on patients has provided many important data that may relate directly to underlying mechanisms of pathology and can lead to novel treatments. However, this is usually descriptive, since any interventions must be considered in the context of overriding clinical priorities and the well-being of the patient. Data derived from patients also suffer from diversity of the extent of injury, the time of onset, concurrent therapies and variations on the normal physiology (e.g. age, sex, underlying pathological considerations). A number of these problems can be addressed by the use of scoring systems that grade either the amount of tissue damage (e.g. the Injury Severity Score), the physiological response to an injury (e.g. the Revised Trauma Score, Glasgow Coma Scale) or a combination of the local and general responses (e.g. the Sepsis Score). The health status of the patient before 'injury' is included in the Apache system, used most commonly in intensive care units. These problems are further exacerbated when CNS responses to trauma are studied; in humans such studies almost always rely on indirect measures. Controlled research on experimental animals therefore represents a feasible approach to study CNS control of responses to trauma. Nevertheless, the limitations of data obtained on animals and their relevance to clinical conditions must be recognised.

## Study of trauma in experimental animals

A wide variety of experimental methods has been used to cause tissue damage (see Table 3.1) in numerous species. For practical, financial and ethical reasons the majority of these have employed rodents (e.g. rats, mice) or rabbits, although studies have been undertaken on larger species, particularly the dog, cat, pig and, in very limited cases, primates.

Many early studies used 'models' that were almost as complex as the injuries seen clinically, with the result that the apparently laudable aim of achieving realism added little to our knowledge of the mechanisms of the response to injury. It should, therefore, be axiomatic that the nature of the injury must be accurately identified, its size must be measurable

Table 3.1. *Experimental models of injury in laboratory animals*

| |
|---|
| *Peripheral* |
| Long-bone fracture (usually femur) |
| Scald or burn injury |
| Laparotomy |
| Penetrating or gunshot wounds |
| Sterile abscess (intramuscular, subcutaneous injection of turpentine) |
| Skin and surface-tissue cuts |
| Limb ischaemia (tourniquet) |
| Haemorrhage |
| *Head injury* |
| Fluid percussion |
| Stab or penetrating wounds |
| Freezing |
| Cerebral ischaemia (focal or global, temporary or permanent, hypoxic or thrombo-embolism) |
| Subdural haematoma |
| Mechanical lesions (electrolytic, radio-frequency) |
| Pharmacological lesions – e.g. injections of excitotoxins |

and controllable, and it must be reproducible. If these criteria are met, then the number of animals used can be kept to the minimum compatible with good science. Overwhelming injuries, which may fit well into the working day, should not be used, as they may mask any potential benefits offered by putative treatments. The limitations of a simple model such as haemorrhage should also be realised. There is a plethora of data on the responses to haemorrhage to a fixed blood volume or arterial blood pressure but little is clinically relevant. An uncomplicated haemorrhage is not common clinically; most often it is accompanied by tissue damage (and associated nociceptive afferent stimuli), the presence of which can markedly alter the physiological response to haemorrhage.

The choice of injury model is also influenced by the question asked, for example, the role of the central nervous system (CNS) in mediating the general (systemic) responses to a peripheral injury or the general responses elicited by a direct injury to the CNS. It is also important to differentiate between the local and general responses induced by an injury and the time courses of the responses. The great benefit of animal experiments is that the acute early changes can be studied in the absence of treatment, but they are generally less valid as models of the delayed 'flow' phase responses.

The use of animals for the study of trauma offers considerable experimental and ethical advantages, but reservations and limitations of extrapolating data from these studies to clinical situations must also be considered. Experimentally induced injury allows clear definition of the type, severity and time of trauma, control of variables such as age, genetic background and physiological status (e.g. nutritional and hormonal status), and interventions that would not be possible in the clinical setting. Thus, studies on animals provide the only valid means of directly testing hypotheses and investigating mechanisms contributing to overall outcome after trauma by controlled intervention and observation. Whereas animal experimentation overcomes most of the moral, ethical and legal problems associated with human research, such considerations are now, quite rightly, imposed on animal studies in most countries, and are particularly relevant to the study of trauma. Clear scientific justification, good experimental design, direct clinical relevance and limitations of the degree of pain and suffering imposed are therefore all important prerequisites for animal research. Studies on those species that might be most relevant to humans (e.g. primates) are subject to the most severe restraints, and in addition pose severe financial problems.

It might be argued that the very factors described above, which offer advantages to animal research, also limit their clinical relevance. For example, experimental studies rarely involve multiple trauma, resuscitation or intensive pharmacological management. They are usually restricted to young animals without the underlying factors that may contribute to outcome (e.g. diabetes, hypertension, obesity, alcoholism, infections, etc.), and fail to highlight genetic influences. However, with regard to the latter point, both inter-colony and inter-strain as well as inter-species variations have been reported for many animal studies.

In almost all animal studies injury is, quite correctly, inflicted under surgical anaesthesia. However, it is important that the effects of the anaesthetic agents themselves are taken into account. They can modify both homeostatic reflex activity and the interactions between injury and such reflexes. The modifications can also be selective and not simply a reflection of a general depression of CNS activity. In humans accidental injury occurs in the absence of such anaesthesia, although acute ethanol intoxication is common and can modify the metabolic and physiological response to injury. In this context it must be acknowledged that much has been learned from studies of the responses to surgical injury inflicted under either general or regional anaesthesia.

Certain aspects of trauma research on animals carry specific problems when data are translated to humans. Perhaps most obvious are the problems associated with assessing the mechanisms and control of pain and behavioural responses in lower mammals. For example, studies on behavioural changes following injury or illness in rodents usually rely on assessments such as food-seeking activity, responses to novel environments and learning tasks. Although these have provided much valuable information, it is difficult to equate results with findings in humans.

Thermoregulatory and metabolic studies are directly influenced by the small size of most experimental animals. This influence of species on the relative importance of thermoregulatory effector mechanisms is well illustrated by the confusion raised over the definition of the acute response to tissue injury – the 'ebb' phase. Injury inhibits the neural pathways controlling both heat loss and heat production. In the rat, heat production is the dominant regulated variable, and after tissue ischaemia there is a fall in both heat production and body temperature at environmental temperatures below the thermoneutral zone. However, in humans heat loss is the dominant variable and its inhibition after injury can lead to what may appear to be a paradoxical increase in body temperature and metabolic rate.

In addition to its effects on thermoregulation, the increase in the ratio of surface area to volume in small animals compared to humans can also influence the rate of energy turnover, and relative effective drug doses in animals are usually much higher than in humans. Some animals show markedly varied sensitivities to interventions, most apparent in the high resistance to endotoxin and various forms of infection noted in the rat. The small size of experimental animals can also pose serious limitations on tissue or blood sampling, particularly where repeated samples are required.

However, in spite of these reservations and drawbacks, many aspects of research into trauma can *only* be undertaken on experimental animals. Investigation into CNS control and mechanism is perhaps the most obvious of these, where research on animals can utilise a wide variety of sophisticated techniques for influencing and assessing CNS function.

### *Methods for studying CNS function in animals*

Analysis of enzyme activities, metabolites, neurotransmitters and neuropeptide concentrations, receptor density and mRNA expression in post-mortem brain samples is one of the most readily available and widely applied means of studying CNS function in humans. The same techniques can be used in animals, but with important refinements and improvements.

Post-mortem delay, which is usually inevitable in patient studies, can influence the measurement of many molecules. Such delay is avoided in animal experiments and post-mortem breakdown of particularly labile molecules (e.g. specific enzymes, cAMP, cGMP, mRNAs) can be further diminished by rapid microwave-induced death or by snap-freezing. Histological, immunohistochemical and molecular measurements can be facilitated by rapid perfusion fixation of brain tissue.

Single point measurements of the brain content of putative mediators or their receptors may provide important descriptive information, but this is difficult to relate to a functional or causal role in physiological or pathological events. The value of such measurements can be greatly enhanced in animal experiments by direct comparison with appropriate controls (including sham-operated or vehicle-treated animals), or by studying the time course after insults or interventions. The turnover of some potential mediators can be estimated by blocking transmitter synthesis, re-uptake or release with specific pharmacological agents prior to sacrifice.

*In vivo* assessments of synthesis or release of molecules in the brain can, in some cases, be derived from analysis of cerebrospinal fluid. However, this is not appropriate for factors that are released only locally into brain tissue or are rapidly degraded. Push–pull perfusion allows continuous sampling of extracellular fluid in specific brain regions of anaesthetised and conscious free-moving animals. However, push–pull perfusion causes some local tissue damage even at low ($\approx 1$ µl/min) flow rates. Damage is minimised by the use of dialysis, whereby no fluid directly enters the brain, but molecules (of a molecular weight determined by the cutoff size of the dialysis membrane around the probe) pass from the extracellular fluid into the dialysate. This technique is most appropriate for low molecular weight, hydrophilic molecules such as amino acids, glucose and neurotransmitters (e.g. acetylcholine, 5-hydroxytryptamine, noradrenaline). Continuous dialysis in free-moving animals can be linked directly to on-line 'real-time' analysis, usually by connection to high pressure liquid chromatography. (HPLC).

*In vivo* recording of electrical activity in animals may be achieved at the single-cell level using either extracellular or intracellular electrodes, with simultaneous multiple injections of substances in minute and precisely controlled amounts (e.g. by iontophoretic application of a few molecules). More detailed electrophysiological data can be obtained from rapidly dissected brain slices where patch–clamp analysis has now been successfully applied. Growth of specific populations of neurones in primary culture allows the study of single cells, although extrapolation of data from cultures may be limited by the fact that foetal or neonatal tissues, from which cultures are derived, may be very different from those of adults *in vivo*. Primary neuronal cultures have now been successfully grown from human foetal brain tissue, but in some countries their use is subject to legal restrictions.

The greatest advantage of animal research into CNS function and its control of other systems lies in the ability to make direct experimental interventions. Stereotaxically located injections can be made into cerebral ventricles or specific brain regions by direct injection via indwelling guide cannulae in conscious animals, and now by dialysis to limit local tissue damage. Thus, the activity of neuronal pathways can be selectively influenced by administration of naturally occurring neuromodulators, receptor agonists and antagonists, agents to modify synthesis, release, re-uptake or intracellular signal transduction mechanisms or neutralising antibodies to specific neuropeptides.

Electrical stimulation of brain pathways is achieved via acutely or chronically implanted electrodes, and a wide variety of techniques is now available for chronic destruction of specific neurones or fibre tracts. Electrolytic or radio-frequency lesions cause non-selective destruction of brain tissue, but transection of fibre tracks or deafferentation of brain structures can be made by stereotaxic knife cuts. More selective destruction of neurochemical pathways can be achieved by injection of neurotoxic agents. For example, injection of 5-hydroxytryptamine causes lesions to serotonergic pathways (provided that uptake in noradrenergic neurones is blocked), whereas kainic acid destroys cell bodies but leaves fibres intact. Development of techniques to induce 'immunotoxic lesions' offers considerable potential for studies on neuropeptide systems within the brain. Local injections into specific brain regions of a toxin (usually ricin) conjugated to an antipeptide antibody allow the toxin to be selectively taken up into neurones that synthesise the peptide, and are subsequently destroyed. This technique has already proved valuable in the investigation of activations of vasopressin and corticotrophin-releasing factor in the brain.

The extensive and continually expanding range of techniques available for research into the CNS in animals is of value not only in elucidating mechanisms and highlighting potentially valuable interventions, but also in validation of less invasive methods that can be used in humans. In animals, therefore, it is possible to determine whether analysis of molecules in the cerebrospinal fluid correlates with local brain production, or to compare non-invasive imaging techniques with more direct measures of brain activity. Unfortunately, the availability of such techniques does not necessarily result in valid scientific experimentation with readily interpretable data. A large number of data now exist on the effects of injecting or inhibiting the actions of a vast array of molecules in the brain on local or systemic functions. While many of these have led to considerable advances in understanding neuronal physiological processes and responses to insults, in some cases it may be difficult to distinguish pharmacological effects from those that reflect endogenous mechanisms.

## Study of trauma in humans

Despite the limitations imposed by the necessity for treatment, useful data can be obtained during the very early phase of the response to injury in humans. Such studies can be considered *observational*, whereas at later times after resuscitation and stabilisation *interventional* studies can be made.

The observational approach has been dismissed by some as 'data dredging' or 'trawling'. However, it has an important role in providing data from which hypotheses can be deduced for later testing in interventional studies. This approach has a number of other advantages – the measurements and/or samples can be taken quickly (often before resuscitation starts and subsequently at hiatuses in treatment), a large number of patients can be recruited quickly, and there are few ethical objections, as no intervention or disruption to treatment is involved. The most valid objection to observational studies is that there are many variables that cannot be controlled (e.g. age, severity and type of injury, pre-existing disease, nutritional status, time of day, time after injury, etc.). However, provided such information is collected from a large enough number of patients, it can prove highly valuable. Such analysis is greatly enhanced by the inclusion of a numerical scale for grading the severity of injury. Relationships with severity of injury can therefore be sought within the group of injured patients rather than by comparison of a group of injured patients with a group of controls. The development and general acceptance of such severity scales or scores using easily obtained data allow meaningful comparisons of results from different centres. The large number of patients needed for observational studies can be reduced if the study is longitudinal. Patients are studied shortly after injury and again once they have recovered (obviously allowances must be made for deaths if the injuries are very severe).

During the later, delayed phase of the response to injury, interventional studies can be made. These often involve testing the ability of an injured patient to respond to a superimposed stress, such as a glucose tolerance test or a change in either posture (active or passive) or ambient temperature. A strict experimental protocol where all extraneous influences can be controlled is imposed on the new steady-state established by injury. A major advantage of this approach is that only a small number of patients have to be studied to disprove most hypotheses; however, there are a number of disadvantages. The studies are very demanding on resources and it is difficult to ensure that the patients selected for study are representative. It is also often difficult to dispel fears that the patients are being experimented on.

Another important use of interventional studies is the evaluation of new treatments. This is, however, often more difficult than expected because of the problems of defining the end-point by which efficacy can be judged. The least controversial end-point is death, but unless the expected mortality rate is very high and the treatment remarkably effective, large numbers of patients have to be recruited to the study to demonstrate an effect.

In addition to studies on injured patients, it is possible to mimic aspects of the response to injury in control subjects. In this way the relative importance of different features of tissue damage (e.g. afferent nociceptive stimulation and blood loss) in mediating the response to real injuries can be assessed. A major advantage of this approach is that the subjects act as their own controls with measurements being made before and after 'injury'. It is also possible to manipulate factors such as diet, and nutritional and hormonal status before the studies are done. The 'injuries' that have been studied, with appropriate ethical approval, include limb ischaemia to generate afferent nociceptive impulses, haemorrhage of up to 20% of blood volume or until syncope, and the application of negative pressure to pool blood in the lower extremities, thereby reducing central blood volume. The latter manoeuvre has the advantage over haemorrhage in that it can be quickly reversed. Infusions of counter-regulatory hormones (either alone or combined) have also been used to reproduce a number of the metabolic responses to injury. The ability of subjects to generate pyrexial and/or hypermetabolic states and the physiological/ metabolic responses to such states can be studied by the intravenous injection or infusion of endotoxin or bacteria or by inoculation with, for example, typhoid vaccine.

**Summary**

Progress in understanding the mechanisms underlying responses to trauma and direct application of these findings to the patient clearly requires research on both experimental animals and humans. An important goal is to sustain and enhance dialogue and interactions between scientists and clinicians in order to elucidate fundamental mechanisms while maintaining clinical relevance. The limitations of direct extrapolation from research on animals to human pathology are manifold and must be sensibly considered. Nevertheless, research in animals over the last decade has already led to a host of new and exciting potential therapies such as novel antiischaemic drugs, cytokine inhibitors and specific dietary interventions. In spite of these successes, our current ignorance about many aspects of the responses to trauma means that animal research frequently offers the only appropriate means available for research into this field.

# 4

# Neurohormonal control of cytokines during injury

ISTVAN BERCZI and EVA NAGY

## Introduction

Hans Selye (1936*a*) was the first to report that a variety of noxious agents cause a profound involution of the thymus, spleen and lymph nodes, and the enlargement of the adrenal gland. In subsequent experiments, Selye found that these changes were mediated by the activation of the pituitary–adrenal axis and that glucocorticosteroids were responsible for the lymphoid involution (Selye, 1936*b*). The physical, chemical, or emotional *stimuli* that could evoke this neuroendocrine response, were termed 'stress' by Selye, and the body's reaction to stress was termed the 'general adaptation syndrome'. During stress, the initial alarm reaction is followed by a period of adaptation, when the organism shows resistance towards the stressor and the endocrine and other parameters return to normal. Eventually, with lasting stress, breakdown due to exhaustion can occur, which can lead to death (Selye, 1946, 1955). Selye (1949) was the first to describe the endocrine regulation of inflammation and observed with his colleagues that immune reactions are also subject to stress-induced alterations (Karady *et al.*, 1938). He also demonstrated the influence of sex hormones on lymphoid organs (Selye, 1943). It is only now that the pathophysiological pathways are beginning to emerge for Selye's observations, and this, no doubt, will lead to a wider understanding and appreciation of his teachings.

## Terminology

For some time, a confusion of terminology has prevailed with regards to the definition of soluble mediators, which are called hormones, growth factors, lymphokines and cytokines, and may also be classified under various other names, such as interleukins, interferons, prostaglandins, etc.

By now, it is quite clear that the so-called classical hormones, neurotransmitters and immune mediators are all produced in many organs and tissues (Geenen *et al.*, 1989; Blalock, 1989; Berczi, 1990; Koenig, 1991; Ohalloran *et al.*, 1991), and for this reason it is no longer possible to categorize a single molecule as a hormone, neurotransmitter, or cytokine. Nevertheless, one may suggest a categorization of 'mediator functions', which should be useful to clear the current conceptual confusion. For the purpose of our discussions, the following classifications will be adopted.

### *Hormones*

Hormones are chemical messenger molecules that are always present in the blood and may be present also in other biological fluids. Characteristically they have a long half-life in the plasma, and they regulate distant target tissues and organs, which express specific and high-affinity receptors for their regulatory hormones.

### *Acute phase hormones*

These hormones appear in the circulation during the acute phase response to trauma, sepsis and shock. Normally, most of these mediators have an autocrine/paracrine function in various organs and tissues, and their level in the blood is low to undetectable. They have a short half-life in the circulation and act on their target tissues/cells through specific and high-affinity receptors.

### *Cytokines*

Cytokines are cellular/tissue hormones typically engaged in short-range paracrine/autocrine regulation. They are produced in minute quantities, act through specific and high-affinity receptors and normally are not present in the circulation. If applied systemically, the half-life of cytokines in the circulation is short.

### *Neurotransmitters*

Neurotransmitters are secreted by nerve terminals and are designed for short-range transmission of messages to other nerve cells or cells of various tissues and organs. Typically, neurotransmitters are produced in small quantities and have a short half-life. Neurotransmitters act on specific low-affinity receptors, which allows repeated and frequently reversible stimulation.

## The response to injury

### *Types of injury and pathways of cytokine–endocrine response*

In a broad sense, the agents capable of causing injury may be classified as physical, chemical or biological.

#### *Injury due to physical agents*

*Ultraviolet radiation* Ultraviolet (UV)* irradiation of the skin has mutagenic, carcinogenic and immunosuppressive effects in experimental animals (Stern, 1989; Ullrich *et al.*, 1989). Keratinocytes treated with UVB radiation were found to release interleukin-1 (IL-1) (Robertson *et al.*, 1987), contra-IL-1 (Schwarz *et al.*, 1987), IL-1 receptor antagonist (Haskill *et al.*, 1991), contact hypersensitivity inhibiting factor (Schwarz *et al.*, 1986), and prostaglandin $E_2$ ($PGE_2$) (Jun *et al.*, 1988). UV radiation has also been found to activate antigen-specific suppressor cells (Horio & Yokamoto, 1982; Horio & Okamoto, 1983; Kripke *et al.*, 1983).

The susceptibility of UV-irradiated mice was increased significantly to infection with *Mycobacterium bovis* BCG (Jeevan *et al.*, 1992), *Leishmania major* (Giannini, 1986) and to Herpes simplex virus type 1 (Hayashi & Aurelian, 1987; Yasumoto *et al.*, 1987; Howie *et al.*, 1988).

*X-irradiation* X-rays activate a programmed suicide pathway (apoptosis) in damaged cells (Baxter & Lavin, 1992). Apoptosis triggers phagocytosis, but inflammatory and immune reactions are not activated. Because of the damage to the gut mucosa and the profound immunosuppression caused by X-irradiation, intestinal infections leading to sepsis are frequent complications of radiation injury (Wells *et al.*, 1990). The administration of anti-IL-6 antibody to irradiated mice greatly increased mortality, blocked the IL-1-induced increase in adrenocorticotropic hormone (ACTH) in plasma, and exacerbated hypoglycemia induced by tumor necrosis factor (TNF), but did not reduce IL-1-induced hypoglycemia (Neta *et al.*, 1992).

* A list of abbreviations is given at the end of this chapter.

*Cold injury* Frostbite leads to inflammation or, in serious cases, to necrosis (Killian, 1981). Mast cell degranulation and diminution occur 30 min after cold injury to rat skin, whereas the adrenergic nerves are intact. Fluid extravasation, ischemia, thrombosis and necrosis follow. Degenerative changes occur in adrenergic nerves at 16 h. The increased vascular permeability is due, at least in part, to substances liberated from mast cells (Waris & Kyösala, 1982). Abnormal hypersensitivity of mast cells to cold leads to cold urticaria (Bentley-Phillips *et al.*, 1976).

*Burn injury* Severe burns are associated with profound immunosuppression, and reduced serum levels of immunoglobulin, complement and properdin. Serum levels of glucocorticoids (GC) and histamine are elevated and the secretion of adrenalin is increased for the first 24 h, after which it may subside in uncomplicated cases. Serum levels of androgens are suppressed and may not normalize, even after complete healing (Birke *et al.*, 1957; Howerton & Kolmen, 1972; Asko-Seljavaara, 1974; Bjornson *et al.*, 1977; Chithara & Feierabend, 1981; Heideman, 1981).

In patients with major burns, increasingly high levels of IL-2 and the alpha chain of the IL-2 receptor (IL-2R$\alpha$) were observed (Teodorczyk-Injeyan *et al.*, 1989; Teodorczyk-Injeyan *et al.*, 1991). Serum IL-6 levels were maximal in burn patients in the first 3 days, returning to normal by day 30–50 in survivors, and increasing continuously in non-survivors until death occurred due to sepsis (Schluter *et al.*, 1991). Monocytes of burn patients showed significantly elevated levels of total TNF$\alpha$ and $PGE_2$ after stimulation with suboptimal concentrations of interferon (IFN)-$\gamma$ or muramyl dipeptide 3 days before a septic episode (Takayama *et al.*, 1990).

Burned rats infected with *Pseudomonas aeruginosa* had a 100% increase in hepatic TNF$\alpha$ messenger RNA (mRNA) (Marano *et al.*, 1988).

*Trauma* Tissue damage and bleeding activate the coagulation, kallikrein–kinin, fibrinolytic and complement systems. The complement split products, C3a and C5a, activate mast cells and fibroblasts and attract neutrophilic granulocytes and macrophages (Nuytinck *et al.*, 1986; Heideman, 1989; Yurt & Lowry, 1990; Billiau & Vandekerckhove, 1991). Cytokines and other mediators released by platelets, mast cells, macrophages, neutrophils and activated endothelial cells (Tables 4.1–4.5) play a major role in the local inflammatory response to injury.

Table 4.1. *Cytokines and enzymes released by tissue mast cells and basophils*

| Discharges | Cytokines/hormones | Enzymes |
|---|---|---|
| Antigen–IgE complex | Eosinophil chemotactic factor | Cathepsin G |
| β-Endorphin | GM-CSF | Proteases |
| Bradykinin | Heparin | |
| C3a, C5a | Histamine | |
| Calcitonin gene-related peptide | Interleukin-3 | |
| Cold insult | Leukotriene $C_4$ | |
| Dynorphin | Neutrophil chemotactic factor | |
| GM-CSF | Platelet activating factor | |
| Interleukin-3 | Prostaglandin $D_2$, $-D_4$, $-E_4$ | |
| Leu-enkephalin | Serotonin | |
| Lipopolysaccharide | Tumor necrosis factor | |
| Neurotensin | | |
| Oxidative insults | | |
| Somatostatin | | |
| Substance P | | |
| Vasoactive intestinal peptide | | |

It is beyond the scope of this review to discuss all aspects of basophil/mast cell activation and mediator release. Instead the reader is referred to recent reviews on the subject by Haak-Frendscho *et al.* (1988); Wodnar-Filipowicz *et al.* (1989); Galli *et al.* (1990).
C3a, C5a, complement components; GM-CSF, granulocyte/monocyte colony stimulating factor.

Bleeding of mice induced a significant elevation of serum TNF (Ayala *et al.*, 1990). In surgery and trauma patients, circulating IL-6 levels peaked at 4–6 h, followed by the appearance of circulating acute phase proteins (APP), which arose during a 30 h period following injury. TNF was not detectable (Pullicino *et al.*, 1990). After surgical trauma, an early and short-lived rise of IL-1β, followed by a rise in IL-6, was seen. TNFα and IFN-γ were not detected (Baigrie, *et al.*, 1991). CD3- and CD4-positive T cells were reduced in trauma patients, whereas macrophages and immunoglobulin levels were elevated. The production of IL-1, IL-2 and IFN-γ was reduced. Monocytes of trauma patients produced more IL-6 than did control cells *in vitro* after FcγRI stimulation. This response could be downregulated by IL-4 (Faist *et al.*, 1989; Szabo *et al.*, 1991*a*, *b*).

In surgery patients, ACTH, growth hormone, prolactin, GC and estrone were elevated, whereas androgens and progesterone were diminished. The endocrine response to abdominal surgery could be prevented by spinal

Table 4.2. *Mediators produced by activated monocytes–macrophages*

| Stimulus/activators | Cytokines/hormones | Enzymes/proteins |
|---|---|---|
| Ag–Ab complex (IgG1, IgG3) | Angiogenesis factor | Arginase |
| C3a, C5a | Fibroblast growth factor | Cathepsin |
| C-reactive protein | G-CSF, GM-CSF, M-CSF | Coagulation factors |
| Interleukin-4, -6 | IP-10 | Collagenase |
| Interferon | Interferon | Complement components |
| Lipopolysaccharide | Interleukin-1, -6, -8 | Elastase |
| Oxidative insults | Leukotrienes | Fibronectin |
| Transforming growth factor-$\beta$ | MCAF | Inhibitors of enzymes and cytokines |
| Tumor necrosis factor | PDGF | Lipoprotein lipase |
| | Prostaglandin $E_2$ | Lysozyme |
| | Platelet activating factor | Plasminogen activator |
| | Sterol hormones | Reactive oxygen intermediates |
| | Transforming growth factor-$\beta$ | Tissue factor |
| | Thromboxane $A_2$ | |
| | Tumor necrosis factor-$\alpha$ | |

An exhaustive discussion of monocyte/macrophage-activating agents and mediator release is beyond the scope of this chapter. For reviews on the subject, please see Wieser *et al.* (1989), Douglas & Hassam (1990), Oppenheim *et al.* (1991) and text for further references.
Ag–Ab complex, antigen–antibody complex; C3a, C5a, complement components; MCAF, macrophage chemoattractant and activating factor; PDGF, platelet-derived growth factor.

anesthesia. Major surgical trauma had a rapid, profound and long-lasting inhibitory effect on gonadal activity (Newsome & Rose, 1971; Noel *et al.*, 1971; *Adami et al.*, 1982; Lindh *et al.*, 1992). In trauma, a similar endocrine response was found. In addition, endorphins (END), arginine vasopressin (AVP), erythropoietin (EPO), and catecholamines, epinephrine, and norepinephrine were also elevated and no change or decrease was found in the level of thyroid-stimulating hormone (TSH), triiodothyronine and thyroxin, with no change in alpha melanocyte stimulating hormone ($\alpha$-MSH). In patients with severe trauma, growth hormone was usually not elevated and the levels of ACTH and GC could be subnormal. Insulin was low in relation to the hyperglycemia present. Glucagon, catecholamine

Table 4.3. *Mediators released by neutrophilic granulocytes*

| Stimulus | Cytokines | Enzymes and other molecules |
|---|---|---|
| C5a, C3b | Leukotriene $B_4$ | Acid hydrolases |
| C-reactive protein | Monocyte chemoattractant | C5a cleaving enzyme |
| Formyl peptide | Platelet activating factor | Cathepsin G |
| Interleukin-8 | Prostaglandin $E_2$ | Collagenase |
| Kallikrein | Transforming growth factor-$\beta$ | Defensins |
| Leukotriene $B_4$ | | Elastase (stimulates generation of C3a, C5a) |
| Platelet activating factor | | Histaminase |
| Substance P | | Lysozyme |
| Tumor necrosis factor | | Oxygen metabolites |
| | | PKC inhibitor |
| | | Plasminogen |
| | | Plasminogen activator |

The stimuli and released mediators listed here are for the purposes of our discussion. Readers interested in more information are referred to Curnutte & Babior (1990) and Smolen & Boxer (1990).
C5a, C3b, complement components; PKC, protein kinase C.

arginine vasopressin and aldosterone were all elevated, whereas triiodothyronine and thyroxin were usually subnormal. The initially high catecholamine levels decreased in survivors, but increased greatly before death. Thyroid releasing hormone (TRH) stimulation affected TSH levels minimally or not at all in dying patients, in whom the catecholamine and triiodothyronine/thyroxin levels were inversely related (Baue, 1989).

*Chemical agents causing injury*

A vast amount of chemicals have the potential to cause inflammation by irritation, to induce necrosis or apoptosis, and even to trigger immune mechanisms by altering self proteins. The cytokine response to chemical insults can be mediated by neurogenic pathways, by those outlined above, under 'trauma', and by antigen-mediated activation of the immune system (Barnetson & Gawkroger, 1989; Sinha *et al.*, 1990; Eastman & Barry, 1992).

Table 4.4. *Platelet-derived mediators*

| Activators | Cytokines/hormones | Other mediators |
|---|---|---|
| ADP | β-Thromboglobulin | Acid hydrolases |
| Ag–IgG complex | Chemotactic factor | ATP, ADP, GTP, GDP |
| Bacteria | Interleukin-8 | Calcium |
| Collagen | Mitogenic factor | Factors V, VIII |
| Epinephrine, norepinephrine | Platelet activating factor | Fibrinogen |
| Fibrinogen | PDGF | Fibronectin |
| Lipopolysaccharide | PF-4 | Proteins |
| Platelet activating factor | Prostaglandins | Thrombin |
| Serotonin | Serotonin | von Willebrand factor |
| Thrombin | Transforming growth factor-β | |
| Thromboxane $A_2$ | Thromboxanes ($A_2$) | |
| Tumor cells | | |
| Vasopressin | | |
| Viruses | | |

The data listed in this table are for the purposes of this discussion only. Readers interested in more information are referred to reviews by Packham & Mustard, 1984; Holmsen, 1990; Oppenheim *et al.*, 1991.
ADP, adenosine diphosphate; ATP, -triphosphate; GTP, guanosine triphosphate; GDP, -diphosphate; Ag, antigen; PDGF, platelet-derived growth factor; PF-4, basic platelet factor.

Table 4.5. *Cytokines produced by the endothelium*

| Releasing factors | Cytokines/hormones | Other molecules |
|---|---|---|
| C-reactive protein | Endothelin | Factor VIII |
| G-CSF | GM-CSF | Fibrinolysis inhibitor |
| GM-CSF | Interleukin-1 | Plasminogen activators |
| Interferon-γ | Interleukin-8 | von Willebrand factor |
| Interleukin-1 | IP-10 | |
| Injury | Platelet activating factor | |
| Lipopolysaccharide | PDGF | |
| Thrombin | Prostaglandin $E_2$ | |
| Tumor necrosis factor | Prostacyclin (PG12) | |

For review, please see Mohammad *et al.* (1984), Oppenheim *et al.* (1991), Malone *et al.* (1988), Bussolino *et al.* (1989) and Broudy *et al.* (1986).
G(M)-CSF, granulocyte (monocyte)-colony stimulating factor; PDGF, platelet-derived growth factor.

***Biological injury***

*Infection and parasitic infestation* Infections frequently occur in immunocompromised patients, including the elderly, those on immunosuppressive therapy, and those suffering from cancer, severe trauma, or shock. The immune system is designed to control infections locally. The penetration of infectious agents or their products into the bloodstream frequently elicits an acute phase response. Many pathogenic microorganisms are capable of polyclonal lymphocyte activation (Banck & Forsgren, 1978), which leads to excess cytokine production.

Insulin, glucagon, epinephrine, norepinephrine and cortisone are all elevated during infection (Curnow *et al.*, 1976; Iochida *et al.*, 1989; Lang & Dobrescu, 1989, 1991). Glucocorticoids are increased shortly before the onset of fever. The circadian rhythm is lost if the infection becomes subacute or chronic and glucocorticoid levels generally fall to values below normal (Beisel, 1975). Patients with subclinical GC deficiency succumb to infection sooner than those with a normal GC response (Sibbald *et al.*, 1977; Rothwell, 1991).

In sheep, bacteremia caused a surge of plasma $\beta$-END, followed by increases in prolactin and growth hormone and a depression of plasma LH. Only the growth hormone response was inhibited by naloxone (Leshin & Malven, 1984). Septic patients with suppressed basal insulin levels and elevated glucagon levels did not respond to treatment with human growth hormone by raising serum levels of insulin-like growth factor 1 (IGF-1) (Dahn *et al.*, 1988).

*The response to bacterial endotoxin* The cell wall of Gram-negative microorganisms contains a lipopolysaccharide (LPS) component that is released after the death of bacteria. LPS induces a lethal shock in higher vertebrates, but not in the fish or frog (Berczi *et al.*, 1966*a*). It is the major pathogenic factor during Gram-negative infections (Berczi *et al.*, 1966*b*, 1968; Nagy *et al.*, 1968). Bile acids present in the gastrointestinal tract detoxify endotoxin. Oral intoxication is possible only if the bile is diverted from the gut (Bertok, 1977).

LPS activates B lymphocytes polyclonally for proliferation and immunoglobulin secretion, activates monocyte/macrophages for the production of various cytokines, triggers mediator release from mast cells, basophils and endothelial cells, and affects neutrophilic granulocytes. LPS also activates the complement and coagulation cascades (Müller-Eberhard, 1975; Fujiwara *et al.*, 1980; Burrell, 1991).

Several receptor molecules may be involved in the mediation of the biological effect of LPS. An LPS-binding glycoprotein (LBP) of $M_r$ 60 000, which was isolated from human and rabbit serum, rose significantly during the acute phase response. It was suggested that LBP activated the complement system after combining with LPS and stimulated monocytes via CD14; however, B lymphocytes do not process CD14, yet they responded to stimulation by LPS (Raetz *et al.*, 1991). LPS receptors and their signalling pathways are the subject of current enquiry.

*Cytokine and acute phase hormone response to LPS* Peripheral administration of LPS to rats induced immunoreactive IL-1$\beta$ in macrophages and ramified microglial cells in the meninges, choroid plexus, brain blood vessels and brain parenchyma (Van Dam *et al.*, 1992).

High but transient TNF$\alpha$ peaks were observed in mice after bolus intravenous (i.v.) challenges with LPS or bacteria (*Escherichia coli* 0111). In contrast, TNF$\alpha$, IL-1 and IL-6 levels increased progressively during lethal bacterial peritonitis to 50–100-fold lower than the peak values observed after i.v. challenge and remained constant until death. Anti-TNF$\alpha$ antibodies protected mice only after i.v. challenge with LPS, whereas anti-LPS antibodies were protective also in the peritonitis model. This protection was accompanied by a striking reduction of bacterial numbers and levels of TNF$\alpha$, IL-1 and IL-6 in the serum (Zanetti *et al.*, 1992).

In rats and mice, serum TNF levels were maximally elevated at 1–2 h after LPS injection and returned to normal by 4 h. Adrenalectomy led to an exaggerated production of TNF and high mortality, which could be counteracted by GC treatment (Waage, 1987; Parant *et al.*, 1991; Ramachandra *et al.*, 1992). Macrophages from hypophysectomized rats exerted a poor TNF$\alpha$ response to stimulation *in vitro* with LPS. Treatment of hypophysectomized animals with growth hormone partially corrected this deficiency (Edwards *et al.*, 1991).

Normal mice did not respond to repeated LPS injections with increased serum levels of TNF (endotoxin tolerance), whereas adrenalectomized mice did respond. Glucocorticoid treatment restored the ability of adrenalectomized mice to develop tolerance. Mice sensitized to LPS by the intoxication of the liver using galactosamine similarly lacked the ability to develop endotoxin tolerance, even though these animals exerted a normal elevation of serum GC in response to LPS (Evans & Zuckerman, 1991). Spleen cells of rats infused with a non-lethal dose of LPS for 2 weeks showed an impaired IL-1 and TNF response to LPS *in vitro.*

IFN-$\alpha$, -$\beta$ and -$\gamma$, induced by concanavalin A (Con A), were also suppressed (Friedman *et al.*, 1992).

In 12 healthy human volunteers given a 5-min i.v. infusion of purified LPS, plasma TNF was significantly elevated at 75–90 min, END rose at 1 h and cortisol at 1–5 h after infusion (Richardson *et al.*, 1989). Histamine release by human basophilic leukocytes in response to anti-IgE, specific antigens, or the calcium ionophore A23187 was enhanced by LPS (Clementsen *et al.*, 1990).

Mice injected with LPS showed a significant elevation of colony stimulating factors (CSF) at 45 min, which was further increased after 2 h (Quesenberry *et al.*, 1972).

In rats, LPS stimulated the synthesis of platelet activating factor (PAF), particularly in the lung, and this could be prevented by pretreatment with dexamethasone (DEX) (Ibbotson & Wallace, 1989).

*Neuroendocrine response to LPS* Wexler and coworkers (1957) discovered in rats that the injection of LPS stimulated the release of endogenous ACTH. Macrophage-derived cytokines, especially IL-1, play an important role in the ACTH response to LPS, although the underlying mechanism is complex and other, as yet unidentified, factors and pathways appear to be involved. LPS is capable of inducing elevated levels of serum glucocorticoids in hypophysectomized rats (Suzuki *et al.*, 1986, Rivier *et al.*, 1989; Derijk & Berkenbosch, 1991; Derijk *et al.*, 1992; Elenkov *et al.*, 1992). Circulating $\alpha$-MSH increased significantly in rabbits after LPS injection (Martin & Lipton, 1990).

In mice, serum prolactin levels increased five-fold 1 h after LPS injection, returning to normal by 90 min. Adrenalectomy had no effect on this response (Ramachandra *et al.*, 1992). Low doses of LPS given to lactating sows decreased prolactin concentrations and increased cortisol levels in the plasma (Smith & Wagner, 1984, 1985). Human volunteers injected with 4 ng/kg LPS responded with elevated growth hormone and cortisol secretion (Elin & Csako, 1989).

A non-lethal dose of i.v. LPS given to male rats induced large increases of estrogen, progesterone and corticosterone, and decreased serum testosterone, with maximal responses at 2 h (Christeff *et al.*, 1987).

A single subtoxic dose of LPS given to newborn rats decreased the level of serum thyroxin and led to an impaired thyroid response to TSH in adulthood, associated with somatic retardation. Treatment of adult rats with a shock-inducing dose of LPS induced a similar thyroid deficiency (Bertok & Nagy, 1984; Nagy & Bertok, 1990).

Endotoxin induced hyperglycemia and elevated insulin levels in rats. The level of plasma insulin was elevated only in conscious, but not in anesthetized rats. LPS decreased the inhibitory effect of epinephrine on insulin levels (Jones & Yelich, 1987; Yelich, 1990; Yelich *et al.*, 1991). Pretreatment of rats with DEX 1 h before LPS administration prevented hyperinsulinemia and hyperglycemia (Yelich *et al.*, 1987). In LPS-treated dogs, the elevation of plasma methionine-enkephalin (M-ENK) and $\beta$-END, but not of leucine-ENK (L-ENK), preceded the onset of hyperinsulinism (Merrill & Anderson, 1987). Plasma levels of epinephrine and norepinephrine increased in conscious adult rats with both the dose of LPS and with time, and did not correlate with heart rate or blood pressure (Jones & Romano, 1989).

The sympathetic nervous system activity was increased in the heart, liver, brown adipose tissue, and gastrocnemius muscle 26 h after LPS injection in rats (Arnold *et al.*, 1990). LPS activated noradrenergic, dopaminergic and epinephrine-containing neurones in the hypothalamus and dopaminergic neurones in other parts of the brain in rats. Prostaglandin synthesis played an important role in the catecholamine response to LPS in all brain regions examined (Masana *et al.*, 1990). In rats treated with LPS, plasma levels of endothelin (ET)-1 were increased sevenfold and ET-3 levels two-fold. Similar increases of ET-1 and ET-3 were observed in liver lymph (Vemulapalli *et al.*, 1991).

*Endotoxic shock* Geller *et al.* observed in 1954 that the administration of cortisone to mice prior to, or simultaneously with, a lethal dose of LPS protected the majority of the animals from death, but there was no protection when cortisone was administered after LPS. A transient bacteremia occurred in some animals a few hours after the injection of LPS. This could be suppressed by antibiotic treatment, but without protection. Injection of streptomycin or penicillin in animals previously treated with cortisone resulted in significantly higher mortality rates than in animals given cortisone alone. The protective effect of GC against endotoxic shock has since been observed repeatedly in various species and is attributed to the ability of these hormones to suppress leukocyte activation and excess cytokine production (Izumi & Bakhle, 1988; Jansen *et al.*, 1991).

Mice and baboons could be protected against a lethal dose of LPS or septicemia induced by *E. coli* by pretreatment with anti-TNF antibodies. However, anti-TNF antibodies did not improve the survival of mice nor reduced serum IL-1 and IL-6 levels after intraperitoneal (i.p.) bacterial challenge or after cecal ligation and puncture (Beutler *et al.*, 1985*a*; Tracey *et al.*, 1987; Eskandari *et al.*, 1992; Zanetti *et al.*, 1992).

No correlation was found between TNF serum levels and the lethal effects induced by different types of LPS in rats (Sanchez-Cantu *et al.*, 1991). The cotreatment of rats with low doses of TNF and LPS resulted in the rapid demise of the animals, leading to 100% mortality within 4 h (Myers *et al.*, 1990; Ciancio *et al.*, 1991). Pretreatment of rats with a single low i.v. dose of TNF prevented subsequent death from a lethal dose of TNF 24 h later and also provided protection against the lethal effects of LPS or cecal ligation and puncture applied 24 h later (Sheppard *et al.*, 1989).

Treatment of dogs given LPS at $LD_{80}$ doses i.v. with naloxone prevented the characteristic bloody diarrhea and reduced mortality (Ganes *et al.*, 1987). Treatment of rats with indomethacin reduced LPS-induced mortality, which was further diminished by dopamine infusion following indomethacin, but dopamine alone was ineffective (Goto & Griffin, 1988). Rabbits treated with an $LD_{80}$ dose of LPS were protected by additional treatment with IL-1 receptor antagonist (Ohlsson *et al.*, 1990). In mice pretreated with monoclonal antibodies to IFN-$\gamma$, mortality was significantly reduced after LPS treatment, although there was only a minor effect on serum TNF levels (Heinzel, 1990). In contrast, mice treated with neutralizing antibodies to murine TNF$\alpha$ serum IFN levels were reduced, and protection was afforded. Doses of TNF$\alpha$ and IFN-$\gamma$, which were well tolerated when given individually, were lethal when combined, and induced higher levels of IL-6 than did either cytokine alone (Doherty *et al.*, 1992). Treatment of rabbits with IFN-$\gamma$ and LPS led to a significant increase in toxicity (Jurkovich *et al.*, 1991). PAF plays a pathogenic role in endotoxic shock and the pharmacological inhibition of PAF has a preventive effect (Myers *et al.*, 1990; Crespo & Fernandez-Gallardo, 1991).

*Immunological injury* Substances that are otherwise harmless to the body may cause severe injury if there is an abnormal immune response directed against them (hypersensitivity). Tissue injury may be mediated by IgE antibodies (immediate hypersensitivity, allergy, asthma, anaphylaxis), by sensitized T lymphocytes (delayed hypersensitivity, contact dermatitis, etc.), by immune complexes, and by phagocyte cells activated either by antibodies or cytokines. Humoral or cell-mediated immune reactions may also be directed against self antigens and could lead to autoimmune disease. A detailed discussion of these mechanisms is beyond the scope of this review. Instead, the reader is referred to some key references (Talal,

1977; Brostoff & Hall, 1989; Barnetson & Gawkroger, 1989; Hay, 1989; Paul, 1989; Sinha *et al.*, 1990; Derijk & Berkenbosch, 1991; Homo-Delarche *et al.*, 1991; Berczi *et al.*, 1993).

The immune system has an elaborate internal regulatory network and has been regarded until recently as a self-regulating autonomous system in the body. However, it has become apparent during the past 15 years or so that a number of hormones are required for the normal development and function of the immune system and that even mild antigenic stimulation, which has no obvious pathological consequences, will activate the hypothalamus–pituitary–adrenal axis (Berczi, 1968*a*, 1990; Berkenbosch *et al.*, 1990; Ader & Cohen, 1991). An overwhelming body of evidence now supports the pathophysiological importance of this feedback regulatory interaction.

### *The acute phase response*

Wannemacher *et al.* (1975) described a proteinaceous secretion from leukocytes, termed leukocytic endogenous mediator (LEM), which stimulated the uptake of amino acids by the liver in adrenalectomized, hypophysectomized, thyroidectomized or diabetic rats. Similar stimulation could not be duplicated by pharmacological doses of a large variety of hormones. RNA synthesis was also augmented by LEM, which enhanced the hepatic production of a number of acute phase plasma globulins.

The acute phase response is the reaction of the body to injury caused by a variety of agents, including infectious disease. Clinically, it is characterized by fever, loss of appetite, inactivity and sleepiness. The reaction is mediated by cytokines, which appear in the circulation and function as acute phase hormones affecting the central nervous system (CNS), the neuroendocrine system and the function of virtually every other tissue and organ in the body. IL-6, TNF, and IL-1 have been identified as major mediators of the endocrine and metabolic changes characteristic of the acute phase response. However, several other cytokines have recently been found to be inducers of the acute phase response and, with the increase of our knowledge of new cytokines, it is likely that additional acute phase hormones will be identified (Jamieson *et al.*, 1987; Berczi, 1990; Spangelo & MacLeod, 1990; Akira & Kishimoto, 1992). ACTH, GC, epinephrine, norepinephrine, glucagon, AVP and aldosterone are elevated during the acute phase response, whereas growth hormone, estrogens, androgens, insulin and thyroid hormones may be either elevated or suppressed, depending on the severity of the condition (Table 4.6) (Baue, 1989).

Table 4.6. *Neuroendocrine response to injury*

| Hormone | Burn[a] | Trauma[b] | Surgery[c] | Infection[d] | Endotoxin[d] | APR[a] |
|---|---|---|---|---|---|---|
| ACTH | | ↑ | ↑ | | ↑ | ↑ |
| Glucocorticoids | ↑ | ↑ | ↑ | ↑ | ↑ | ↑ |
| Growth hormone | | ↑ | ↑ | ↑↓ | ↑ | ↑↓ |
| Prolactin | | | ↑ | ↑ | ↑↓ | |
| LH | 0 | ↓ | | ↓ | | |
| FSH | | ↓ | | | | |
| Estrogen | | | ↑ | | | ↑↓ |
| Androgen | ↓ | | ↓ | | | ↑↓ |
| Progesterone | | | ↓ | | | |
| TSH | | 0↓ | | | | |
| Thyroxine | | ↓ | | | ↓ | ↑↓ |
| Triiodothyronine | | ↓ | | 0↑ | | ↑↓ |
| Insulin | | | | ↑ | ↑ | ↑↓ |
| Glucagon | | | | ↑ | ↑ | ↑ |
| MSH | | 0 | | | ↑ | |
| Endorphin | | ↑ | | ↑ | ↑ | |
| Epinephrine | ↑ | ↑ | | ↑ | ↑ | ↑ |
| Norepinephrine | ↑ | ↑ | | ↑ | ↑ | ↑ |
| Dopamine | | | | | ↑ | |
| Histamine | ↑ | | | | | |
| AVP | | ↑ | | | ↑ | ↑ |
| Aldosterone | | | | | | ↑ |
| EPO | | ↑ | | | | |

↑, Increased serum/plasma level; ↓, decreased level; ↑↓, level may be either increased or decreased; 0, no change.
ACTH, adrenocorticotropic hormone; APR, acute phase response; AVP, arginine vasopressin; EPO, erythropoietin; FSH, follicle stimulating hormone; LH, luteinizing hormone; MSH, α-melanocyte stimulating hormone; PRL, prolactin; TSH, thyroid stimulating hormone.
[a] Birke *et al.*, 1957; Lephart *et al.*, 1987.
[b] Baue, 1989.
[c] Noel *et al.*, 1971; Adami *et al.*, 1982; Newsome & Rose, 1971; Lindh *et al.*, 1992.
[d] Please see text for references.

An alteration of protein synthesis by the liver is most characteristic for the acute phase response. A synthesis of new proteins, the so-called acute phase reactants, is initiated, whereas the synthesis of some normal serum constituents such as albumin and transferrin is decreased. The concentration of acute phase serum proteins (APP) increases dramatically. For example, in humans, C-reactive protein (CRP) and serum amyloid A (SAA) may increase over 1000-fold in cases of severe reaction. Fibrinogen,

$\alpha_1$-antitrypsin and certain complement and properdin components (factor B and C3) show a more moderate increase.

CRP has the capacity to combine specifically with phosphocholine and possibly also with some polysaccharides containing galactose, and with some biological polycations such as protamine, poly-L-lysine, and myelin basic protein. These moieties are frequent cell surface components on bacteria, fungi, parasites and damaged cells. CRP was found to localize *in vivo* at sites of inflamed, damaged tissue. After complexing with a specific ligand, CRP acquires the capacity to activate complement by the classical pathway, to activate neutrophils and monocytes for chemotaxis and enhanced phagocytosis, to induce tumoricidal activity in macrophages, which is complement-dependent, to stimulate the synthesis of IL-1 and TNF$\alpha$, and to potentiate the cytotoxic activity of T lymphocytes, natural killer cells and platelets. CRP also has the capacity to bind and block the activity of PAF. Therefore, CRP has the capacity to recognize foreign pathogens and damaged cells and to trigger their containment or elimination. IL-6 was effective in inducing CRP synthesis by human liver cells *in vitro*, but other cytokines were not. However, the production of CRP is modulated by IL-1, TNF$\alpha$, TGF$\beta$, and 1FN-$\gamma$. DEX potentiated the production of both CRP and SAA. The clinical determination of CRP has diagnostic value for infectious and inflammatory diseases. Similar proteins have been identified in all mammals, chicken, fish and even crabs (Ballou & Kushner, 1992).

The LBP that was isolated from human and rabbit serum also showed a 100-fold increase (from 0.5 to 50 μg/ml) during an acute phase response. LBP is capable of opsonizing LPS-bearing particles, and thus may be required for the activation of complement by endotoxin through the alternate pathway. LBP–LPS complexes were also potent stimulators of cytokines from monocytes and macrophages after combining with CD14 on the surface of the cells (Raetz *et al.*, 1991).

A number of other APPs are proteinase inhibitors, such as $\alpha_2$-macroglobulin, $\alpha_1$-acid glycoprotein, antithrombin III, $\alpha_1$-acute phase globulin, and $\alpha_1$-proteinase inhibitor, which are abundant in the rat. Turpentine injection into rats elicited an enhanced secretion of APP including $\alpha_2$-macroglobulin. Hypophysectomized rats did not show a similar response unless treated with DEX together with turpentine. Tissue culture medium conditioned by Kupffer cells induced a dose-dependent stimulation of $\alpha_2$-macroglobulin by hepatocytes in the presence of DEX at $10^{-9}$ mol/l (Bauer *et al.*, 1984).

Other APP have roles in blood clotting (fibrinogen) and healing.

Alpha-macrofetoprotein ($\alpha$-MFP) was found to be a strong inhibitor of inflammatory mediators, such as histamine, bradykinin, serotonin and $PGE_2$ and to inhibit polymorphonuclear cell chemotaxis. Catecholamines and GC induced $\alpha$-MFP in normal rats. The levels induced by catecholamines were very high, comparable to those observed in the post-injury phase, whereas the effect of GC was moderate. Since catecholamines activate the adrenal cortex *in vivo*, a synergistic effect has been suggested for these two kinds of adrenal hormone. In adrenalectomized rats the effect of catecholamines on $\alpha$-MFP synthesis was greatly diminished, whereas the moderate effect of GC was maintained. The combination of GC and catecholamines induced extremely high levels also in adrenalectomized animals. Other acute phase reactants, such as haptoglobin and $\alpha_1$-major APP, were affected differently by these hormones (Van Gool *et al.*, 1984).

Treatment of mice with LPS, TNF, and IL-1 decreased cytochrome P-450 in the liver, increased plasma fibrinogen and induced hypoferremia. Only IL-1, and not TNF or LPS, depressed cytochrome P-450 in cultured hepatocytes. Pretreatment of mice with DEX protected against the depression of liver cytochrome P-450 by LPS or TNF, but not by IL-1, and DEX had no influence on the increase of plasma fibrinogen and decrease of plasma iron levels (Bertini *et al.*, 1989). IL-1 and TNF can initiate a full range of APP *in vivo*, but only a limited number of APP were induced by these cytokines in cultured liver cells compared with crude cytokine preparations from macrophages. This led to the discovery of IL-6 as a major inducer of APP synthesis. Recently, additional cytokines, namely IFN-$\gamma$, leukemia inhibitory factor, TGF$\beta$ and oncostatin M, were found to be active as direct inducers of APP from liver (Akira & Kishimoto, 1992).

A protein purified and cloned from rat sciatic nerve was found to have neurotropic properties and was named ciliary neurotropic factor (CNTF). CNTF induced the APP genes haptoglobin and $\alpha_1$-antichymotrypsin in human hepatoma cells (HepG2), and $\alpha_2$-macroglobulin and $\beta$-fibrinogen in primary rat hepatocytes, with a time-course and dose response comparable to that of IL-6. CNTF has so far been found intracellularly in large quantities in the central and peripheral nervous system and in non-neural cells, but it is not clear whether or not it can be secreted. The physiological relevance of these observations is not resolved. It is possible that CNTF is released during injury and thereby can participate in the initiation of a systemic response. Because APP are synthesized not only in the liver, but also in the choroid plexus and placenta, CNTF may be involved in the regulation of APP synthesis in the choroid plexus (Schooltink *et al.*, 1992).

IL-6 activates the genes of APP through the DNA binding protein called NF-IL-6. Consequently, NF-IL-6 may be a pleiotropic mediator of many inducible genes involved in the acute, immune and inflammatory responses, similarly to another DNA binding protein, NFkB. Both NF-IL-6 and NFkB binding sites are present in the inducible genes, such as IL-6 , IL-8 and several acute phase genes (Akira & Kishimoto, 1992).

Adrenalin evokes a high level of IL-6 in rats and this can be antagonized by propranolol. When IL-6 release is blocked in this way, the fast reacting APP $\alpha_2$-macroglobulin and cysteine protease inhibitor are strongly depressed. Isoprenalin, which is a $\beta_2$ adrenergic receptor agonist, also causes very high levels of IL-6, indicating that $\beta_2$ receptors are involved (Van Gool *et al.*, 1990).

## Neural and endocrine regulation of cytokines

### *Regulation by hormones*

#### *Growth and lactogenic hormones*

Growth hormone and prolactin are essential for the function of the bone marrow and thymus, and for the maintenance of immunocompetence (Nagy & Berczi, 1989, 1991; Berczi *et al.*, 1991). These observations imply that there must be a relationship between growth hormone and prolactin action and the cytokine network in all lymphoid organs that somehow regulates lymphoproliferation and function in harmony. However, few details of this interaction have been elucidated to date.

Under proper conditions, a direct mitogenic effect of growth hormone on lymphocytes and augmentation of IL-2 production can be demonstrated. Growth hormone also stimulates the production of IL-1 and superoxide anions and potentiates the induction of TNF$\alpha$ by LPS in mononuclear phagocytes (Edwards *et al.*, 1988, 1991; Schimpff & Repellin, 1990). Growth hormone stimulated neutrophilic leukocytes for lysosomal enzyme production and oxidative metabolism, primed for superoxide production, promoted adhesiveness and inhibited chemotaxis (Rovensky *et al.*, 1985; Spadoni *et al.*, 1990; Fu *et al.*, 1991; Wiedermann *et al.*, 1991*a, b*).

The production of IFN-$\gamma$ by T lymphocytes and lymphocyte proliferation in response to mitogens was depressed in spleen cells of mice treated with bromocriptine. These deficiencies could be reversed by additional treatment with prolactin (Bernton *et al.*, 1988). Prolactin induced the expression of IL-2 receptors by spleen cells of rats, but did not induce IL-2 secretion. This response was dependent on the concentration of prolactin and was observed with splenocytes from ovariectomized rats or from rats in diestrus, whereas spleen cells from estrogen-treated ovariectomized rats or rats in estrus did not respond (Mukherjee *et al.*, 1990).

A murine helper T-cell clone responded to stimulation with IL-2 only in the presence of prolactin. The cells internalized prolactin from the culture medium, and the prolactin translocated from the cytoplasm to the nucleus after stimulation with IL-2. These data suggest that extracellular prolactin is required for T-cell proliferation and that prolactin renders T cells competent to respond to IL-2 by acting on the nucleus (Clevenger *et al.*, 1990).

### *The ACTH–adrenal axis*

*Proopiomelanocortin-derived peptides* Although most of the effect of ACTH on the immune system is due to the stimulation of GC hormone secretion by the adrenal cortex, a direct action of ACTH on lymphocytes has also been demonstrated. ACTH potentiated the induction of IL-6 and TNF$\alpha$ by LPS, as discussed above. $\alpha$-MSH has been found to antagonize several effects of IL-1 , including pyrogenicity, thymocyte proliferation, neutrophilia, the induction of APP, depression of TNF and contact sensitivity, and induction of prostaglandin E in fibroblasts. These effects are not mediated by classical $\alpha$-MSH receptors. Much of the antagonism takes place at the level of the CNS (Glyn-Ballinger *et al.*, 1983; Murphy *et al.*, 1983; Cannon *et al.*, 1986; Robertson *et al.*, 1988; Sundar *et al.*, 1989).

$\beta$-END, L-ENK and $\beta$-neoendorphin potentiated IL-1 production by murine bone marrow-derived macrophages after stimulation by either LPS or silica. $\alpha$-END, M-ENK and $\alpha$-neoendorphin were ineffective in this respect (Apte *et al.*, 1990). $\beta$-END enhanced significantly the IL-1 induced IL-2 production by the murine lymphoid cell line EL-4. These effects were seen with both IL-1$\alpha$ and IL-1$\beta$, and it was completely abolished by naloxone. Other opioid peptides, including $\gamma$-END and ENK, elicited similar effects. The enhancing effect was associated with higher levels of IL-2 mRNA (Bessler *et al.*, 1990). $\beta$-END also enhanced the production of IL-2 by unfractionated murine splenocytes after mitogen stimulation. This enhancement was irreversible by naloxone (Gilmore & Weiner, 1988). Rats were infused with $\beta$-END, and IL-2 production by their spleen cells was examined *in vitro* after Con A stimulation. Although the infusion induced a dose-dependent enhancement of the proliferative response of spleen cells to Con A, suppressed if the rats were also treated with naloxone, neither treatment influenced IL-2 production after 48 h in culture. When spleen cells were treated with β-END *in vitro*, with or without naloxone, Con A-induced proliferation was enhanced by β-END ($10^{-12}$ to $10^{-9}$ mol/l) and abrogated by naloxone ($10^{-6}$ mol/l) (Kusnecov *et al.*, 1987).

β-END may either enhance or suppress the production of IFN-γ by mitogen-stimulated human peripheral blood lymphocytes (PBL) *in vitro*. Considerable variation was observed on the effect of β-END on IFN production in individuals who underwent multiple testing. Suppression was significantly greater in 16 male donors than in 8 female donors upon preincubation of PBL for 3 h with β-END followed by Con A stimulation for 72 h in 20% (v/v) fetal bovine serum (FBS). Lowering the concentration of FBS resulted in increased production of IFN-γ in PBL exposed to β-END. β-END did not alter IFN-γ production in culture medium containing 3% autologous serum. Neither did arachidonic acid, but a significant suppression resulted when the two agents were added together (Brummitt *et al.*, 1988). β-END and M-ENK enhanced IFN-γ production by Con A-stimulated human mononuclear cells from the majority of donors tested at concentrations between $10^{-14}$ and $10^{-10}$ mol/l. Some cells did not respond. There is not an absolute correlation between an enhanced response to β-END and M-ENK, suggesting the presence of multiple receptor types for opioids on these cells. Naloxone had no significant influence on the opioid effect (Brown & Van Epps, 1986).

β-END induced a dose-dependent release of histamine from rat peritoneal mast cells (PMC) at $10^{-6}$ mol/l (Sydbom, 1988). Human volunteers reacted with positive immediate-type skin reactions to testing with morphine, codeine, meperidine, dynorphin, L-ENK, and morphiceptin. The order of potency for inducing wheal-and-flare reactions was dynorphin > β-END = morphiceptin. Mast cell degranulation was demonstrated by electron microscopy at the reaction sites and experiments with naloxone suggested that both opioid and non-opioid receptors were involved (Casale *et al.*, 1984).

*Glucocorticoids* Virtually all the functions of the monocyte–macrophage cell series are inhibited by GC. These include cell metabolism, chemotaxis, cytotoxic reactions and the capacity to present antigen, to secrete cytokines, and to produce enzymes and other factors (Berczi, 1986*b*).

Hydrocortisone at pharmacological concentration ($10^{-5}$ mol/l) markedly suppressed IL-1 secretion by fresh human monocytes after stimulation with LPS. IFN-$\gamma$ enhanced IL-1 secretion when applied alone, but suppression resulted when it was combined with hydrocortisone (Haq, 1988). GC markedly decreased IL-1$\beta$ mRNA levels in the human promonocytic cell line U-937 after induction with phorbol ester and LPS. Both the transcription of the IL-1 gene and a selective decrease in stability of IL-1$\beta$ mRNA has been observed (Lee *et al.*, 1988). The importance of GC in the regulation of IL-1 and its biological activity is illustrated by the observation that adrenalectomy sensitizes mice to the lethal effect of IL-1, which could be prevented by pretreatment with DEX (Bertini *et al.*, 1988). The expression of IL-1 receptor by human peripheral blood monocytes was increased by both physiological and pharmacological concentrations of GC, whereas progesterone, 17$\beta$-estradiol and testosterone had no effect. Maximum enhancement was seen 6 h after treatment and it was dose-dependent, with half the maximum effect elicited by 100 nmol prednisolone/l. Glucocorticoids also induced the expression of IL-1 receptor on normal human fibroblasts and on a large granular lymphocyte cell line YT (Akahoshi *et al.*, 1988).

Human monocytes were stimulated to produce TNF by LPS, phorbol myristate acetate (PMA), silica quartz, and anti-human IgG antibody. Prednisolone and budenoside strongly inhibited secretion of TNF induced by LPS and anti-human IgG, and more weakly after silica induction. Minimum inhibition was present when PMA was used as an inducer. Inhibition could not be overcome by increasing the cell activating stimulus, and the presence of corticosteroids during the phase of cell activation was necessary (Debets *et al.*, 1989). The tumoricidal activity of macrophages from murine peritoneal exudate, and activated by IFN-$\gamma$ and LPS, was markedly inhibited in a dose-dependent fashion when GCs were added simultaneously, but inhibition was suboptimal if GCs were added 24 h later. Sex hormones had no effect (Hogan & Vogel, 1988).

The injection of LPS i.v. (25 μg) for 9 days in mice bearing the SA1 sarcoma, resulted in extensive necrosis of the core of this tumor, which was followed by complete regression. This was associated with TNF production in the tumor tissue. Such hemorrhagic necrosis and regression failed to occur in mice that were given subcutaneous (s.c.) cortisone acetate or DEX 12 h before being given LPS. GC had no effect, however, on the ability of TNF injected i.v. to cause tumor hemorrhagic necrosis and regression (North & Havell, 1989). Adrenalectomy rendered mice susceptible to the lethal effect of TNF, which could be prevented with DEX (0.3 mg/kg) (Bertini *et al.*, 1988).

High concentrations of circulating TNF were detected in cancer patients undergoing immunotherapy with IL-2. When such patients were given DEX, in most cases TNF levels remained below the threshold of detectability by radioimmunoassay. Treatment also prevented the elevation of CRP and the development of the neutrophil chemotactic defect that is characteristic of IL-2 recipients (Mier *et al.*, 1990).

GCs prevented the transcription of the IL-6 gene in human peripheral blood mononuclear cells (Zanker *et al.*, 1990). On the other hand, DEX upregulated the expression of IL-6 receptors on a human epithelial cell line (UAC) and on two hepatoma cell lines (HepG2 and Hep3B). The enhancing effect was due to an increase in mRNA expression (Snyers *et al.*, 1990).

In human lung fibroblasts, TNF induces the expression of IL-6, IL-8, GM-CSF and M-CSF. DEX (1 μmol/l) repressed GM-CSF, IL-6 and IL-8, mRNA and protein levels, but did not affect M-CSF production (Tobler *et al.*, 1992).

The helper, suppressor, and killer function of T lymphocytes and their production of interleukins are inhibited by GC (Berczi, 1986*b*). DEX and 6α-methylprednisolone blocked the mitogen-induced IL-2 gene expression in human PBL. The antiproliferative effect of these GC could not be antagonized by IL-1, -2, -3, -4, -5, -6, TNFα, -β, and IFN-γ when applied individually. A combination of IL-1 plus IL-6 plus IFN-γ (25–50 U/ml each) totally abrogated this antiproliferative effect (Almawi *et al.*, 1991). At low concentrations, GC inhibited IL-2 production by murine T lymphocytes, whereas IL-4 production was increased in *in vivo* experiments. Similar changes in the pattern of the production of these interleukins was observed following short pulses with low-dose GC *in vitro* and the steroid-induced depression in IL-2 production could be reversed or inhibited by treatment with the steroid antagonist RU486 (Daynes & Araneo, 1989).

Hydrocortisone ($10^{-9}$–$10^{-6}$ mol/l) inhibited the antigen induced, but not the IL-2-mediated proliferative response of human influenza virus immune T-cell clones. The production of IL-2 by these clones was inhibited in both situations. Hydrocortisone had no effect on the induction of tolerance by antigen (Moss *et al.*, 1984). Exposure of the murine cytotoxic T-cell line clone CTLL-2 to DEX induced apoptosis. The presence of a saturating concentration of IL-2 during the treatment of CTLL-2 with GC prevented cell death (Nieto & Lopez-Rivas, 1989).

The production of IL-2, IFN-γ and CSF by long-term alloreactive murine T-cell lines after Con A stimulation was suppressed by physiological concentrations ($10^{-8}$–$10^{-6}$ mol/l) of GC. An additional cytokine, macrophage activating factor (MAF), was also suppressed under these conditions. Pre-exposure and removal of DEX before Con A stimulation inhibited MAF release. The growth inhibitory effect of DEX could be dissociated from its action on lymphokine secretion (Kelso & Munck, 1984). Hydrocortisone inhibited the production of IFN-$\gamma$ by rat spleen cells in a dose-dependent manner ($5.5 \times 10^{-10}$–$5.5 \times 10^{-8}$ mol/l concentrations being effective) *in vitro* without affecting cell survival. This inhibitory effect could be blocked by RU38486 (Jiayi *et al.*, 1989).

The expression of Fc receptors for IgG by human monocytes (FeR$\gamma$I) was increased by IFN-$\gamma$, and the effect was maximal when the cells were cotreated with DEX. A newly discovered surface antigen of monocytes identified with monoclonal antibody showed a similar enhancement of expression when both agents were used; however, this moiety was inhibited or unaffected by treatment with IFN-$\gamma$ alone (Morganelli & Guyre, 1988). Exposure of the murine macrophage cell line RAW264.7 to murine IFN-$\gamma$ significantly increased the number of GC receptors (GC-R) with the doubling time of 24 h and maximal levels at 36 h. A twofold increase in GC-R activity was also found. These results suggest that IFN-$\gamma$ may increase the sensitivity of macrophages to feedback inhibition by GC (Salkowski & Vogel, 1992). DEX (200 nmol/l) increased twofold the number of IFN-$\gamma$ receptors on human monocytes *in vitro*. This effect was noted if the concentration of DEX was greater than 50 nmol/l and could be observed as early as after 18 h of treatment (Strickland *et al.*, 1986). Physiological and therapeutic concentrations of GC decrease the number of Fc$\gamma$R on human monocyte-like cells, whereas IFN-$\gamma$ increases receptor expression. When cultures of monocytes were incubated with both GC and IFN-$\gamma$ for 18 h the number of Fc$\gamma$R was significantly higher than on monocytes treated with IFN-$\gamma$ alone. Treatment with GC alone did not consistently decrease monocyte Fc$\gamma$R levels after either 18 or 42 h of exposure. Other steroids tested had no effect on IFN-$\gamma$ action. Other types of IFN were ineffective (Girard *et al.*, 1987).

DEX increased polymeric IgA and antigen-specific IgA antibody levels in the serum of rats. This response to DEX coincided with declining IgA and IgG levels in the saliva and vaginal secretions. A protein called secretory component (SC) functions as the receptor responsible for the transportation of IgA from blood and tissue into bile and external secretions. SC binds to IgA molecules to form dimers. DEX-treated rats had increased SC levels in the serum and saliva, and an increased SC production rate in the liver (Wira & Rossoll, 1991).

In recent years, a family of chemotactic proinflammatory cytokines has been described that also exert reparative activities. All have molecular masses of 8–10 kDa and exhibit 20–45% homology. Five, including IL-8, platelet factor 4 (PF-4), $\beta$-thromboglobulin ($\beta$-TG), IP-10 and melanoma growth stimulating factor or GRO, can be assigned to a subfamily encoded on chromosome 4. The genes of the second subset (LD78, ACT-2, I-309, RANTES, and macrophage chemotactic and activating factor (MCAF)) are closely linked on human chromosome 17. PF-4 and $\beta$-TG have so far been detected only in platelets, whereas IL-8, IP-10, GRO, MCAF and the murine JE are produced by leukocytes and non-leukocytic cells in response to a wide variety of endogenous stimuli as well as exogenous agents, such as lectins, bacterial products, viruses, and injurious agents, such as silica or sodium urate crystals. The inflammatory cytokines, such as IL-1, IFN, TNF, epidermal growth factor (EGF), and platelet derived growth factor (PDGF), are potent inducers of some of these chemotactic proinflammatory cytokines. GC and TGF$\beta$ have so far been identified as suppressing agents. IL-8 is also suppressed by IL-4 and 1,25$(OH)_2$-vitamin $D_3$ (Hirashima *et al.*, 1985; Oppenheim, 1991). GC potentiated the synergistic stimulatory effect of IL-1 and IL-6 on immunoglobulin production by activated B cells (Emilie *et al.*, 1988). Thymic hormones, IL-1, IL-2, and IFN all antagonize the inhibitory effect of GC on lymphoid tissue (Berczi, 1986*b*; Fuggetta *et al.*, 1988; Nieto & Lopez-Rivas, 1989).

Preincubation of mouse bone marrow-derived mast cells with DEX for 24 h inhibited granule secretion, the IgE-dependent biosynthesis and release of leukotrienes $LTC_4$ and $LTB_4$ significantly increased the release of prostaglandin $D_2$, and decreased the number of IgE-Fc receptors by 55% (Robin *et al.*, 1985). The release of arachidonic acid metabolites from rat PMC by Con A, the antigen ovalbumin, and anti-IgE antibody, was markedly reduced by overnight preincubation with hydrocortisone. However, GC pretreatment did not alter arachidonic acid release stimulated by somatostatin, compound 48/80, or the calcium ionophore A32187 (Heiman & Crews, 1984).

Cutaneous mast cells were depleted in humans by the topical application of two corticosteroids, clobetasol-17-propionate and fluocinonide. A greater than 85% decrease was found in histamine content after 6 weeks of treatment, whereas in treatment with betamethasone valerate, there was a 68% decrease. After the cessation of treatment, it took 3 months for histamine levels to return to normal (Lavker & Schechter, 1985).

GC induce lipocortins in various target cells and tissues that include macrophages, neutrophils, thymus, spleen, lung and kidney cells. Lipocortins inhibit phospholipase $A_2$, a key enzyme in arachidonic acid production, and through this, the secretion of prostaglandins and leukotrienes is reduced. Lipocortins are not involved in the regulation of inflammation by mast cells. They are members of a calcium-binding protein family that is distinct from the calmodulin family. So far, six lipocortin-like proteins have been characterized. At present, they are regarded as intracellular mediators of GC action, and it is doubtful whether lipocortins are secreted (Whitehouse, 1989).

*Catecholamines* Treatment of murine macrophages with norepinephrine or with the $\alpha_2$-adrenergic agonist UK-14304 augmented the production of LPS-stimulated TNF. This effect could be inhibited by the $\alpha_2$-antagonist yohimbine. The greatest increase in TNF production occurred at lower LPS concentrations. UK-14304 increased LPS-induced TNF mRNA accumulation, which could also be blocked by yohimbine (Spengler *et al.*, 1990). The production of TNF by human blood monocytes and THP-1 cells stimulated by LPS was inhibited by epinephrine and isoproterenol. This effect of epinephrine was prevented by a $\beta$-receptor antagonist, but not by an $\alpha$-receptor antagonist. The levels of TNF mRNA were not reduced by epinephrine and the inhibitory effect of TNF was observed only if the cells were exposed to epinephrine or isoproterenol at about the same time as to LPS. When THP-1 cells were incubated with isoproterenol for 24 h before LPS stimulation, the TNF response was dramatically increased, and could not be suppressed by a second dose of isoproterenol. Intracellular cAMP levels were increased by epinephrine and isoproterenol when TNF production was inhibited, whereas after prolonged incubation of THP-1 cells with isoproterenol, a depression of cAMP was found (Severn *et al.*, 1992).

Epinephrine and norepinephrine blocked the capacity of IFN-$\gamma$ to activate murine macrophages to kill target cells infected with herpes simplex virus. ACTH, dopamine, serotonin and $\beta$-END had no effect in this regard. Treatment with dibutyryl cAMP blocked the induction of macrophage-mediated cytotoxicity, suggesting that the catecholamines were modulating macrophage function through the adrenergic receptor (Koff & Dunegan, 1986).

The incubation of human PBL for 1 h with the $\beta$-adrenergic receptor antagonist, propranolol ($10^{-6}$ mol/l), resulted in an increase of low affinity IL-2 receptor-positive cells. Propanolol also augmented the induction of IL-2 receptors by phytohemagglutinin (PHA) (Malec & Nowak, 1988). The $\beta$-adrenergic receptor agonist isoproterenol blocked the expression of IL-2 receptors on mitogen-stimulated human lymphocytes and on IL-2-dependent T-lymphocyte cell lines. Only low affinity receptors were affected; no significant effect on high-affinity IL-2 receptor sites could be detected in the system (Feldman *et al.*, 1987). Histamine release from sensitized human leukocytes by antigen was inhibited by $\beta$-adrenergic agonists (Assem & Schild, 1973).

### *Sex hormones*

Mice were infused continuously for 15 days with a daily dose of $6.6 \times 10^{-10}$ mol/l of one of the following compounds: prednisone, testosterone, 17$\beta$-estradiol ($E_2$), diethylstilbestrol, progesterone and ethisterone. The production of IL-1 by peritoneal macrophages was stimulated in the animals treated with $E_2$ and diethylstilbestrol, progesterone and ethisterone, but not by GC or testosterone. The same hormones also stimulated the expression of MHC-II antigens by macrophages (Flynn, 1986). The activity of the IFN-$\gamma$ promoter in lymphoid cells that expressed the appropriate hormone receptor was increased markedly by 17$\beta$-estradiol. This effect was mediated by sequences in the 5′ flanking region of the gene and can augment the effect of T-cell-activating agents. The short-term exposure of Con A-treated murine spleen cells to $E_2$ increased the level of IFN-$\gamma$ mRNA (Fox *et al.*, 1991). The production of IFN by human leukocytes was reduced slightly by $E_2$, but only in pharmacological concentrations. Progesterone had a modest effect at pharmacological levels, but only when Con A was the inducer. Testosterone did not affect IFN titers at any concentration. None of the sex steroids affected IFN-$\alpha$ production (Le *et al.*, 1988).

Uterine epithelial cells isolated from immature, diestrous and estrous stage mice produced similar amounts of IL-6. The addition of $E_2$ to these cultures markedly inhibited total IL-6 secretion. Uterine stromal cells in culture also secreted IL-6, which was inhibited by $E_2$ and physiological concentrations of progesterone. There was a synergistic effect when the two hormones were applied together. The secretion of IL-6 by stromal, but not by epithelial, cells was stimulated by IL-1$\alpha$. Messenger RNA was detected in stromal cells for IL-6 and IL-1$\alpha$, but not IL-1$\beta$. TNF$\alpha$ mRNA was present only after culture with IL-1$\alpha$ (Jacobs *et al.*, 1992).

*Other hormones*

Nerve growth factor (NGF) is synthesized in the submandibular gland and in the CNS by various cells including hypothalamic nuclei, and is present in the bloodstream. NGF has an influence on the hematopoietic and immune systems. Rat PMC, preincubated with NGF, responded with a marked enhancement of histamine release upon challenge with antigen when compared with the release induced by antigen alone. NGF increased the initial rate of release at 15 s, but did not prolong the overall duration of release. The simultaneous addition of antigen and NGF did not cause enhanced release. A minimum of 5 min was necessary for preincubation and the effect lasted 1 h. NGF enhanced histamine release induced by Con A, compound 48/80, and calcium ionophore A23187. NGF also caused mast cell hyperplasia, which in the case of connective tissue mast cells was dependent on the ability of NGF to cause degranulation, whereas in the case of mucosal mast cells it was independent of degranulation. Histamine release by human umbilical cord blood cells induced by IL-3 was significantly enhanced in serum-free cultures by NGF and IL-4 (Tomioka *et al.*, 1988; Levi-Montalcini *et al.*, 1990; Marshall *et al.*, 1990; Richard *et al.*, 1992).

Calcitonin inhibited the ability of human macrophages to produce $H_2O_2$ in response to IFN-$\gamma$ or to act as antigen presenting cells (Nong *et al.*, 1989).

***Neural and neuropeptide regulation of cytokines***

*Macrophages*

Substance P, neurokinin A, neurotensin, bombesin, gastrin-releasing peptide, END, ENK and somatostatin are all capable of up- or down-regulating macrophage activity. These interactions may play a role in the regulation of local immunity and inflammatory response in tissues with dense neuropeptidergic innervation (Hartung, 1988). Substance P and its carboxy terminal peptides, SP4-11 and substance K, induce the release of IL-1, TNF$\alpha$ and IL-6 from human blood monocytes. This effect occurs at low concentrations, can be inhibited by a substance antagonist and requires *de novo* protein synthesis (Lotz *et al.*, 1988). Neurotensin enhanced the release of IL-1 from rat alveolar macrophages after induction by LPS, muramyl dipeptide or zymosan. The effect was dose dependent and was observed at $10^{11}$–$10^{-6}$ ml/l of concentrations (Lemaire, 1988). Calcitonin gene related peptide (CGRP) inhibited antigen presentation and IFN-$\gamma$ induced $H_2O_2$ production by human macrophages (Nong *et al.*, 1989).

Intracerebroventricular (i.c.v.) injections of IL-1 in rats produced a dose-dependent increase in plasma corticosterone and ACTH and suppression of the secretion of IL-1 in splenic macrophages following LPS stimulation *in vitro*. Macrophage TGF$\beta$ secretion was not affected. In adrenalectomized animals, i.c.v. IL-1$\beta$ injection resulted in stimulation of IL-1 secretion, indicating that the suppression was mediated by corticosterone. However, denervation of the spleen also prevented the macrophage suppressive signal after i.c.v. IL-1$\beta$ administration. In adrenalectomized rats with spleen denervation, secretion of IL-1 by splenic macrophages after stimulation with i.c.v. IL-1$\beta$ was greater than in those with either adrenalectomy or splenic nerve section alone (Brown *et al.*, 1991).

### *T lymphocytes*

Substance P synergized with PMA in a dose-dependent manner to induce IL-2 production by the murine T-cell lines EL-4.IL-2 and LBRM-TG6. This effect was inhibited by spantide and physalaemin, which have affinity for SP receptors (Rameshwar *et al.*, 1992). The expression of IL-2 mRNA and secretion of IL-2 by the human T cell lines Jurkat and HUT78, and by peripheral blood human T cells activated by PHA plus PMA was enhanced by substance P. The cosignal activity was carried by the C terminal portion of substance P and optimal effects were observed with concentrations of $10^{-12}$–$10^{-10}$ mol/l. The increase of IL-2 was inhibited by a substance P antagonist (Calvo *et al.*, 1992).

Corticotropin releasing factor (CRF) increased the proliferation of human lymphocytes in the absence or the presence of T-cell mitogens, such as Con A and PHA. CRF also enhanced the expression of IL-2 receptors on activated T cells in culture after 3–5 days of incubation (Singh, 1989). Somatostatin and vasoactive intestinal peptide (VIP) reduced the production of IFN-$\gamma$ by human peripheral blood mononuclear cells activated by staphylococcal enterotoxin A (Muscettola & Grasso, 1990).

### *Tissue mast cells and basophils*

Substance P induces mediator release from rat PMC and intestinal mucosal mast cells (IMC). This release can be inhibited by antiallergic drugs, microtubule-inhibiting agents and calmodulin inhibitors. The profile of responsiveness to a panel of antiallergic drugs was similar for both PMC and IMC to what was reported previously for immunologically induced mast cell discharge. Thus, cromoglycate, theophylline, and Ro22-3747 inhibited peptide-induced secretion from PMC, but not from IMC. Doxantrazole was effective against both PMC and IMC (Shanahan *et al.*, 1986; Mio *et al.*, 1991).

Somatostatin suppressed mediator release from unpurified human basophils challenged with antibody to IgE, but had no influence on mediator release elicited by the calcium ionophore A23187. Similar results were obtained with rat basophil leukemia cells (Goetzl & Payan, 1984). Isolated rat PMC released histamine after stimulation with somatostatin. PMC prepared from mice and hamsters were noticeably less reactive, whereas human basophils and tissue mast cells of the guinea pig were essentially unreactive to somatostatin (Kassessinoff & Pearce, 1988). Human mast cells associated with mucosal surfaces did not respond to substance P, VIP or somatostatin with histamine release, whereas skin mast cells did (Church *et al.*, 1991).

A variety of basic, sensorineuropeptides (substance P, CGRP, somatomedin, VIP, neurokinin A and B, peptide histidine–methionine) induced the release of histamine from rat PMC. However, a wide range of other polycationic agents, such as 48/80, the mast cell degranulating peptide from bee venom, and polylysine, also induced discharge. Species- and tissue-specific differences were observed. The compounds tested were most active against rat serosal mast cells. Tissue mast cells of the rat and PMC of other rodents showed graded responses, whereas guinea pig and human mast cells were unreactive (Pearce *et al.*, 1989).

### *Neutrophilic granulocytes*

Substance P activated the respiratory burst and the secretion of specific and azurophilic granules by granulocytes. The SP (4-11) fragment was much more stimulating than the entire molecule, whereas the SP (1–4) fragment was inactive (Serra *et al.*, 1988). Substance P ($10^{-7}$–$10^{-9}$ mol/l) caused neutrophilic and eosinophilic infiltration in the skin of mice 6 h after injection. SP (1-9) ($10^{-5}$–$10^{-4}$ mol/l) also caused granulocyte infiltration, which was associated with mast cell degranulation. In contrast, SP (6-11) ($10^{-7}$–$10^{-4}$ mol/l), which was found to increase vascular permeability, induced no significant granulocyte infiltration or mast cell degranulation. However, SP (6-11) enhanced SP (1-9)-induced granulocyte infiltration in the skin without any significant increase in mast cell degranulation (Iwamoto *et al.*, 1992). Treatment of neonatal rats with capsaicin permanently destroyed primary afferent unmyelinated nerves and depleted the skin and organs of substance P. These animals had a reduced capacity to mount an inflammatory response to injury. Neutrophils from such capsaicin-treated rats showed normal chemotaxis induced by substance P *in vitro*, indicating that these granulocytes were not affected by the capsaicin treatment (Helme *et al.*, 1987).

*Platelets*

Apart from their role in the initiation of blood coagulation and reaction to injury, platelets also participate in an IgE- or lymphokine-dependent killing of parasites and other targets. Substance P and its carboxy-terminal fragment SP (4-11) ($10^{-8}$ mol/l) induced the cytotoxic activity of platelets towards larvae of *Schistosoma mansoni*, whereas the modified C-terminal SP, the substance P-free acid, was ineffective in this respect. The effect was specific, as revealed by inhibition with the antagonist D/SP. Preincubation of platelets with myeloma human IgE or with AP2 monoclonal antibodies, which inhibit IgE-dependent killing by platelets, led to a dramatic decrease of SP-induced cytotoxic activity (Damonneville *et al.*, 1990).

*Astrocytes*

Astrocytes carry receptors for SP. When rat astrocytes were treated with $10^{-10}$–$10^{-8}$ mol/l SP, the formation of PGE and thromboxane $B_2$ ($TXB_2$) was induced in a dose-dependent manner. The carboxy-terminal peptide sequence of SP was responsible primarily for this biological activity (Hartung *et al.*, 1988).

**Defense mechanisms against injury**

Although there are numerous gaps in our knowledge with regard to the response of the body to injury, it is now possible to outline the general pathways that are involved and to construct hypotheses that can be tested. The body is constantly bombarded by a variety of insults that could result in injury and the hallmark of a healthy organism is to be able to mount adequate defense/compensatory mechanisms so that health (homeostasis) is maintained. It is likely that the cytokine network constantly interacts harmoniously with the neuroendocrine system and with other tissues and organs at a subclinical level, which is a prerequisite of being in good health. Much remains to be investigated in this area.

***The local inflammatory response to injury***

Sensory nerves may be regarded as the first line of defense against injury by having the function of alerting the CNS about unpleasant stimuli (e.g. heat, cold, mechanical or chemical insult, etc.) so that the organism can react before things have gone too far. That sensory nerves also have the capacity to induce inflammation has been discovered by Jancso and coworkers (1967). The insult is sensed by the nerve endings (polymodal nociceptors) and the information is transmitted towards the CNS, but such impulses pass antidromically into other branches of the neurone to cause the release of SP and other neuropeptides, which induce inflammation either directly or indirectly by degranulating mast cells. In addition to SP, somatostatin and neurokinin A have been localized in sensory nerves which form neuroeffector junctions with mast cells. The depletion of sensory neuropeptides in lung and skin by capsaicin prevents the inflammatory changes and bronchial constriction induced by nerve stimulation or by chemical or dermal stimuli (Foreman, 1987).

In patients, neurogenic inflammation could be elicited by treatment with mustard oil in normally innervated skin, but not in skin areas affected by herpes zoster or in a patient suffering from congenital analgesia. If a skin area was treated repeatedly with capsaicin, desensitization occurred towards neurogenic inflammatory stimuli that lasted for several days. In the desensitized area, chemical pain sensation was strongly reduced, whereas threshold for warmth and heat pain sensations were significantly elevated. Local capsaicin desensitization of the skin prevented whealing, flaring and itching in patients with acquired cold and heat urticaria (Jancso *et al.*, 1985).

Inflammation was produced in rats by the intraarticular injection of 2% (w/v) carrageenan, 20 μg SP, 1% (v/v) formalin and 2% (w/v) urate. Surgical denervation of the joint significantly inhibited the inflammatory response to carrageenan and formalin. Pretreatment of the joint with 1% (w/v) capsaicin about 1 week prior to challenge significantly reduced the inflammatory response to all agents except formalin. In animals that received long-term pretreatment with reserpine (which depletes sympathetic nerve endings and their transmitters) a significant reduction occurred in the inflammatory response to SP and urate. The intraarticular injection of compound 48/80 produced a marked inflammatory response, which was reduced significantly in animals pretreated with capsaicin (Lam & Ferrell, 1991). Mast cells were not involved in the initial response to the electrical stimulation of the saphenous nerve in rats, which caused increased vascular permeability and vasodilation. However, when the electrical stimulation was extended to 30 min, the degranulation of mast cells and the depletion of the histamine content of the skin was also observed (Kowalski & Kaliner, 1988; Kowalski *et al.*, 1990).

Mice given 100 mg capsaicin/kg s.c. and tested 1–2 weeks later, exhibited insensitivity to chemically induced irritation, but contact sensitivity reactions and delayed-type hypersensitivity (DTH) were enhanced (Girolomoni & Tigelaar, 1990).

In normal rats injected with urate crystals into the hind paw, the inflammatory response was reduced by $\beta$-END, somatostatin, and $\alpha$-MSH, and increased by neurotensin and SP when injected along with the irritant. Intramuscular treatment with calcitonin inhibited inflammation. In rats deficient in essential fatty acids and thereby in prostaglandins, $\beta$-END nullified the proinflammatory activity of $PGE_2$ (Denko & Gabriel, 1985).

Hypophysectomy, but not adrenalectomy, decreased the inflammatory response in anesthetized rats to thermal injury. When such rats were treated with $\alpha$-helical CRF(9-41), which is a competitive antagonist of CRF (92 μg/kg i.v. given 10 min before or immediately after heat exposure), the insensitive state of hypophysectomized animals to burn injury was reversed (Wei *et al.*, 1990). Treatment of rats i.p. with rabbit anti-CRF serum caused the suppression of inflammatory exudate volume and cell concentration to chemically induced aseptic inflammation. CRF was detected in the inflamed area but not in the systemic circulation. Immunoreactive CRF is produced in peripheral inflammatory sites, where it acts as an autocrine or paracrine inflammatory cytokine (Karalis *et al.*, 1991).

A role for neurogenic inflammation has been demonstrated in the airways of several species and this mechanism may contribute to the inflammatory response in asthmatic airways. SP, CGRP and neurokinin A released from sensory nerves in the airways cause bronchial constriction, vasodilation, plasma exudation and mucous secretion. Sensory nerves may become sensitized by inflammatory products and triggered by mediators such as bradykinin, which leads to exaggerated inflammation. The effects of tachykinins may be further amplified by loss of the major degrading enzyme, neutral endopeptidase, from epithelial cells (Barnes, 1991). VIP inhibits T-cell and macrophage function and can protect tissues against inflammatory injury in the airways. Injured lungs release relatively large amounts of VIP (Ottaway, 1987; Berisha *et al.*, 1990; Said, 1990).

Pulmonary inflammation was induced in rats sensitized to the nematode *Nippostrongylus brasiliensis* by exposure to the specific antigen. The bilateral decentralization of the superior cervical ganglia attenuated the inflammatory response. The bilateral removal of these ganglia also reduced the anaphylaxis-induced accumulation of inflammatory cells in the lungs. The removal of the submandibular gland did not modify the severity of the pulmonary inflammation but abolished the protective effect of decentralization. It was suggested that cervical sympathetic nerves tonically inhibit the release of antiinflammatory factors from the submandibular glands (Mathison *et al.*, 1992). The production of an immunosuppressive factor by the submandibular gland in the rat was found to be under endocrine control (Nagy *et al.*, 1992).

SP and CGRP play a role in gastrointestinal inflammation, where they affect the vasculature and influence the priming of the immune system. Eosinophils have also been shown to produce SP in liver granulomas, which raises the possibility that some of the SP in inflammatory tissue may be of immune origin. Inflammatory mediators, such as prostaglandin, bradykinin and histamine, can excite afferent nerve endings in the intestine, and this potentially gives rise to reflex responses modulating postganglionic sympathetic neurones. Sympathetic activation through peripheral or central reflexes may cause release of mediators such as prostaglandins from sympathetic endings and so set up a positive feedback loop. The primary efferents may release their transmitters locally and activate efferent receptors, induce inflammation and act on blood vessels. This system is therefore capable of chronic excitation of efferent fibers, and maintains the local inflammatory response. Enteroendocrine cells may release their contents in response to luminal stimulation, which could also activate the intestinal efferents. Finally, cytokines may influence the release of peptides or the constitution of these peptides from primary efferent nerves (Sharkey, 1992).

### *Cytokines and local defense*

The recently discovered family of chemotactic and proinflammatory cytokines may be regarded as important and standard mediators of the body's response to injury. They also illustrate the importance of the inflammatory response in host defense by their related nature, overlapping functions and the variety of cells that can produce them (macrophages, monocytes, T cells, B cells, fibroblasts, endothelial cells, keratinocytes, platelets, neutrophils, hepatocytes, chondrocytes, synovial cells, and smooth muscle cells) (Oppenheim *et al.*, 1991). There can be little doubt that additional cytokines mediating the response to injury will be found. The stimuli that can induce chemotactic proinflammatory cytokines are diverse and include mitogens (PHA, Con A, LPS), cytokines (IL-1$\alpha$, IL-1$\beta$, TNF$\alpha$, IL-3, IFN-$\gamma$, IL-2), growth factors (PDGF, EGF), microorganisms (viruses, *Listeria monocytogenes*), and chemical irritants (phorbol esters, sodium urate crystals, hydroxyurea, silica) (Oppenheim *et al.*, 1991), which makes them truly ubiquitous mediators for all sorts of insults that can induce injury. IL-8 which is the best studied member of this group, has been shown to have a chemotactic, activating and degranulating effect on neutrophilic leukocytes. Moreover, IL-8 is also chemotactic for T lymphocytes, basophils and monocytes, and stimulates keratinocytes for proliferation. Five other peptides were shown to have a chemotactic and/or activating effect on neutrophils, four on monocytes, one on T lymphocytes, two on fibroblasts, and one on endothelial cells. Little is known about the inhibitors of these cytokines other than those of IL-8, which can be inhibited by TGF$\beta$, IL-4 and 1,25$(OH)_2$ vitamin $D_3$, all of which may be locally produced/released by various cells in the inflammatory tissue (Oppenheim *et al.*, 1991).

The type of insult and the nature of responding tissue may lead to differences in the cytokine/inflammatory response. For instance, in UV-induced skin injury, the keratinocyte is regarded as the major cytokine-producing cell, which secretes proinflammatory (IL-1), chemotactic, and immunosuppressive cytokines at the same time. The systemic immunosuppression induced by UV radiation is believed to be due to the immunosuppressive cytokines primarily produced by keratinocytes. Some preliminary evidence suggests that neurogenic inflammation and possibly endothelium-derived mediators initiate the response to cold injury, which is followed by massive infiltration by neutrophilic leukocytes. In thermal injury the activation of the complement system, and elevated levels of IL-1, IL-2 and IL-6 have been observed, which suggest the involvement of monocytes/macrophages and T lymphocytes. Surgical and other forms of mechanical trauma elicit similar responses. An inflammatory response in the brain usually has devastating effects and there is a special vascular barrier to prevent the entry of inflammatory cells into the CNS. The brain, however, still responds to injury by IL-1 and TNF production. The interaction of microglia, extrinsic macrophages and glial cells appears to initiate the response. Glial cells proliferate and probably seal the brain fairly soon after injury, before T- and B-cell infiltration takes place. Patients with head injury had surprisingly high serum levels of TNF compared to those in many other disease states, which did not correlate strongly with nitrogen wasting. Some evidence suggests that immunosuppressive therapy may be beneficial to block the CNS inflammatory response to injury and improve the recovery of motor strength after ischemic damage to the spinal cord (Giulian, 1990; Goodman *et al.*, 1990; Berkenbosch, 1992).

Bacterial infections often activate the complement system non-specifically (e.g. with the aid of CRP or endotoxin binding protein), stimulate chemotaxis and phagocytosis non-specifically and release chemotactic and inflammatory cytokines at the site of infection. This may be followed by a strong humoral immune response, where antibodies lyse bacteria by activating the complement cascade, or opsonize them, which amplifies their engulfment and destruction by phagocytes that are stimulated through their Fc and complement receptors. Neutrophilic leukocytes and monocyte/macrophages play a fundamental role in host defense against bacteria. Certain bacteria that live intracellularly, such as the tubercle bacillus, leprosy bacillus or brucella, preferentially stimulate cell-mediated immunity, which protects the host, whereas antibody formation is weak and irregular and contributes little to host defense. Cell-mediated immunity also plays an important role in defense against viruses, as the infected cells have to be destroyed in order to get rid of the virus. However, antibodies are needed to neutralize virus particles in the circulation. Cell-mediated immunity (delayed-type hypersensitivity) is the first line of defence against fungal infections. IgE antibodies, mast cells, basophilic leukocytes and eosinophilic leukocytes participate in the host defense against parasitic infestation (Rook, 1989; Taverne, 1989). Natural antibodies and natural killer cells also participate in the host defense against infections (Drutz & Graybill, 1987; Heyeman & McKerrow, 1987; Rook, 1989; Taverne, 1989). Since phagocytic cells have the capacity to recognize foreign materials and tissues, microorganisms are frequently engulfed by this mechanism, but may not be destroyed unless the cell is activated. The generation of chemotactic proinflammatory cytokines by infectious agents is probably important to attract inflammatory cells to the infection site and to activate them for phagocytosis and destruction of the pathogens.

Inflammation is an important local defense reaction, which involves the activation of tissue cells (e.g. mast cells, endothelium, fibroblasts, etc.) and the attraction of inflammatory cells to the site (granulocytes, macrophages, lymphocytes), which are also activated either non-specifically or specifically. The increased delivery of serum factors (complement components, natural antibodies, hormones, nutrients, etc.) through vasodilation and increased permeability is also important. These changes are aimed at the restriction, destruction, and elimination of the foreign material/infectious agent from the site of invasion. In mammals, the regional lymph nodes provide further barriers to the spread of infectious agents. If the inflammatory agent is immunogenic, an immune response is also mounted in the regional lymph node, which results in systemic immunity in 7–10 days.

It is inevitable that host tissues/cells become damaged during an inflammatory response, either by the irritant/infectious agent or by enzymes and toxins released from damaged cells and by various phagocytes. Macrophages appear to play an important role in wound healing by the stimulation of angiogenesis and of fibroblasts to proliferate and produce collagen. Several new growth factors (e.g. alveolar macrophage-derived growth factor, macrophage-derived growth factor, fibroblast activating factor) have been detected, which may play important roles in healing. TGF$\beta$ is also released from platelets and macrophages. T lymphocytes migrate to the wounds where they secrete growth factors such as TGF$\beta$. In the circulation, TGF$\beta$ is biologically inactive or latent, due to its non-covalent association with a 75 kDa glycosylated latency-associated protein that is covalently linked to a 235 kDa binding protein. The latent complex binds to IGF-II receptors and, after binding, becomes susceptible to protease activation by plasmin and cathepsin. These enzymes are released at inflammatory sites by various leukocytes. The half-life of the latent form in the serum is more than 90 min, whereas active TGF$\beta$ is cleared from the circulation within a few minutes. TGF$\beta$ has been shown to augment its own secretion in many cells and its mRNA appears most abundant during active inflammation and cell-mediated immune reactions. TGF$\beta$, at picomolar concentrations, increases monocyte mRNA levels for IL-1, TNF, PDGF, basic fibroblast growth factor, and IL-6. In addition, TGF$\beta$ induces Fc$\gamma$RIII on newly recruited monocytes. Therefore, TGF$\beta$ plays a critical role in the early phase of inflammation, which is also illustrated by the fact that locally administered TGF$\beta$ exacerbates an ongoing inflammatory response. This action of TGF$\beta$ is self limiting and reversible, which could be due to the short half-life, the down-regulation of receptors, and the fact that TGF$\beta$ cannot prevent leukocyte apoptosis. During wound healing, TGF$\beta$ regulates many processes including angiogenesis, chemotaxis, fibroblast proliferation and controlled synthesis of the extracellular matrix necessary for repair. It induces PDGF and its receptors. The production of fibroblast collagen, fibronectin, and glycosaminoglycan are upregulated by TGF$\beta$. Both IFN-$\gamma$ and TNF counteract the proliferative activity of TGF$\beta$ (Wahl, 1992).

In several models of inflammatory disease, which include arthritis induced by adjuvant and bacterial cell walls, experimental allergic encephalomyelitis, graft rejection and reperfusion-induced injury, systemically administered TGF$\beta$ downregulates organ inflammation. This occurs in the absence of generalized immune suppression and may be related to the differential effect of TGF$\beta$ on target cells in different stages of differentiation. Therefore, TGF$\beta$ is released early during inflammation and functions to promote the inflammatory response, by its stimulating effect on immature monocytes and T cells. However, once these cells differentiate and become activated, they become susceptible to phenotypic modulation and functional inhibition by TGF$\beta$. This transition from pro- to antiinflammatory responsiveness occurs with minimal disruption of the homeostasis of host cells and tissues. This antiinflammatory effect may be supported by other cytokines, such as IL-4, IL-5, and IL-10. TGF$\beta$ also rapidly diminishes the IL-1- or TNF-induced hepatocyte APP synthesis (Barbul, 1989; Wahl, 1992). This dual function is not unique to TGF$\beta$, as TNF$\alpha$ has also been shown to be an important T cell-derived growth factor for human B cells (Kehrl *et al.*, 1987). Certain neuropeptides, such as AVP, VIP and somatostatin may also moderate the inflammatory response.

In the intestinal tract, mast cells alert the nervous system when invading organisms, toxins, or allergens are present. The nervous system will then respond to eliminate the noxious molecules/organisms from the gut lumen, which manifest in intestinal malaise and sudden-onset diarrhea (Wood, 1992). There is evidence to indicate that IMC are innervated and that the density of this cell type changes significantly in nematode-infected rats. Jejunal mucosal nerves remodel after *Nippostrongylus brasiliensis* infection, first with degenerative and later with regenerative phases during the acute and recovery stages of inflammation, respectively. Seven weeks after infection, there is a net increase in the density and number of mucosal nerves (Stead, 1992). The function of enteric nerves is also altered in nematode-infected rats, and is mediated by IL-1. Identical changes can be induced by exogenous IL-1 and the response can be attenuated by IL-1 antagonist. Macrophage-like cells are present in the myenteric plexus and produce IL-1 locally, which in turn modulates neural membranes (Collins *et al.*, 1992).

## *Systemic defense mechanisms*

### *The role of acute-phase hormones*

Severe injury, regardless of the nature of the insult, will elicit the appearance in the circulation of tissue-derived acute-phase hormones, which initiate the defense response of the host through interaction with the neuroendocrine system and with practically every tissue and organ in the body. The nature of the injury will determine to some extent the type of response elicited. Thus, for instance, in patients undergoing elective surgery, IL-1 appeared briefly in the circulation, followed by IL-6, but other cytokines, such as TNF$\alpha$ or IFN-$\gamma$, were not detected. Similarly, in burn injury, TNF$\alpha$ and PGE were elevated only if sepsis also occurred (Pullicino *et al.*, 1990; Takayama *et al.*, 1990). TNF is invariably elevated, however, if endotoxemia is associated with the injury. In patients with burn injury, both serum IL-2 and IL-2R$\alpha$ are elevated for long periods of time (Teodorczyk-Injeyan *et al.*, 1989, 1991), whereas in trauma there is a consistent depression of IL-2 (Faist *et al.*, 1989). Colony stimulating factors (e.g. GM-CSF) may also be elevated in the serum, especially during infections or endotoxemia. Several other factors can also have significant systemic effects, especially in endotoxic shock.

Interleukin-1$\alpha$ and -$\beta$ induce fever, release ACTH and possibly other pituitary hormones, antagonize opioid receptors in the brain, promote slow-wave sleep, decrease appetite, stimulate APP in the liver, promote proteolysis in muscle, inhibit thyroglobulin gene expression, stimulate thyroid growth, stimulate insulin release (though in high doses the effect is inhibitory), inhibit steroid synthesis by the gonads and adrenals, and stimulate bone resorption (Dinarello, 1988; Rivier & Vale, 1989; Yamashita *et al.*, 1989; Besedovsky *et al.*, 1991; Berkenbosch *et al.*, 1992). IL-1$\alpha$ and -$\beta$ have been reported to affect the release of a number of other hormones in the rat that include gonadotrophin-releasing hormone (GnRH), luteinizing hormone (LH), TSH, growth hormone and prolactin, but some of these observations are controversial and need further clarification.

TNF$\alpha$ (cachectin) and TNF$\beta$ (lymphotoxin) have many overlapping functions with IL-1, including pyrogenicity, promotion of slow-wave sleep, a strong catabolic effect, release of ACTH, GnRH, blocking of growth hormone release, T- and B-cell activation, and stimulation of bone resorption. Neutrophils, eosinophils and macrophages are also activated by TNF. In addition, TNF is cytotoxic for certain tumors and other targets by the activation of the suicide pathway and causes inflammation, hemorrhage and shock, if produced in excess. TNF plays a major role in the multiple endocrine and metabolic changes associated with trauma and sepsis. IL-1 and TNF inhibit the $\beta$-adrenergic responsiveness of cardiac myocytes (Beutler *et al.*, 1985*b*; Beutler & Cerami, 1988; Gulic *et al.*, 1989; Sharp *et al.*, 1989; Bernardini *et al.*, 1990; Yamaguchi *et al.*, 1990*b*; Besedovsky *et al.*, 1991; Elsasser *et al.*, 1991). TNF, IL-1 and other

Table 4.7. *Cytokines derived from T lymphocytes*

| Inducers | Cytokines |
|---|---|
| Antigen | GM-CSF |
| Epinephrine | IFN-$\gamma$ |
| IFN-$\gamma$ | IL-2, -3, -4, -5, -6, -10 |
| IL-1 | TGF-$\beta$ |
| IL-2 | TNF-$\alpha$, -$\beta$ |

LPS-induced mediators enhance non-specific resistance to bacterial, viral and parasitic infections, autoimmune disease and radiation sickness (Koff & Fann, 1986; Urbaschek & Urbaschek, 1987; Gordon *et al.*, 1989). Moreover, IL-1 given to rats, either i.v. or into the cerebrospinal fluid, inhibited gastric injury induced by a variety of experimental agents such as stress, aspirin and ethanol. This protection was mediated by the inhibition of acid secretion and PG release (Tache & Saperas, 1992). TNF stimulates the production of numerous inflammatory mediators by its ability to activate a variety of inflammatory cell types (Tables 4.2, 4.3 and 4.5).

IL-6 promotes the terminal differentiation of B-lymphocytes, supports the multipotential colony formation of hematopoietic stem cells, induces APP in the liver, plays a role in the differentiation and activation of T cells and macrophages and contributes to neural differentiation (Akira & Kishimoto, 1992). IL-6 has been shown to release ACTH and $\beta$-END from mouse pituitary adenomas *in vitro* (Woloski *et al.*, 1985; Fukata *et al.*, 1989), to stimulate the release of ACTH and inhibit TSH release by acting on the hypothalamus in the rat, and to inhibit ACTH release by acting directly on rat pituitary glands *in vitro* (Vankelecom *et al.*, 1990; Lyson *et al.*, 1991). However, IL-6 has been shown to act as a locally produced cytokine in the pituitary gland of rats and therefore it may also function as a paracrine regulator of prolactin release (Yamaguchi *et al.*, 1990*a*). Nevertheless, IL-6 stimulated ACTH and corticosterone output when given to freely moving rats (Besedovsky *et al.*, 1991).

IL-2 is a product of T lymphocytes (Table 4.7) and it functions primarily as a growth factor for T cells and activator of natural killer (NK) and lymphokine-activated killer (LAK) cells. When given in high doses to animals or patients, IL-2 exerts a neurotoxic effect, which in rats coincided temporarily with the induction of serum TNF (Denicoff *et al.*, 1987;

Ellison & Merchant, 1991). IL-2 was reported to inhibit growth hormone, LH and follicle stimulating hormone (FSH) release and to promote ACTH, TSH and prolactin release from pituitary glands of rats and mice (Smith *et al.*, 1989; Karanth & McCann, 1991). In humans, IL-2 treatment increased ACTH, β-END, growth hormone and prolactin in the circulation (Denicoff *et al.*, 1989; Lissoni *et al.*, 1990).

IFN-γ is the product of T lymphocytes and macrophages and was recognized first for its antiviral effect. Now it is known to be a major regulator of cytokine production by monocytes/macrophages and T lymphocytes (Tables 4.2 and 4.7). IFN-γ is also known to activate NK cells for cytotoxicity. IFN-γ has the capacity to induce GC receptors in murine monocytes and act in conjunction with GC to initiate the expression of FcRγI receptors on human monocytes (Morganelli & Guyre, 1988; Salkowsky & Vogel, 1992). IFN-γ was reported to release ACTH and to inhibit growth hormone and TSH release by the hypothalamus in rats. By treating rat pituitary glands with IFN-γ *in vitro*, some investigators found the inhibition of ACTH production and release as well as the inhibition of prolactin and growth hormone release, whereas others observed increased release of ACTH, LH, FSH, growth hormone and prolactin. IFN-γ released ACTH from human pituitary adenomas (Malarkey & Zvara, 1989; Pang *et al.*, 1989; Gaillard *et al.*, 1990; Gonzalez *et al.*, 1990, 1991; Vankelecom *et al.*, 1990).

The colony stimulating factors G-CSF, M-CSF, and GM-CSF play an important role in the maturation of granulocytes and macrophages in the bone marrow, as well as being important activators of these cells during infection and inflammation (Metcalf, 1991). G-CSF released ACTH *in vitro* from human pituitary adenomas (Malarkey & Zvara, 1989).

PAF is a lipid chemical mediator that can be produced by most mammalian cells. It is a major inflammatory mediator with vasoactive properties and it plays a role in arterial thrombosis, endotoxic shock, acute allergic disease, embryo implantation, parturition and fetal lung development (Hanahan, 1992). PAF released ACTH and β-END in rats by acting on the hypothalamus, and released growth hormone and prolactin through direct action on the pituitary gland (Bernardini *et al.*, 1989; Camoratto & Grandison, 1989; Rougeot *et al.*, 1990).

PDGF released prolactin from rat pituitary adenoma *in vitro* (Sullivan & Tashjian, 1983), bradykinin also stimulated prolactin release from rat pituitary glands (Drouhault *et al.*, 1987; Jones *et al.*, 1989), and histamine released ACTH, β-END and prolactin in rats by acting on the hypothalamus (Knigge *et al.*, 1988; Kjaer *et al.*, 1990). TGFβ stimulated the basal secretion of growth hormone and inhibited the basal secretion of prolactin, and TSH mediated prolactin release from rat pituitary glands and also inhibited prolactin gene expression in rat pituitary adenoma (Delidow *et al.*, 1991; Murata & Ying, 1991).

Whether or not the elevation of acute-phase hormones in the circulation is the result of release from various tissues after injury, or the consequence of the massive activation of leukocytes in the circulation, remains to be elucidated. The observation that in mice the TNF produced locally during bacterial peritonitis did not readily enter the circulation, whereas LPS did (Eskandari *et al.*, 1992; Zanetti *et al.*, 1992) suggests that the pathogenic agents (e.g. bacteria, bacterial products, or viruses) and not the cytokines, enter the circulation under these conditions. Similar problems exist with regard to the extravasation of circulating cytokine hormones into brain tissue, where a vascular barrier exists. The production of a number of cytokines, including IL-1, IL-6 and TNF, has already been detected in the CNS (Rothwell, 1991). However, the fact remains that after peripheral injection, these acute-phase hormones have the capacity to alter brain function, hormone secretion and influence nearly every organ and tissue in the body.

Normally, if the cytokine-hormones are kept within tolerable limits, they help recovery and healing. For instance, IL-1 is indispensable for the induction of the immune response, and acts in conjunction with the presentation of antigen to B and T lymphocytes. IL-2, -4, -5 and -6 are also essential growth factors involved in the induction of the immune response. TNF and IFN-$\gamma$ protect against bacterial and viral infections non-specifically. The CSFs do not only enhance the activity of phagocytes, but also stimulate their production by the bone marrow.

Although our knowledge is still very deficient with regard to the complex regulatory interaction of the cytokine network, it is clear that as soon as induction takes place, inhibitory cytokines are also produced. These include the IL-1 inhibitor, IL-1 receptor antagonist, TNF inhibitor, etc. Furthermore, IL-4 inhibits the action of IL-6, TGF$\beta$ antagonizes TNF$\alpha$, and IL-5 and IL-10 have antiinflammatory effects. The existence of these regulatory circuits may explain the observation that the kinetics of TNF production in adrenalectomized mice are no different from intact animals after LPS induction, even though these animals show an exaggerated response (Ramachandra *et al.*, 1992) (Figure 4.1). The dual action of TGF$\beta$ in promoting local inflammation, but exerting a systemic immunosuppressive and antiinflammatory effect, appears to be most important in relation to damage localization and control during injury.

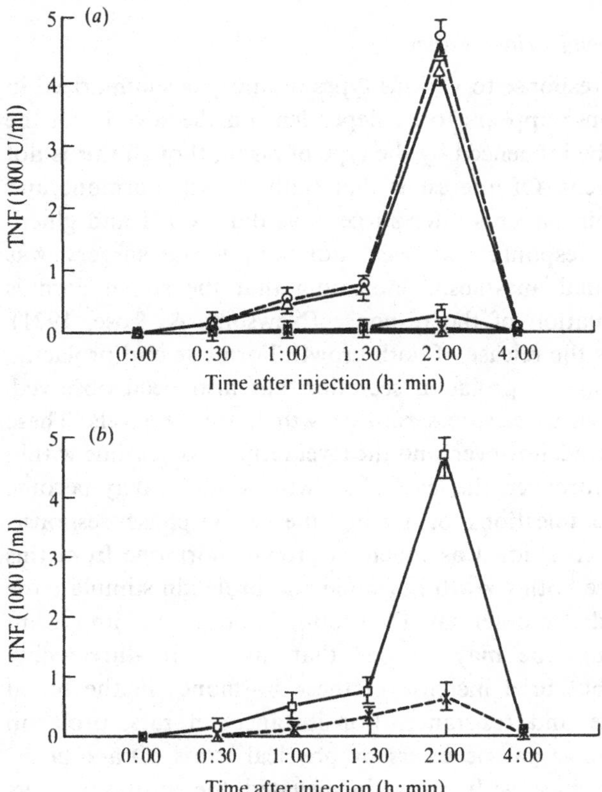


Figure 4.1. TNF response (*a*) after lipid A at 2.5 μg/kg (× and △) or 10 μg/kg (□ and ○) in intact (× and □) and adrenalectomized (△ and ○) mice. Student's *t*-test showed intact and adrenalectomized mice significantly different ($p < 0.001$) 2 h after injection; (*b*) after dexamethasone (3.0 mg/kg once a day for 5 days) followed by lipid A (10 μg/kg i.v. 30 min after the last dexamethasone injection) in four adrenalectomized mice (×), significantly lower ($p < 0.001$) than in an untreated adrenalectomized group (□). (From Ramachandra *et al.*, 1992.)

The complement split product C3a shows similar properties (Heideman, 1981, 1989). The elaborate internal regulatory pathways of the immune system, which involve soluble mediators and suppressor cells, are inadequate to control excess cytokine production, even during deliberate immunization, as is illustrated by the death of adrenalectomized animals after stimulation with complete Freund's adjuvant (Perretti *et al.*, 1991). The neuroendocrine system acts as the ultimate regulator of immune/inflammatory activity and coordinates the response in the interest of survival, as discussed below.

*The role of the neuroendocrine system*

The neuroendocrine response to various types of injury is summarized in Table 4.6. The response appears to be dependent on the severity of the injury and may also be influenced by the type of insult, though this is not entirely clear at present. Of interest is that both growth hormone and prolactin levels rose in patients after surgery, as did ACTH and glucocorticoid levels. No response was seen, however, if the surgery was performed under spinal anesthesia, indicating that the spinal cord is involved in the mediation of the response (Newsome & Rose, 1971). Endotoxin stimulates the release of both growth hormone and prolactin, although the inhibition of prolactin secretion has also been observed. Trauma is also known to elevate serum growth hormone levels. These responses are short-lived, however, and the level returns to baseline within a matter of hours. Moreover, the level of growth hormone may become subnormal in severe infections or during the acute phase response. Prolactin has not been studied as much as growth hormone from this point of view. Because both growth hormone and prolactin stimulate the immune response and also potentiate the production of several important cytokines (Table 4.8), one may suggest that, in non-life-threatening situations, a sharp but brief increase of these hormones in the blood elevates host defense and resistance. For instance, in rats, prolactin reduced the induction of gastric ulcers by physical stress (Drago *et al.*, 1989). Treatment of mice with prolactin elevated the antibody titers against rotavirus in serum and milk (Ijaz *et al.*, 1990). In severe situations, however, when excess cytokine production is life threatening, the subnormal levels of these hormones appear to serve as one of the control mechanisms to limit the production of inflammatory mediators.

The ACTH–adrenal axis serves as the highest and most powerful neuroendocrine control pathway of immune/inflammatory reactions in the hierarchy of regulators. The level of GC increases in the circulation proportionally to the severity of injury. In addition to the hypothalamus–pituitary–adrenal pathway, there is indication of direct release of GC from the adrenal gland by inflammatory mediators. The extreme sensitivity of adrenalectomized animals to LPS, TNF or IL-1, which can be reversed by treatment with GC, illustrates the vital importance of this neuroendocrine regulatory system. GC are powerful suppressors of the immune response, due to their ability to inhibit the production of all cytokines with the possible exception of IL-4 and IL-6 (Table 4.8).

One may suggest that during injury the alteration of self antigens readily

Table 4.8. *The effect of hormones on cytokine secretion*

| | Cytokines | | | | |
|---|---|---|---|---|---|
| Hormone | IL-1 | TNFα | IL-6 | IFN-γ | IL-2 |
| ACTH | | ↑ | ↑ | | |
| Glucocorticoids | ↓ | ↓ | 0↓ | ↓ | ↓ |
| Growth hormone | ↑ | ↑ | | | |
| Prolactin | | | | ↑ | |
| $\beta$-Endorphin | ↑ | | | ↑↓ | |
| Enkephalin | ↑ | | | ↑ | ↑ |
| Estrogen | ↑ | | ↓ | ↓ | |
| Progesterone | ↑ | | ↓ | | |
| Insulin | | ↑ | ↑ | | |
| Catecholamines | | ↑↓ | ↑ | | |

↑, Increased serum/plasma level; ↓ decreased level; ↑↓, level may be either increased or decreased; 0, no change.
IL, Interleukin; TNF, tumor necrosis factor; IFN, interferon; ACTH, adrenocorticotropic hormone.
Glucocorticoid also inhibits platelet activating factor, IL-8, granulocyte–macrophage colony-stimulating factor and chemotactic–proinflammatory factor secretion, has no effect on macrophage colony-stimulating factor and stimulates the production of IL-4. Please see the details and relevant references for this table in the text.

takes place and, since the specific immune response is known to be initiated by altered self molecules of the major histocompatibility complex, bodily injuries could trigger autoimmune reactions in immunocompetent hosts. There is at least some evidence to indicate a role for trauma in rheumatoid arthritis and systemic lupus erythematosus (Wallace, 1987). Therefore, the profound suppression of a specific immune response under these conditions may be a necessity for survival. The profound thymolitic action of GC by their ability to induce apoptosis in thymocytes (Crompton & Cidlowski, 1992) may serve as a preventive measure for the release of potentially autoreactive T lymphocytes during injury and thus decrease the risk of autoreactivity.

Many pathogenic microorganisms have the capacity to activate the immune system non-specifically (for example, with LPS or superantigens), and this leads to life-threatening excess production of toxic cytokines. Invariably this situation must lead to a powerful GC response if the host is to survive. That this may help the pathogen is illustrated by the observation that LPS can trigger bacterial invasion in animals (Geller *et al.*, 1954). However, GC have no effect on the response of memory T cells, which are capable of proliferating in an autocrine fashion after exposure to the specific antigen. This mechanism is likely to allow for the maintenance of at least some anamnestic immune responses during injury when the primary response is profoundly inhibited. Preformed antibodies are also protective under these conditions. Moreover, some cytokines have the ability to antagonize the antiproliferative effect of GC on T lymphocytes (Claman, 1987; Schwartz, 1990; Almawi *et al.*, 1991).

In contrast to the downregulation of cytokines by GC, IL-1 receptors on monocytes and fibroblasts, IL-6 receptors on hepatocytes and epithelial cells, IFN-$\gamma$ receptors and Fc$\gamma$I receptors on monocytes are all upregulated by GC (Robin *et al.*, 1985; Akahoshi *et al.*, 1988; Morganelli & Guyre, 1988; Snyers *et al.*, 1990). These effects may be regarded as the potentiation of specific immune and non-specific host defense mechanisms by GC.

GC are required for the induction of APP synthesis by cytokines in the liver. This is an additional example of boosting non-specific defense mechanisms by GC. As already pointed out, the production of CRP and endotoxin-binding protein, which have the ability to activate the complement system and trigger the destruction of microorganisms by phagocytes, may be regarded as a rapid host defense response. The elevation of these proteins and of complement components in the serum takes hours instead of the 7–10 day period which is necessary for the development of specific immunity. The elevated serum level of fibrinogen during the acute phase response may serve to isolate the noxious/infectious agent by thrombosis of microvessels in affected tissues, whereas the enzyme inhibitors curb the damage caused by enzymes inadvertently released by dying cells and by phagocytes at sites of injury and also intravascularly during systemic disease. The antiinflammatory $\alpha$-macrofetoprotein is likely to inhibit tissue damage inflicted by inflammatory mediators. The observation that endotoxin tolerance does not develop in animals that are adrenalectomized or, alternatively, in which the liver is intoxicated by galactosamine, may indeed illustrate the interaction of GC and APP in the regulation of cytokine production, as suggested by Evans & Zuckerman (1991). Endotoxin-tolerant animals also show increased resistance to various insults.

Another characteristic response to severe trauma, infection or shock is the elevation of catecholamines in the circulation. Cytokines appear to elevate catecholamines, although hemodynamic and metabolic changes under these conditions certainly contribute to the catecholamine response. Catecholamines are moderators of inflammation, as illustrated by the inhibition of asthma and anaphylactic shock by $\beta$-adrenergic agents.

Catecholamines also have an inhibitory effect on other immune phenomena, including neutrophil activation and macrophage cytotoxicity. Variable effects have been found on the antibody response (Berczi, 1986*b*; Sanders & Munson, 1985). However, epinephrine is capable of stimulating IL-6 production and it appears that catecholamines in conjunction with GC can induce an acute phase response without the presence of injury.

Insulin is elevated in endotoxicosis and during infection, whereas, during the acute phase response, it may be either elevated or decreased. Glucagon is always elevated, usually in proportion to the severity of the condition. Although insulin has an influence on the production of cytokines, such as IL-6 and TNF$\alpha$, and in turn cytokines (IL-1, TNF) regulate insulin secretion, the role of these hormones is likely to be more important in the metabolic response to injury than in the direct regulation of cytokines.

Thyroid function is invariably suppressed by various forms of injury, which again may be related to the metabolic alterations in these conditions. The observation that lasting impairment of thyroid function may be induced if newborn rats are treated with LPS (Bertok & Nagy, 1984; Nagy & Bertok, 1990) may point to an important facet of the developmental interaction of the endocrine system with cytokines.

The general trend for the levels of sex hormones (estrogens, androgens and progestogens) is a state of depression during injury, with the possible exception of estrogens, which may show a brief period of elevation. Estradiol is known to cause bone marrow deficiency and thymic involution and to inhibit various T-lymphocyte functions, which include regulatory (helper and suppressor) and effector (killer and delayed hypersensitivity) T-cell mechanisms. Natural killer cells, neutrophils and mast cell degranulation are also inhibited by $E_2$. However, phagocytosis, humoral immune reactions and certain autoimmune diseases are enhanced by $E_2$ in laboratory animals (Raveche & Steinberg, 1986; Nelson & Steinberg, 1987; Stimson, 1987). Estrogens augment IL-1 and suppress IL-6 and IFN-$\gamma$ production (Table 4.8), which is in accord with their immunoregulatory influence. Progesterone also stimulates IL-1 and suppresses IL-6. The stimulation of phagocytic activity by estrogens may in fact be advantageous, as it boosts non-specific defense and thus fits into the strategy of the acute phase reaction. The long-term suppression of androgens, especially after burn injury, may aid recovery of the immune system, as androgens are generally immunosuppressive (Raveche & Steinberg, 1986).

$\beta$-END is invariably elevated during injury. Numerous experiments on the immunomodulatory effect of $\beta$-END, and of opioids in general, indicate that they may enhance and/or suppress various immune functions, probably dependent on physiological variants present in various cell donors at the time of sampling. These observations suggest that ENDs are capable of amplifying both stimulatory and suppressive signals to lymphocytes. This is reflected in the effect of $\beta$-END on the production of IFN-$\gamma$, which may be enhanced or suppressed depending on the condition. $\beta$-END boosts IL-1, which should be beneficial for mounting an acute phase response. The role of systemically released ENK during injury is rather uncertain at the present time.

AVP shows a consistent elevation during injury and it probably plays an important role in the regulation of blood vessels under these conditions. However, it also has an antiinflammatory effect and hence its systemic elevation during an acute phase response may indeed be helpful to control non-specific damage to the organism.

The metabolic alterations during injury are proportional to the severity of the condition and are the result of the coordinated action of acute phase hormones with the nervous and endocrine systems. In general, catabolism (loss of muscle protein, body fat, decrease of the synthesis of regular proteins such as albumin in the liver) prevails, whereas the activity of leukocytes, of the bone marrow and the synthesis of APP, primarily by the liver, are enhanced. Fever, which is the result of the action of several acute-phase hormones on the brain is beneficial to the host, as elevated temperatures enhance the activity of specific and non-specific immune mechanisms and are also likely to accelerate the production of APP, which are in high demand under these conditions. The metabolic and thermal response is under the ultimate control of the CNS (Van Dijk & Rademaker, 1985; Andersson *et al.*, 1987; Jepson *et al.*, 1988; Morimoto *et al.*, 1988; Kawasaki *et al.*, 1989; Lin *et al.*, 1989; Rothwell, 1989).

The recent findings that classical hormones and a number of neuropeptides are produced by various cells of the immune system (reviewed by Blalock, 1989) proves that mediators are shared by the neuroendocrine and immune systems. However, the quantities of these mediators produced in lymphoid tissue are small, which suggests that they fulfil local paracrine/autocrine regulatory functions, as cytokines. Mediator sharing is not unique to the nervous and immune systems, but rather is a general phenomenon. Numerous cytokine mediators with paracrine/autocrine functions are present, even in the pituitary gland itself (Ohalloran *et al.*, 1991). While at present there is a lot of evidence for the regulatory influence of classical hormones on immune and inflammatory reactions, there is no compelling evidence for a systemic role for 'classical hormones' produced by lymphocytes. It is clear, however, that shared mediators act on nerve terminals that play a constant regulatory role in the local inflammatory/immune response. Through this interaction, the endocrine response to injury may be modulated. On the other hand, centrally acting cytokine-hormones may modulate immune/inflammatory processes locally by modulating the delivery of neurotransmitters. Much remains to be clarified about the nature of this neurohormonal-immune/inflammatory regulatory interaction, which is vital for everyday survival of higher organisms. The importance of the immune system for survival is also illustrated by the many alternative molecules, cells and pathways that can perform similar functions, so that the probability of failure is minimal.

Emotional or physical stress elicits a neuroendocrine response without the presence of injury, which is similar to the one seen after injury (Dantzer & Kelley, 1989; Jasmin & Chentin, 1991). In general, though not always, stressed animals are immunosuppressed, whereas the production of APP may be stimulated, as outlined earlier. This may be an important adaptive response aimed at enhancing the chances of survival in anticipation of danger. However, if the stress effect is prolonged, the long-term metabolic alterations and excess production of certain APP, such as fibrinogen, for instance, may elevate the risk of heart disease, stroke and thrombosis (Markowe *et al.*, 1985; Keller *et al.*, 1991; Shavit, 1991). The risk of infectious disease is also higher, due to the inhibition of the primary immune response under these conditions. Yet another phenomenon that may have defensive value is the conditioning of immune responses. Here, immune reactivity may be either enhanced or diminished upon repeated exposure to the same antigenic stimulus if paired with 'conditioning' sensory stimuli (Ader & Cohen, 1991).

### *Severe trauma, sepsis and shock*

The acute phase response is an emergency reaction where the host regulatory system is still trying to boost non-specific immune and inflammatory reactions, while controlling the systemic activation of destructive immune/inflammatory mechanisms. After the local and specific immune mechanisms have failed, this emergency reaction still has a good chance of succeeding and assuring host survival. The danger is, however, that pathogenic microbes take advantage of the suppression of specific immunity, which is proportional to the extent of injury, and invade the organism, usually from the gastrointestinal tract.

The critically injured patient is normally stable or shows improvement for 2–3 days, when a septic response may follow, with the failure of several organs, especially the lung; at around day 10, bacteriological evidence of sepsis develops, which is refractory to antibiotic treatment, and the patient succumbs, usually to pneumonia. Endotoxin and tissue degradation products released into the circulation under these conditions may cause diffuse intravascular coagulation, the systemic activation of the complement system by both pathways and the release of hormones and cytokines with immunosuppressive potential. The systemic release of C3a and C5a is immunosuppressive and may impair chemotaxis. The activation of phagocytic cells, especially neutrophils, by these complement split products may lead to vascular damage, increased permeability with edema, and impaired microvascular flow, and may ultimately contribute to multiorgan failure. The release of cytokines and other biologically active substances from basophils, mast cells and platelets may further aggravate the situation. The production of IL-1, IL-2 and IFN-$\gamma$ is depressed, whereas the level of $PGE_2$ is excessively elevated throughout the course of disease. TNF was present in the plasma of 27 out of 74 patients with septic shock, and in 1 of 12 patients with shock due to other causes. TNF was detected with equal frequency in patients with shock from Gram-negative or from Gram-positive bacillary sepsis. The levels of TNF were highest in the initial sample and decreased significantly over the subsequent 24 h. Normally, the rise in serum GC and catecholamine levels is proportional to the severity of the septic condition. Patients with subclinical hypocortisolism are more susceptible to death during sepsis than are those with normal adrenal function. In severely traumatized or septic patients, there is a lack of skin reactivity to recall antigens, monocyte/macrophage function is depressed, and there is increased production of PGE. Chemotaxis, phagocytosis, chemiluminescence and the intracellular killing activity of neutrophils are also suppressed. There is decreased NK and LAK function, long-term T-cell depression with increased T-suppressor activity and reversal of the T helper/T suppressor ratio (Bjornson *et al.*, 1977; Nuytinck *et al.*, 1986; Border *et al.*, 1987; Faist *et al.*, 1989; Heideman, 1989; Ninneman, 1989; Marks *et al.*, 1990).

The pathological process during severe trauma, sepsis and shock may start by various pathways and snowball into the septic state, multiple organ failure and death. In patients suffering from shock with subsequent resuscitation, some organs such as the gut or liver may be critically injured by oxygen free radicals. If a significant amount of devitalized tissue is left in place it may activate the complement system and phagocytic cells in a massive way. The complement and coagulation systems may also be activated by infectious agents along with massive cytokine production. A correlation could be shown between the intensity of complement activation and the blood levels of elastase with the severity of injury, the development of adult respiratory distress syndrome, multiple organ failure and fatal outcome. Septic patients with detectable TNF also had a higher incidence and severity of the adult respiratory distress syndrome and a higher mortality rate (Nuytinck *et al.*, 1986; Border *et al.*, 1987; Marks *et al.*, 1990).

Animal experiments revealed that TNF, IL-1, IFN-$\gamma$, PAF, opioids and prostaglandins all contribute to the fatal outcome of endotoxic shock. During infection, the destructive effect of microorganisms growing in various tissues or in the blood, the consumption of essential nutrients by these pathogens, and the toxicity of their metabolic byproducts are additional factors that complicate the situation. By the time septic shock developed, enough damage had been done to kill the individual and hence it is not surprising that treatment with GC has no beneficial effect (Sprung *et al.*, 1984; Bone *et al.*, 1987; Veterans Coop. Study, 1987; Marks *et al.*, 1990). Such therapy could be expected to be beneficial in a minority of patients who may be GC deficient, whereas in the majority with an adequate response, additional high-dose GC therapy may inflict additional damage, by inhibition of the rapid growth of intestinal cells, for instance (Mochizuki *et al.*, 1984), and by the aggravation of immunosuppression. Preventive measures, such as early enteric protein feeding and the prompt removal of devitalized tissue from severely traumatized patients, are most important, as these measures tend to prevent or decrease the severity of the septic state (Border *et al.*, 1987; Ninneman, 1989). Treatment with antibiotics has not been excessively useful in the past because of the development of resistance and, in the case of Gram-negative organisms, such treatment accelerated the release of endotoxin, which in turn aggravated the disease (Johnston & Griesman, 1984; Shenep *et al.*, 1988). Pharmacological treatment with cortisol, lidocain and calcium blockers reduced the release of bioactive complement components. Plasmapheresis has been used for the removal of anaphylatoxins from the blood (Heideman, 1989).

Ideally, one would like to prevent the systemic activation of complement and coagulation pathways and of the excess release of cytokines during trauma/infection. A simple and inexpensive measure to prevent the absorption of endotoxin from the gastrointestinal tract during liver failure would be to apply bile acids, which would detoxify LPS in the gut (Bertok, 1977). Although proven experimentally, this has not yet been evaluated in the clinical setting. The administration of antibodies to LPS or to its toxic moiety, lipid A, can also be done with benefit. This approach is being studied experimentally and there are ongoing clinical trials. Human and murine anti-lipid A monoclonal antibodies improved the survival rate and facilitated the recovery of patients suffering from Gram-negative bacteremia and septic shock (Greenman *et al.*, 1991; Ziegler *et al.*, 1991).

Animal studies have shown that lipid A-specific monoclonal antibodies are capable of protecting the host against lethal endotoxic shock only if given prior to or simultaneously with endotoxin. No protection could be achieved if the antibody were administered 2 h after LPS injection (Ramachandra *et al.*, 1993). The apparent reason for this is that the initiation of excess TNF/cytokine production takes place shortly after injection of endotoxin, TNF reaching maximum levels within 2 h, which in turn initiates the cytokine cascade. Endotoxin is therefore not required for the development of the shock beyond this time (Ramachandra *et al.*, 1992). Once the cytokine response is under way, TNF is not required either, as it returns to baseline levels within 4 h or so, and the host does not respond with elevation of TNF to additional LPS injection. Therefore, the use of specific anti-TNF antibodies (Beutler *et al.*, 1985*a*) also has limitations, as discussed earlier. The use of specific antibodies to IL-1 and TNF, with the naturally occurring cytokine IL-1 receptor antagonist, and with soluble TNF and IL-1 receptors as additional inhibitors, may have further advantages. The application of PAF antagonists is an additional possibility (Crespo & Fernandez-Gallardo, 1992; Dinarello, 1991).

While the above therapeutic approaches should be studied further in the interest of improving patient care, there is a danger that they are based on a gross oversimplification of the pathomechanism of sepsis and lethal shock. We have just begun to understand the principles by which the complex interaction of virtually all cells and tissues of the body take place in response to injury. This reaction enables the organism to cope with a variety of injuries, whether inflicted by physical, chemical or biological agents. As we progress with our understanding of this defense system, our insights into the pathomechanism of trauma, sepsis, shock and possibly also of other diseases with underlying immune/inflammatory mechanisms, will improve, which should result in better approaches for treatment.

## Conclusions

The central nervous system plays an important role in the prevention/avoidance of injury by a variety of agents through sensing the danger or the insult and initiating a response of avoidance. During the insult, irritation or pain will also lead to preventive measures, such as avoidance or expulsion (e.g. cough, diarrhea, etc.) from various cavities. If the insult cannot be eliminated without tissue damage, local inflammation develops, which is a general reaction of host defense. Inflammation may be initiated by sensory nerves acting on blood vessels, tissue mast cells, and neutrophilic granulocytes. Substance P and CGRP are the major neuropeptides mediating the inflammatory response.

Injured cells release a number of chemotactic–proinflammatory cytokines, which will attract inflammatory cells (macrophages, granulocytes, lymphocytes) to the site of injury; the latter then become activated and cause an inflammatory response. If bleeding takes places, the coagulation and kinin systems also become activated, and they in turn will activate the complement system non-specifically. The complement split products, C3a and C5a, function as chemotactic factors and activators for mast cells and basophils, monocytes and macrophages, and granulocytes, and again, inflammation develops as the result. Finally, specific immune mechanisms can also initiate inflammation by the degranulation of tissue mast cells (immediate hypersensitivity), by the activation of the complement system (Arthus reaction), and by antigen-specific effector T cells (DTH). The nature of inflammation depends to some extent on the underlying mechanism of induction. Frequently, however, more than one mechanism is involved in the inflammatory response. The purpose of the inflammatory reaction is to eliminate the irritant/infectious agent and to heal the tissue damage. The ability of the organism to respond rapidly through a neurogenic mechanism is of major significance. This is especially important in the gastrointestinal tract, where the discharge of mast cells, either by immunological or non-immune mechanisms, quickly activates the nervous system, which in turn initiates diarrhea in order to eliminate the noxious agent. The density and number of mucosal nerves increase in the gut after parasitic infestation. There is evidence to indicate that neuropeptides are also involved in the suppression of the inflammatory response, which may be mediated by somatostatin, VIP or CRF.

In addition to the chemotactic and proinflammatory cytokines (which include IL-1, IL-2, IL-6 and IL-8, TNF and IFN-$\gamma$), a number of growth factors, such as PDGF, EGF, and TGF$\beta$ and several others that are under characterization, are also produced at the inflammatory site, and this aids proliferation and healing. TGF$\beta$ plays a role in the local induction of inflammation and initiation of healing, whereas systemically it exerts antiinflammatory properties and thus may be regarded as one of the major coordinators of the inflammatory response. Other antiinflammatory cytokines are IL-4, IL-5 and IL-10.

Mild injury or a sublethal dose of endotoxin elicits a sharp, brief elevation of growth hormone and prolactin in the serum. These hormones are pleiotropic and have a proinflammatory and immunostimulatory effect. In severe trauma, sepsis and shock, growth hormone and prolactin are suppressed, whereas glucocorticoids and catecholamines are elevated. Under these conditions, an acute phase response is initiated by tissue-derived (cytokine) hormones, such as IL-1, IL-6 and TNF$\alpha$ (and several others may be involved), which elicit the neuroendocrine response and initiate major metabolic alterations. There is protein loss from muscles and catabolism in many other tissues and organs, whereas the synthesis of certain proteins, called acute phase proteins in the liver, cell proliferation in the bone marrow, and protein synthesis in leukocytes is elevated. These may be regarded as emergency measures to save the organism after the local immune/inflammatory response has failed to isolate and eliminate the agent causing injury. Under these conditions, the systemic activation of the complement system and of leukocytes releasing enzymes and highly toxic cytokines may seriously threaten survival. Glucocorticoids suppress proinflammatory cytokine production of and greatly potentiate the secretion of the acute phase proteins. Some of these proteins, such as CRP or LPS binding protein, are designed to bind microorganisms and trigger their destruction by the activation of the complement system and phagocytes. The enhanced production of some complement components also strengthens non-specific resistance. Increased production of fibrinogen promotes blood clotting, which can still serve to isolate the invading agent by triggering thrombosis in damaged tissues. A number of enzyme inhibitors are produced as acute phase proteins, which are likely to serve to curb the non-specific damage caused by enzymes released from phagocytes, and possibly other cells, into the circulation. The anti-inflammatory $\alpha$-macrofetoprotein is likely to inhibit damage inflicted by inflammatory cells. Catecholamines are known to inhibit inflammatory responses and have recently been shown to promote, even initiate, the acute phase response.

If the acute phase response fails to control the insult, which is usually bacterial infection and frequently involves endotoxin, shock will develop. Patients with subclinical adrenal insufficiency succumb to septic shock almost invariably if GC therapy is not given. However, GC treatment of patients with normal adrenal function has not been helpful. The use of antibiotics to control infection did not lead to spectacular success either, because of the emergence of resistant strains and the enhanced release of endotoxin by this therapy. The new approaches to prevent and treat septic shock involve the use of antibodies capable of neutralizing the biological effect of endotoxin and of cytokines and the inhibition of cytokine action by antagonist agents.

**Abbreviations**

| | |
|---|---|
| ACTH | adrenocorticotropic hormone |
| APP | acute phase protein |
| AVP | arginine vasopressin |
| CGRP | calcitonin gene related peptide |
| CNS | central nervous system |
| CRF | corticotropin-releasing factor |
| CRP | C-reactive protein |
| CSF | colony stimulating factor |
| DEX | dexamethasone |
| DTH | delayed-type hypersensitivity |
| $E_2$ | $17\beta$-estradiol |
| EGF | epidermal growth factor |
| END | endorphin |
| ENK | enkephalin |
| EPO | erythropoietin |
| ET | endothelin |
| FBS | fetal bovine serum |
| GC | glucocorticoid |
| GC-R | glucocorticoid receptor |
| GRO | melanoma growth-stimulating factor |
| IFN | interferon |
| IGF | insulin-like growth factor |
| IL | interleukin |
| IL-2R$\alpha$ | alpha chain of IL-2 receptor |
| IMC | intestinal mucosal mast cells |
| IP-10 | chemotactic and proinflammatory cytokine |
| LBP | lipopolysaccharide binding protein |
| LEM | leukocytic endogenous mediator |
| L-ENK | leucine-enkephalin |
| LH | luteinizing hormone |
| LPS | lipopolysaccharide |
| MAF | macrophage activating factor |
| MCAF | macrophage chemotactic and activating factor |
| M-ENK | methionine-enkephalin |
| $\alpha$-MFP | alpha-macrofetoprotein |

| | |
|---|---|
| mRNA | messenger RNA |
| α-MSH | alpha melanocyte stimulating hormone |
| NGF | nerve growth factor |
| PAF | platelet activating factor |
| PDGF | platelet-derived growth factor |
| PF-4 | platelet factor 4 |
| PG | prostaglandin |
| PHA | phytohemagglutinin |
| PMA | phorbol myristate acetate |
| PMC | peritoneal mast cells |
| SAA | serum amyloid A |
| SC | secretory component |
| β-TG | beta-thromboglobulin |
| TGF-β | transforming growth factor beta |
| TNF | tumor necrosis factor |
| TRH | thyroid-releasing hormone |
| TSH | thyroid-stimulating hormone |
| $TXB_2$ | thromboxane $B_2$ |
| UV | ultraviolet |
| VIP | vasoactive intestinal peptide |

## References

Adami, H. O., Axelsson, O., Carlstrom, K., Vegelius, J. & Akerstrom, G. (1982). Serum levels of cortisol, dehydroepiandrosterone, dehydroepiandrosterone sulphate, estrone and prolactin after surgical trauma in postmenopausal women. *Uppsala J. Med. Sci.*, **87**, 201–13.

Ader, R. & Cohen N. (1991). The influence of conditioning on the immune response. In *Psychoneuroimmunology*, 2nd edn, ed. R. Ader, D. L. Felten & N. Cohen, pp. 611–46. San Diego: Academic Press.

Akahoshi, T., Oppenheim, J. J. & Matsushima, K. (1988). Induction of high-affinity interleukin 1 receptor on human peripheral blood lymphocytes by glucocorticoid hormones. *J. Exp. Med.*, **167**, 924–36.

Akira, S. & Kishimoto, T. (1992). IL-6 and NF-IL6 in acute-phase response and viral infection. *Immunol. Rev.*, **127**, 26–50.

Almawi, W. Y., Lipman, M. A., Stevens, A. C., Zanker, B., Hadro, E. T. & Storm, T. B. (1991). Abrogation of glucocorticosteroid-mediated inhibition of T cell proliferation by the synergistic action of IL-1, IL-6 and IFN-gamma. *J. Immunol.*, **146**, 3523–7.

Andersson, B., Augustinsson, O., Holst, H. & Jonasson, H. (1987). ACTH-mediated aldosterone hypersecretion during endotoxin-induced fever with apparent influence upon renal sodium excretion. *Acta Physiol. Scand.*, **129**, 451–8.

Apte, R. N., Durum, S. K. & Oppenheim, J. J. (1990). Opioids modulate interleukin-1 production and secretion by bone-marrow macrophages. *Immunol. Lett.*, **24**, 141–8.

Arnold, J., Choo, J. J., Little, R. A. & Rothwell, N. J. (1990). Dopamine beta-hydroxylase inhibition reveals a selective influence of endotoxin on catecholamine content of rat tissues. *Circ. Shock*, **31**, 387–94.

Asko-Seljavaara, S. (1974). Altered cell proliferation in burned mice. *Scand. J. Plast. Reconstr. Surg.*, **A13**, 1–21.

Assem, E. S. K. & Schild, H. O. (1973). β-adrenergic receptors concerned with the anaphylactic mechanism. *Int. J. Allergy Appl. Immunol.*, **45**, 62–9.

Ayala, A., Perrin, M. M., Meldrum, D. R., Ertel, W. & Chaudry, I. H. (1990). Hemorrhage induces an increase in serum TNF which is not associated with elevated levels of endotoxin. *Cytokine*, **2**, 170–4.

Baigrie, R. J., Lamont, P. M., Dallman, M. & Morris, P. J. (1991). The release of interleukin-1-β (IL-1) precedes that of interleukin-6 (IL-6) in patients undergoing major surgery. *Lymphokine Cytokine Res.*, **10**, 253–6.

Ballou, S. P. & Kushner, I. (1992). C-reactive protein and the acute phase response. In *Advances in Internal Medicine*, ed. G. H. Stollerman, J. T. LaMont, J. J. Leonard & M. D. Siperstein, pp. 313–36. St. Louis, MO: Mosby Year Book.

Banck, G. & Forsgren, A. (1978). Many bacterial species are mitogenic for human blood lymphocytes. *Scand. J. Immunol.*, **8**, 347–54.

Barbul, A. (1989). Immune regulation of wound healing. In *Immune Consequences of Trauma, Shock and Sepsis*, ed. E. Faist, J. Ninneman & D. Green, pp. 339–49. Berlin, New York: Springer-Verlag.

Barnes, P. J. (1991). Neurogenic inflammation in airways. *Int. Arch. Allergy Appl. Immunol.*, **94**, 303–9.

Barnetson, St. C. & Gawkroger, D. (1989). Hypersensitivity – type IV. In *Immunology*, 2nd edn, ed. I. Roitt, J. Brostoff & D. Male, pp. 22.1–22.10. London: Gower Medical.

Baue, A. F. (1989). Neuroendocrine response to severe trauma and sepsis. In *Immune Consequences of Trauma, Shock and Sepsis*, ed. E. Faist, J. Ninnemann & D. Green, pp. 17–32. Berlin, New York: Springer-Verlag.

Bauer, J., Birmelin, M., Northoff, G. H., Northemann, W., Tran-Thi, T. A., Ueberberg, H., Decker, K. & Heinrich, P. (1984). Induction of rat α2-macroglobulin *in vivo* and in hepatocyte primary cultures: synergistic action of glucocorticoids and a Kupffer cell derived factor. *FEBS Lett.*, **177**, 89–94.

Baxter, G. D. & Lavin, M. F. (1992). Specific protein dephosphorylation in apoptosis induced by ionizing radiation and heat shock in human lymphoid tumor lines. *J. Immunol.*, **148**, 1949–54.

Beisel, W. R. (1975). Metabolic response to infection. *Ann. Rev. Med.*, **26**, 9–20.

Bentley-Phillips, C. B., Black, A. K. & Greaves, M. W. (1976). Induced tolerance in cold urticaria caused by cold-evoked histamine release. *Lancet*, **2**, 63–6.

Berczi, I. (1986*a*). *Pituitary Function and Immunity*. Boca Raton, FL: CRC Press.

Berczi, I. (1986*b*). The influence of pituitary–adrenal axis on the immune system. In *Pituitary Function and Immunity*, ed. I. Berczi, pp. 49–132. Boca Raton, FL: CRC Press.

Berczi, I. (1990). Neurohormonal immunoregulation. *Endocr. Pathol.*, **1**, 197–219.

Berczi, I., Baintner Jr, K. & Antal, T. (1966*b*). Comparative assay of endotoxin by oral and parenteral administration. *Zbl. Vet. Med. Reihe B*, **13**, 570–5.

Berczi, I., Baragar, F. D., Chalmers, I. M., Keystone, E. C., Nagy, E. & Warrington, R. J. (1993). Hormones in self-tolerance and autoimmunity: a role in the pathogenesis of rheumatoid arthritis. *Autoimmunity* (in press).

Berczi, I., Bertok, L., Baintner Jr, K. & Veress, B. (1968). Failure of oral *Escherichia coli* endotoxin to induce either specific tolerance or toxic syndromes in rats. *J. Path. Bact.*, **96**, 481–6.

Berczi, I., Bertok, L. & Bereznay, T. (1966*a*). Comparative studies on the toxicity of *Escherichia coli* lipopolysaccharide endotoxin in various animal species. *Can. J. Microbiol.*, **12**, 1070–1.

Berczi, I., Nagy, E., Matusik, R. J. & Friesen, H. G. (1991). Pituitary hormones regulate c-*myc* and DNA synthesis in lymphoid tissue. *J. Immunol.*, **146**, 2201–6.

Berisha, H., Foda, H., Sakkakibara, H., Trotz, M., Pakbaz, H. & Said, S. I. (1990). Vasoactive intestinal peptide prevents lung injury due to xanthine/xanthine oxidase. *Am. J. Physiol.*, **259**, L151–5.

Berkenbosch, F. (1992). Macrophages and astroglial interactions in repair to brain injury. *Ann. NY Acad. Sci.*, **650**, 186–90.

Berkenbosch, F., de Rijk, R., Del Rey, A. & Besedovsky, H. (1990). Neuroendocrinology of interleukin-1. In *Circulating Regulatory Factors and Neuroendocrine Function*, ed. J. C. Porter & D. Jezova, pp. 303–14. New York: Plenum Press.

Berkenbosch, F., Van Dam, A.-M., Derijk, R. & Schotanus, K. (1992). Role of the immune hormone interleukin-1 in brain-controlled adaptive responses to infection. In *Stress: Neuroendocrine and Molecular Approaches*, ed. R. Kvetnansky, R. McCarty & J. Axelrod, pp. 623–40. New York: Gordon & Breach Science.

Bernardini, R., Calogero, A. E., Ehrlich, Y. H., Brucke, T., Chrousos, G. P. & Gold, P. W. (1989). The alkyl-ether phospholipid platelet-activating factor is a stimulator of the hypothalamic–pituitary–adrenal axis in the rat. *Endocrinology*, **125**, 1067–73.

Bernardini, R., Kamilaris, T. C., Calogero, A. E., Johnson, E. O., Gomez, M. T., Gold, P. W. & Chrousos, G. P. (1990). Interactions between tumor necrosis factor-α, hypothalamic corticotropin-releasing hormone, and adrenocorticotropin secretion in the rat. *Endocrinology*, **126**, 2876–81.

Bernton, E. W., Meltzer, M. T. & Holaday, J. W. (1988). Suppression of macrophage activation and T-lymphocyte function in hypoprolactinemic mice. *Science*, **239**, 401–4.

Bertini, R., Bianchi, M., Erroi, A., Villa, P. & Ghezzi, P. (1989). Dexamethasone modulation of *in vivo* effects of endotoxin, tumor necrosis factor, and interleukin-1 on liver cytochrome P-450, plasma fibrinogen, and serum iron. *J. Leukocyte Biol.*, **46**, 254–62.

Bertini, R., Bianchi, M. & Ghezzi, P. (1988). Adrenalectomy sensitizes mice to the lethal effects of interleukin 1 and tumor necrosis factor. *J. Exp. Med.*, **167**, 1708–12.

Bertok, L. (1977). Physico-chemical defense of vertebrate organisms. The role of bile acids in defense against bacterial endotoxin. *Perspect. Biol. Med.*, **21**, 70–6.

Bertok, L. & Nagy, S. U. (1984). The effect of endotoxin and radio-detoxified endotoxin on the serum $T_4$ level of rats and response of their thyroid gland to exogenous TSH. *Immunopharmacology*, **8**, 143–6.

Besedovsky, H. O., del Rey, A., Klusman, I., Furukawa, H., Arditi, G. M. & Kabiersch, A. (1991). Cytokines as modulators of the hypothalamus–pituitary–adrenal axis. *J. Steroid Biochem. Mol. Biol.*, **40**, 613–18.

Bessler, H., Sztein, M. B. & Serrate, S. A. (1990). β-Endomorphin modulation of IL-1-induced IL-2 production. *Immunopharmacology*, **19**, 5–14.

Beutler, B. & Cerami, A. (1988). Cachectin (tumor necrosis factor): a macrophage hormone governing cellular metabolism and inflammatory response. *Endocr. Rev.*, **9**, 57–66.
Beutler, B., Milsark, I. W. & Cerami, A. (1985*a*). Passive immunization against cachectin/tumor necrosis factor protects mice from lethal effects of endotoxin. *Science*, **229**, 869–71.
Beutler, B., Milsark, I. W. & Cerami, A. (1985*b*). Cachectin/tumor necrosis factor: production, distribution and metabolic fate *in vivo*. *J. Immunol.*, **135**, 3972–7.
Billiau, A. & Vandekerckhove, F. (1991). Cytokines and their interactions with other inflammatory mediators in the pathogenesis of sepsis and septic shock. *Eur. J. Clin. Invest.*, **21**, 559–73.
Birke, G., Duner, H., Liljedhal, S. O., Pernow, B., Plantin, L.-O. & Troell, L. (1957). Histamine, catecholamines, and adrenocortical steroids in burns. *Acta Chir. Scand.*, **114**, 87–98.
Bjornson, A. B., Altemeier, W. A. & Bjornson, H. S. (1977). Changes in humoral components of host defense following burn trauma. *Ann. Surg.*, **186**, 88–96.
Blalock, J. E. (1989). A molecular basis for bidirectional communication between the immune and neuroendocrine systems. *Physiol. Rev.*, **69**, 1–32.
Bone, R. C., Fisher Jr, C. J., Clemmer, T. P., Slotman, G. J., Metz, C. A. & Balk, R. A. (1987). The Methylprednisolone Severe Sepsis Study Group. A controlled clinical trial of high-dose methylprednisolone in the treatment of severe sepsis and septic shock. *N. Engl. J. Med.*, **317**, 653–8.
Border, J. R., Hassett, J., LaDuca, J., Seibel, R., Steinberg, S., Mills, B., Losi, P. & Border, D. (1987). The gut origin septic states in blunt multiple trauma (ISS = 40) in the ICU. *Ann. Surg.*, **206**, 427–48.
Brostoff, J. & Hall, T. (1989). Hypersensitivity – Type I. In *Immunology*, 2nd edn, ed. I. M. Roitt, J. Brostoff & D. K. Male, pp. 19.1–19.20. London: Gower Medical.
Broudy, V. C., Kaushansky, K., Segal, G. M., Harlan, J. M. & Adamson, J. W. (1986). Tumor necrosis factor type α stimulates human endothelial cells to produce granulocyte/macrophage colony-stimulating factor. *Proc. Nat. Acad. Sci. USA*, **83**, 7467.
Brown, R., Li, Z., Vriend, C. Y., Nirula, R., Janz, L., Falk, J., Nance, D. M., Dyck, D. G. & Greenberg, A. H. (1991). Suppression of splenic macrophage interleukin-1 secretion following intracerebroventricular injection of interleukin-1β: evidence for pituitary adrenal and sympathetic control. *Cell Immunol.*, **132**, 84–93.
Brown, S. L. & Van Epps, D. E. (1986). Opioid peptides modulate production of interferon γ by human mononuclear cells. *Cell. Immunol.*, **103**, 19–26.
Brummitt, C. F., Sharp, B. M., Gekker, G., Keane, W. F. & Peterson, P. K. (1988). Modulatory effects of β-endorphin on interferon-γ production by cultured peripheral blood mononuclear cells: heterogeneity among donors and the influence of culture medium. *Brain Behav. Immun.*, **2**, 187–97.
Burrell, R. (1991). Immunopharmacology of bacterial endotoxin. *EOS-J. Immunol. Immunopharmacol.*, **11**, 85–90.
Bussolino, F., Wang, J. M., Defilippi, P., Turrini, F., Sanavio, F., Edgell, C.-J.S., Aglietta, M., Arese, P. & Mantovani, A. (1989). Granulocyte- and granulocyte–macrophage-colony stimulating factors induce human endothelial cells to migrate and proliferate. *Nature*, **337**, 471–3.

Calvo, C.-F., Chavanel, G. & Senik, A. (1992). Substance P enhances IL-2 expression in activated human T cells. *J. Immunol.*, **148**, 3498–504.
Camoratto, A. M. & Grandison, L. (1989). Platelet-activating factor stimulates prolactin release from dispersed rat anterior pituitary cells *in vitro*. *Endocrinology*, **124**, 1502–6.
Cannon, J. G., Tatro, J. B., Reichlin, S. & Dinarello, C. A. (1986). Alpha melanocyte stimulating hormone inhibits immunostimulatory and inflammatory actions of interleukin 1. *J. Immunol.*, **137**, 2232–6.
Casale, T. B., Bowman, S. & Kaliner, M. (1984). Induction of human cutaneous mast cell degranulation by opiates and endogenous opioid peptides: evidence for opiate and nonopiate receptor participation. *J. Allerg. Clin. Immunol.*, **73**, 775–81.
Chithara, Y. K. & Feierabend, T. C. (1981). Endogenous and exogenous infection with *Pseudomonas aeruginosa* in a burns unit. *Int. Surg.*, **66**, 237–40.
Christeff, N., Auclair, M.-C., Benassayag, C., Carli, A. & Nunez, E. A. (1987). Endotoxin-induced changes in sex steroid hormone levels in male rats. *J. Steroid Biochem.*, **26**, 67–71.
Church, M. K., El-Lati, S. & Caulfield, J. P. (1991). Neuropeptide-induced secretion from human skin mast cells. *Int. Arch. Allergy Appl. Immunol.*, **94**, 310–18.
Ciancio, M. J., Hunt, J., Jones, S. B. & Filkins, J. P. (1991). Comparative and interactive *in vivo* effects of tumor necrosis factor α and endotoxin. *Circ. Shock.*, **33**, 108–20.
Claman, H. N. (1987). Corticosteroids – immunologic and anti-inflammatory effects. In *Hormones and Immunity*, ed. I. Berczi & K. Kovacs, pp. 38–42. Lancaster, UK: MTP Press.
Clementsen, P., Norn, S., Kristensen, K. S., Bach-Mortensen, N., Koch, C. & Permin, H. (1990). Bacteria and endotoxin enhances basophil histamine release and potentiation is abolished by carbohydrates. *Allergy*, **45**, 402–8.
Clevenger, C. V., Russell, D. H., Appasamy, P. M. & Prystowsky, M. B. (1990). Regulation of interleukin 2-driven T-lymphocyte proliferation by prolactin. *Proc. Nat. Acad. Sci. USA*, **87**, 6460–4.
Collins, S. M., Hurst, S. M., Main, C., Stanley, E., Khan, I., Blennerhassett, P. & Swain, M. (1992). Effect of inflammation of enteric nerves. Cytokine-induced changes in neurotransmitter content and release. *Ann. NY Acad. Sci.*, **664**, 415–24.
Crespo, M. S. & Fernandez-Gallardo, S. (1991). Pharmacological modulation of PAF: a therapeutic approach to endotoxin shock. *J. Lipid Mediators*, **4**, 127–44.
Crompton, M. M. & Cidlowski, J. A. (1992). Thymocyte apoptosis. A model of programmed cell death. *Trends Endocrinol. Metab.*, **3**, 17–23.
Curnow, R. T., Rayfield, E. J., George, D. T., Zenser, T. V. & De Rubertis, F. R. (1976). Altered hepatic glycogen metabolism and glucoregulatory hormones during sepsis. *Am. J. Physiol.*, **230**, 1296–301.
Curnutte, J. T. & Babior, B. M. (1990). Composition of neutrophils. In *Hematology*, 4th edn, ed. W. W. Williams, E. Beutler, A. J. Erslev & M. A. Lichtman, pp. 770–4. New York: McGraw-Hill.
Dahn, M. S., Lange, M. P. & Jacobs, L. A. (1988). Insulinlike growth factor 1 production is inhibited in human sepsis. *Arch. Surg.*, **123**, 1409–14.
Damonneville, M., Monte, D., Auriault, C. & Capron, A. (1990). The neuropeptide substance-P stimulates the effector functions of platelets. *Clin. Exp. Immunol.*, **81**, 346–51.

Dantzer, R. & Kelley, K. W. (1989). Minireview: stress and immunity: an integrated view of relationships between the brain and the immune system. *Life Sci.*, **44**, 1995–2008.

Daynes, R. A. & Araneo, B. A. (1989). Contrasting effects of glucocorticoids on the capacity of T-cells to produce the growth factors interleukin-2 and interleukin-4. *Eur. J. Immunol.*, **19**, 2319–25.

Debets, J. M. H., Ruers, T. J. M., Van-Der-Linden, M. P. M. H., Van-Der-Linden, C. J. & Buurman, W. A. (1989). Inhibitory effect of corticosteroids on the secretion of tumor necrosis factor (TNF) by monocytes is dependent on the stimulus inducing TNF synthesis. *Clin. Exp. Immunol.*, **78**, 224–9.

Delidow, B. C., Billis, W. M., Agarwal, P. & White, B. A. (1991). Inhibition of prolactin gene transcription by transforming growth factor-$\beta$ in GH3 cells. *Mol. Endocrinol.*, **5**, 1716–22.

Denicoff, K. D., Durkin, T. M., Lotze, M. T., Quinland, P. E., Lewis, C. L., Listwak, S. J., Rosenberg, S. A. & Rubinow, D. R. (1989). The neuroendocrine effects of interleukin-2 treatment. *J. Clin. Endocrinol. Metab.*, **69**, 402–10.

Denicoff, K. D., Rubinow, D. R., Papa, M. Z., Simpson, C., Seipp, C. A., Lotze, M. T., Chang, A. E., Rosenstein, D. & Rosenberg, S. A. (1987). The neuropsychiatric effects of treatment with interleukin-2 and lymphokine-activated killer cells. *Ann. Intern. Med.*, **107**, 293–300.

Denko, C. W. & Gabriel, P. (1985). Effects of peptide hormones in urate crystal inflammation. *J. Rheumatol.*, **12**, 971–5.

Derijk, R. & Berkenbosch, F. (1991). The immune–hypothalamo–pituitary–adrenal axis and autoimmunity. *Intern. J. Neuroscience*, **59**, 91–100.

Derijk, R. H., Vanrooijen, N. & Berkenbosch, F. (1992). The role of macrophages in the hypothalamic–pituitary–adrenal activation in response to endotoxin (LPS). *Res. Immunol.*, **143**, 224–9.

Dinarello, C. A. (1988). Biology of interleukin-1. *Fed. Am. Soc. Exp. Biol. J.*, **2**, 108–15.

Dinarello, C. A. (1991). The proinflammatory cytokines interleukin-1 and tumor necrosis factor and treatment of the septic shock syndrome. *J. Infect. Dis.*, 163, 1177–84.

Doherty, G. M., Lange, J. R., Langsterin, H. N., Alexander, H. R., Buresh, C. M. & Norton, J. A. (1992). Evidence for IFN-$\gamma$ as a mediator of the lethality of endotoxin and tumor necrosis factor-$\alpha$. *J. Immunol.*, **149**, 1666–70.

Douglas, S. D. & Hassam, N. F. (1990). Morphology of monocytes and macrophages. In *Hematology*, 4th edn, ed. W. W. Williams, E. Beutler, A. J. Erslev & M. A. Lichtman, pp. 859–68. New York: McGraw-Hill.

Drago, F., D'Agata, V., Iacona, T., Spadaro, F., Grassi, M., Valerio, C., Raffaele, R., Astuto, C., Lauria, N. & Vitetta, M. (1989). Prolactin as a protective factor in stress-induced biological changes. *J. Clin. Lab. Anal.*, **3**, 340–4.

Drouhault, R., Abrous, N., David, J. P. & Duffy, B. (1987). Bradykinin parallels thyrotropin-releasing hormone actions on prolactin release from rat anterior pituitary cells. *Neuroendocrinology*, **46**, 360–4.

Drutz, D. J. & Graybill, J. R. (1987). Infectious diseases. In *Basic and Clinical Immunology*, 6th edn, ed. D. P. Stiles, J. D. Stobo & J. V. Wells, pp. 534–81. Norwalk, CT: Appleton & Lange.

Eastman, A. & Barry, M. A. (1992). The origins of DNA breaks – a consequence of DNA damage, DNA repair, or apoptosis. *Cancer Invest.*, **10**, 229–40.

Edwards III, C. K., Ghiasuddin, S. M., Schepper, J. M., Yunger, L. M. & Kelley, K. W. (1988). A newly defined property of somatotropin: priming of macrophages for production of superoxide anion. *Science*, **239**, 769–71.

Edwards, C. K., Lorence, R. M., Dunham, D. M., Arkins, S., Yunger, L. M., Greager, J. A., Walter, R. J., Dantzer, R. & Kelley, K. W. (1991). Hypophysectomy inhibits the synthesis of tumor necrosis factor-α by rat macrophages – partial restoration by exogenous growth hormone or interferon-γ. *Endocrinology*, **128**, 989–96.

Elenkov, I. J., Kovacs, K., Kiss, J., Bertok, L. & Vizi, E. S. (1992). Lipopolysaccharide is able to bypass corticotrophin-releasing factor in affecting plasma ACTH and corticosterone levels – evidence from rats with lesions of the paraventricular nucleus. *J. Endocrinol.*, **133**, 231–6.

Elin, R. J. & Csako, G. (1989). Response of humans to gamma-irradiated reference *Escherichia-coli* endotoxin. *J. Clin. Lab. Immunol.*, **29**, 17–23.

Ellison, M. D. & Merchant, R. E. (1991). Appearance of cytokine-associated central nervous system myelin damage coincides temporarily with serum tumor necrosis factor induction after recombinant interleukin-2 infusion in rats. *J. Neuroimmunol.*, **33**, 245–51.

Elsasser, T. H., Caperna, T. J. & Fayer, R. (1991). Tumor necrosis factor-α affects growth hormone secretion by a direct pituitary interaction. *Proc. Soc. Expl. Biol. Med.*, **198**, 547–54.

Emilie, D., Crevon, M. C., Auffredou, M. T. & Galanaud, P. (1988). Glucocorticosteroid-dependent synergy between interleukin-1 and interleukin-6 for human lymphocyte-B differentiation. *Eur. J. Immunol.*, **18**, 2043–7.

Eskandari, M. K., Bolgos, G., Miller, D., Nguyen, D. T., DeForge, L. E. & Remick, D. G. (1992). Anti-tumor necrosis factor antibody therapy fails to prevent lethality after cecal ligation and puncture of endotoxemia. *J. Immunol.*, **148**, 2724–30.

Evans, G. F. & Zuckerman, S. H. (1991). Glucocorticoid-dependent and glucocorticoid-independent mechanisms involved in lipopolysaccharide tolerance. *Eur. J. Immunol.*, **21**, 1973–9.

Faist, E., Ertel, W., Mewes, A., Alkan, S., Walz, A. & Strasser, T. (1989). Trauma-induced alterations of the lymphokine cascade. In *Immune Consequences of Trauma, Shock and Sepsis*, ed. E. Faist, J. Ninnemann & D. Green, pp. 79–94. Berlin, New York: Springer-Verlag.

Feldman, R. D., Hunninghake, G. W. & McArdle, W. L. (1987). β-Adrenergic receptor-mediated suppression of interleukin 2 receptors in human lymphocytes. *J. Immunol.*, **139**, 3355–9.

Flynn, A. (1986). Expression of Ia and the production of interleukin 1 by peritoneal exudate macrophages activated *in vivo* by steroids. *Life Sci.*, **38**, 2455–60.

Foreman, J. C. (1987). Neuropeptides and the pathogenesis of allergy. *Allergy*, **42**, 1–11.

Fox, H. S., Bond, B. L. & Parslow, T. G. (1991). Estrogen regulates the IFN-γ promoter. *J. Immunol.*, **146**, 4362–7.

Friedman, H., Newton, C., Widen, R., Klein, T. W. & Spitzer, J. A. (1992). Continuous endotoxin infusion suppresses rat spleen cell production of cytokines. *Proc. Soc. Exp. Biol. Med.*, **199**, 360–4.

Fu, Y.-K., Arkins, S., Wang, B. W. & Kelley, K. W. (1991). A novel role of growth hormone and insulin-like growth factor-I. Priming neutrophils for superoxide anion secretion. *J. Immunol.*, **146**, 1602–8.

Fuggetta, M. P., Graziani, G., Aquino, A., D'Atri, S. & Bonmassar, E. (1988). Effect of hydrocortisone on human natural killer activity and its modulation by beta interferon. *Int. J. Immunopharmacol.*, **10**, 687–94.

Fujiwara, M., Kariyone, A. & Kimura, M. (1980). Tolerance inducibility and the elicitation of autoantibodies by LPS in aged NZB mice. *J. Clin. Lab. Immunol.*, **3**, 185–88.

Fukata, J. T., Usui, T., Naitoh, Y., Nakai, Y. & Imura, H. (1989). Effects of recombinant human interleukin-1$\alpha$, -1$\beta$, -2 and -6 on ACTH synthesis and release in the mouse pituitary tumour cell line AtT-20. *J. Endocrinol.*, **122**, 33–9.

Gaillard, R. C., Turnill, D., Sappino, P. & Muller, A. F. (1990). Tumor necrosis factor $\alpha$ inhibits the hormonal response of the pituitary gland to hypothalamic releasing factors. *Endocrinology*, **127**, 101–6.

Galli, S. J., Dvorak, A. M. & Dvorak, H. F. (1990). Morphology, biochemistry and function of basophils and mast cells. In *Hematology*, 4th edn, ed. W. W. Williams, E. Beutler, A. J. Erslev & M. A. Lichtman, pp. 840–5. New York: McGraw-Hill.

Ganes, E., Gurll, N. J. & Reynolds, D. G. (1987). Naloxone pretreatment prevents the bloody diarrhea of canine endotoxic shock. *Proc Soc. Exp. Biol. Med.*, **184**, 267–77.

Geenen, V., Robert, F., Fatemi, M., Martens, H., Defresne, M.-P., Boniver, J., Legros, J. J. & Franchimont, P. (1989). Neuroendocrine–immune interactions in T cell ontogeny. *Thymus*, **13**, 131–40.

Geller, P., Merrill, E. R. & Jawetz, E. (1954). Effects of cortisone and antibiotics on lethal action of endotoxins in mice. *Proc. Soc. Exp. Biol. Med.*, **86**, 716–19.

Giannini, M. S. H. (1986). Suppression of pathogenesis in cutaneous leishmaniasis by UV radiation. *Infect. Immun.*, **51**, 838–43.

Gilmore, W. & Weiner, L. P. (1988). $\beta$-Endorphin enhances interleukin-2 (IL-2) production in murine lymphocytes. *J. Neuroimmunol.*, **18**, 125–38.

Girard, M. T., Hjaltadottir, S., Fejes-Toth, A. N. & Guyre, P. M. (1987). Glucocorticoids enhance the $\gamma$-interferon augmentation of human monocyte immunoglobulin G Fc receptor expression. *J. Immunol.*, **138**, 3235–41.

Girolomoni, G. & Tigelaar, R. E. (1990). Capsaicin-sensitive primary sensory neurons are potent modulators of murine delayed-type hypersensitivity reactions. *J. Immunol.*, **145**, 1105–12.

Giulian, D. (1990). Microglia, cytokines, and cytotoxins: modulators of cellular responses after injury to the central nervous system. *EOS-J. Immunol. Immunopharmacol.*, **10**, 15–21.

Glyn-Ballinger, J. R., Bernardini, G. L. & Lipton, J. M. (1983). Alpha-MSH injected into the septal region reduces fever in rabbits. *Peptides (Fayetteville)*, **4**, 199.

Goetzl, E. J. & Payan, D. G. (1984). Inhibition by somatostatin of the release of mediators from human basophils and rat leukemic basophils. *J. Immunol.*, **133**, 3255–9.

Gonzalez, M. C., Aguila, M. C. & McCann, S. M. (1991). *In vitro* effects of recombinant human $\gamma$-interferon on growth hormone release. *Prog. Neuroendocrinimmunol.*, **4**, 222–7.

Gonzalez, M. C., Riedel, M., Rettori, V., Yu, W. H. & McCann, S. M. (1990). Effect of recombinant human $\gamma$-interferon on the release of anterior pituitary hormones. *Prog. Neuroendocrinimmunol.*, **3**, 49–54.

Goodman, J. C., Robertson, C. S., Grossman, R. G. & Narayan, R. K. (1990). Elevation of tumor necrosis factor in head injury. *J. Neuroimmunol.*, **30**, 213–17.

Gordon, C., Ranges, G. E., Greenspan, J. W. & Wofsy, D. (1989). Chronic therapy with recombinant tumor necrosis-alpha autoimmune NZB/NZW F1 mice. *Clin. Immunol. Immunopathol.*, **52**, 421–34.

Goto, M. & Griffin, A. J. (1988). Adjuvant effects of $\beta$-adrenergic drugs in the indomethacin treatment of highly lethal endotoxic shock. *Res. Commun. Chem. Pathol. Pharm.*, **62**, 133–6.

Greenman, R. L., Schein, R. M. H., Martin, M. A., Wenzel, R. P., MacIntyre, N. R., Emmanuel, G., Chumel, H., Kohler, R. B., McCarthy, M., Plouffe, J. & Russell, J. A., the XOMA Sepsis Study Group. (1991). A controlled clinical trial of E5 murine monoclonal IgM antibody to endotoxin in the treatment of gram-negative sepsis. *J. Am. Med. Assoc.*, **266**, 1097–102.

Gulic, T., Chung, M. K., Pieper, S. J., Lange, L. G. & Schreiber, G. F. (1989). Interleukin 1 and tumor necrosis factor inhibit cardiac monocyte beta-adrenergic responsiveness. *Proc. Natl. Acad. Sci. USA*, **86**, 6753–7.

Haak-Frendscho, M., Arai, N., Arai, K., Baeza, M. L., Finn, A. & Kaplan, A. P. (1988). Human recombinant granulocyte–macrophage colony-stimulating factor and interleukin-3 cause basophil histamine release. *J. Clin. Invest.*, **82**, 17–20.

Hanahan, D. J. (1992). Platelet-activating factor: a novel lipid agonist. *Curr. Topics Cell. Regul.*, **33**, 65–78.

Haq, A. U. (1988). Failure of hydrocortisone to suppress the interferon-gamma-induced augmentation of interleukin-1 secretion of aged human monocytes. *Immunobiology*, **177**, 245–53.

Hartung, H.-P. (1988). Activation of macrophages by neuropeptides. *Brain Behav. Immun.*, **2**, 275–81.

Hartung, H.-P., Heininger, K., Schafer, B. & Toyka, K. V. (1988). Substance P and astrocytes: stimulation of the cyclooxygenase pathway of arachidonic acid metabolism. *Fed. Am. Soc. Exp. Biol. J.*, **2**, 48–51.

Haskill, S., Martin, G., Van Le, L., Morris, J., Peace, A., Bigler, C. F., Jaffe, G. J., Hammerberg, C., Sporn, S. A., Fong, S. *et al.* (1991). cDNA cloning of an intracellular form of the human interleukin 1 receptor antagonist associated with epithelium. *Proc. Natl. Acad. Sci. USA*, **88**, 3681–5.

Hay, F. (1989). Hypersensitivity – Type III. In *Immunology*, 2nd edn, ed. I. M. Roitt, J. Brostoff & D. K. Male, pp. 21.1–21.10. London: Gower Medical.

Hayashi, Y. & Aurelian, L. (1987). Immunity to herpes simplex virus type-2: viral antigen-presenting capacity of epidermal cells and its impairment by ultraviolet irradiation. *J. Immunol.*, **139**, 2788–93.

Heideman, M. (1981). Complement activation by thermal injury and its possible consequences for immune defense. In *The Immune Consequences of Thermal Injury*, ed. J. L. Ninnemann, pp. 127–33. Baltimore, MD: Williams & Wilkins.

Heideman, M. (1989). The role of complement injury. In *Immune Consequences of Trauma, Shock and Sepsis*, ed. E. Faist, J. Ninnemann & D. Green, pp. 215–18. Berlin, New York: Springer-Verlag.

Heiman, A. S. & Crews, F. T. (1984). Hydrocortisone selectively inhibits IgE-dependent arachidonic acid release from rat peritoneal mast cells. *Prostaglandins*, **27**, 335–43.

Heinzel, F. P. (1990). The role of IFN-$\gamma$ in the pathology of experimental endotoxemia. *J. Immunol.*, **145**, 2920–4.

Helme, R. D., Eglezos, A. & Hosking, C. S. (1987). Substance P induces chemotaxis of neutrophils in normal and capsaicin-treated rats. *Immun. Cell. Biol.*, **65**, 267–9.

Heyeman, D. & McKerrow, J. H. (1987). Parasitic diseases. In *Basic and Clinical Immunology*, 6th edn, ed. D. P. Stiles, J. D. Stobo & J. V. Wells, pp. 634–51. Norwalk, CT: Appleton & Lange.

Hirashima, M., Sakata, K., Tashiro, T., Yoshimura, T. & Hayashi, H. (1985). Dexamethasone suppresses concanavalin A-induced production of chemotactic lymphokines by releasing a soluble factor from splenic lymphocytes-T. *Immunology*, **54**, 533–40.

Hogan, M. M. & Vogel, S. N. (1988). Inhibition of macrophage tumoricidal activity by glucocorticoids. *J. Immunol.*, **140**, 513–19.

Holmsen, H. (1990). Composition of platelets. In *Hematology*, 4th edn, ed. W. W. Williams, E. Beutler, A. J. Erslev & M. A. Lichtman, pp. 1182–200. New York: McGraw-Hill.

Homo-Delarche, F., Fitzpatrick, F., Christeff, N., Nunez, E. A., Bach, J. F. & Dardenne, M. (1991). Sex steroids, glucocorticoids, stress and autoimmunity. *J. Steroid Biochem. Mol. Biol.*, **40**, 619–37.

Horio, T. & Okamoto, H. (1983). Immunologic unresponsiveness induced by topical application of hapten to PUVA-treated skin in guinea pigs. *J. Invest. Dermatol.*, **80**, 90–3.

Horio, T. & Yokamoto, M. (1982). The mechanisms of inhibitory effect of 8-methoxypsoralen and longwave ultraviolet light on experimental contact sensitization. *J. Invest. Dermatol.*, **78**, 402–5.

Howerton, E. E. & Kolmen, S. N. (1972). The intestinal tract as a portal of entry of *Pseudomonas* in burned rats. *J. Trauma*, **12**, 335–40.

Howie, S., Norval, M. & Maingay, J. (1988). Exposure to low-dose ultraviolet radiation suppressed delayed-type hypersensitivity to herpes simplex virus in mice. *J. Invest. Dermatol.*, **86**, 125–8.

Ibbotson, G. C. & Wallace, J. L. (1989). Inhibitory effects of dexamethasone in endotoxic shock and its relation to PAF-acether synthesis in the gastrointestinal tract and lung. *J. Lipid Mediator*, **1**, 273–82.

Ijaz, M. K., Dent, D. & Babiuk, L. A. (1990). Neuroimmunomodulation of *in vivo* anti-rotavirus humoral immune response. *J. Neuroimmunol.*, **26**, 159

Iochida, L. C., Tominaga, M., Matsumoto, M., Sekikawa, A. & Sasaki, H. (1989). Insulin resistance in septic rats – a study by the euglycemic clamp technique. *Life Sci.*, **45**, 1567–73.

Iwamoto, I., Tomoe, S., Tomioka, H. & Yoshida, S. (1992). Substance-P-induced granulocyte infiltration in mouse skin – the mast cell-dependent granulocyte infiltration by the N-terminal peptide is enhanced by the activation of vascular endothelial cells by the C-terminal peptide. *Clin. Exp. Immunol.*, **87**, 203–7.

Izumi, T. & Bakhle, Y. S. (1988). Modification by steroids of pulmonary oedema and prostaglandin E2 pharmacokinetics induced by endotoxin in rats. *Br. J. Pharmacol.*, **93**, 955–63.

Jacobs, A. L., Sehgal, P. B., Julian, J. & Carson, D. D. (1992). Secretion and hormonal regulation of interleukin-6 production by mouse uterine stromal and polarized epithelial cells cultured *in vitro*. *Endocrinology*, **131**, 1037–46.

Jamieson, J. C., Lammers, G., Janzen, R. & Woloski, B. M. R. N. J. (1987). The acute phase response to inflammation: the role of monokines in changes in liver glycoproteins and enzymes of glycoprotein metabolism. *Comp. Biochem. Physiol.*, **87B**, 11–15.

Jancso, N., Jancso-Gabor, A. & Szolcsanyi, J. (1967). Direct evidence for neurogenic inflammation and its prevention by denervation and by pretreatment with capsaicin. *Br. J. Pharmacol.*, **31**, 138–51.

Jancso, G., Obal Jr, F., Toth-Kasa, I., Katona, M. & Husz, S. (1985). The modulation of cutaneous inflammatory reactions by peptide-containing sensory nerves. *Int. J. Tiss. Reac.*, **6**, 449–57.

Jansen, N. J. G., Vanoeveren, W., Hoiting, B. H. & Wildevuur, C. R. H. (1991). Methylprednisolone prophylaxis protects against endotoxin-induced death in rabbits. *Inflammation*, **15**, 91–101.

Jasmin, G. & Chentin, M. (eds) (1991). *Stress Revisited 1: Neuroendocrinology of Stress. Methods and Achievements in Experimental Pathology*, vol. 14. Basel: Karger.

Jeevan, A., Evans, R., Brown, E. L. & Kripke, M. L. (1992). Effect of local ultraviolet irradiation on infections of mice with *Candida albicans*, *Mycobacterium bovis*, BCG, and *Schistosoma mansoni*. *J. Invest. Dermatol.*, **99**, 59–64.

Jepson, M. M., Millward, D. J., Rothwell, N. J. & Stock, M. J. (1988). Involvement of sympathetic nervous system and brown fat in endotoxin-induced fever in rats. *Am. J. Physiol.*, **255**, E617–20.

Jiayi, D., Shikun, Y. & Renbao, X. (1989). The inhibitory effect of hydrocortisone on interferon production by rat spleen cells. *J. Steroid Biochem.*, **33**, 1139–41.

Johnston, C. A. & Griesman, S. E. (1984). Endotoxemia induced by antibiotic therapy: a mechanism for adrenal corticosteroid protection in Gram-negative sepsis. *Trans.. Assoc. Am. Physicians*, **97**, 172–81.

Jones, S. B. & Romano, F. D. (1989). Dose- and time-dependent changes in plasma catecholamines in response to endotoxin in conscious rats. *Circ. Shock*, **28**, 59–68.

Jones, S. B. & Yelich, M. R. (1987). Simultaneous elevation of plasma insulin and catecholamines during endotoxicosis in the conscious and anesthetized rat. *Life Sci.*, **41**, 1935–43.

Jones, T. H., Brown, B. L. & Dobson, P. R. M. (1989). Bradykinin stimulates phosphoinositide metabolism and prolactin secretion in rat anterior pituitary cells. *J. Mol. Endocrinol.*, **2**, 47–53.

Jun, B.-D., Roberts, L. K., Cho, B.-H., Robertson, B. & Daynes, R. A. (1988). Parallel recovery of epidermal antigen-presenting cell activity and contact hypersensitivity responses in mice exposed to ultraviolet irradiation: The role of prostaglandin-dependent mechanism. *J. Invest. Dermatol.*, **90**, 311–16.

Jurkovich, G. J., Mileski, W. J., Maier, R. V., Winn, R. K. & Rice, C. L. (1991). Interferon-$\gamma$ increases sensitivity to endotoxin. *J. Surg. Res.*, **51**, 197–203.

Karady, S., Selye, H. & Brownie, J. S. L. (1938). The influence of the alarm reaction on the development of anaphylactic shock. *J. Immunol.*, **35**, 335.

Karalis, K., Sano, H., Redwine, J., Listwak, S., Wilder, R. L. & Chrousos, G. P. (1991). Autocrine or paracrine inflammatory actions of corticotropin-releasing hormone *in vivo*. *Science*, **254**, 421–3.

Karanth, S. & McCann, S. M. (1991). Anterior pituitary hormone controlled by interleukin-2. *Proc. Natl. Acad. Sci. USA*, **88**, 2961–5.

Kassessinoff, T. A. & Pearce, F. L. (1988). Histamine secretion from mast cells stimulated with somatostatin. *Agent Action*, **23**, 211–13.

Kawasaki, H., Moriyama, M., Ohtani, Y., Naitoh, M., Tanaka, A. & Nariuchi, H. (1989). Analysis of endotoxin fever in rabbits by using a monoclonal antibody to tumor necrosis factor (cachectin). *Infect. Immun.*, **57**, 3131–5.

Kehrl, J. H., Alvarez-Mon, M., Delsing, G. A. & Fauci, A. S. (1987). Lymphotoxin is an important T cell-derived growth factor for human B cells. *Science*, **238**, 1144–6.

Keller, S. E., Schleifer, S. J. & Demetrikopoulos, M. K. (1991). Stress induced changes in immune function in animals: hypothalamo–pituitary–adrenal influences. In *Psychoneuroimmunology*, 2nd edn, ed. R. Ader, D. L. Felten & N. Cohen, pp. 771–87. San Diego: Academic Press.

Kelso, A. & Munck A. (1984). Glucocorticoid inhibition of lymphokine secretion by alloreactive T lymphocyte clones. *J. Immunol.*, **133**, 784–91.

Killian, H. (1981). *Cold and Frost Injuries – Rewarming Damages. Biological, Angiological and Clinical Aspects.* Berlin: Springer-Verlag.

Kjaer, A., Knigge, U. & Warberg, J. (1990). The prolactin releasing effect of histamine is unrelated to its vascular action. *Acta Endocrinol.*, **122**, 49–54.

Knigge, U., Bach, F. W., Matzen, S., Bang, P. & Warberg, J. (1988). Effect of histamine on the secretion of pro-opiomelanocortin derived peptides in rats. *Acta Endocrinol.*, **119**, 312–19.

Koenig, J. L. (1991). Presence of cytokines in the hypothalamic–pituitary axis. *Prog. Neuroendocrinimmunol.*, **4**, 143–53.

Koff, W. C. & Dunegan, M. A. (1986). Neuroendocrine hormones suppress macrophage-mediated lysis of herpes simplex virus-infected cells. *J. Immunol.*, **136**, 705–9.

Koff, W. C. & Fann, A. V. (1986). Human tumor necrosis factor-alpha kills herpes virus-infected but not normal cells. *Lymphokine Res.*, **5**, 215–21.

Kowalski, M. L. & Kaliner, M. A. (1988). Neurogenic inflammation, vascular permeability, and mast cells. *J. Immunol.*, **140,** 3905–11.

Kowalski, M. L., Sliwinska-Kowalski, M. & Kaliner, M. A. (1990). Neurogenic inflammation, vascular permeability, and mast cells. II. Additional evidence indicating that mast cells are not involved in neurogenic inflammation. *J. Immunol.*, **145**, 1214–21.

Kripke, M. L., Morison, W. & Parrish, J. A. (1983). Systemic suppression of contact hypersensitivity in mice by psoralen plus UVA radiation (PUVA). *J. Invest. Dermatol.*, **81**, 87–92.

Kusnecov, A. W., Husband, A. J., King, M. G., Pang, G. & Smith, R. (1987). *In vivo* effects of $\beta$-endorphin on lymphocyte proliferation and interleukin-2 production. *Brain Behav. Immun.*, **1**, 88–97.

Lam, F. Y. & Ferrell, W. R. (1991). Neurogenic component of different models of acute inflammation in the rat knee joint. *Ann. Rheum. Dis.*, **50**, 747–51.

Lang, C. H. & Dobrescu, C. (1989). Sepsis-induced changes in *in vivo* insulin action in diabetic rats. *Am. J. Physiol.*, **257**, E301–8.

Lang, C. H. & Dobrescu, C. (1991). Gram-negative infection increases noninsulin-mediated glucose disposal. *Endocrinology*, **128**, 645–53.

Lavker, R. M. & Schechter, N. M. (1985). Cutaneous mast cell depletion results from topical corticosteroid usage. *J. Immunol.*, **135**, 2368–73.

Le, N., Yousefi, S., Vaziri, N., Carandang, G., Ocariz, J. & Cesario, T. (1988). The effect of beta-estradiol, progesterone and testosterone on the production of human leukocyte derived interferons. *J. Biol. Regul. Homeost. Agent*, **2**, 199–204.

Lee, S. W., Tsou, A.-P., Chan, H., Thomas, J., Petrie, K., Engui, E. M. & Allison, A. C. (1988). Glucocorticoids selectively inhibit the transcription of the interleukin 1$\beta$ gene and decrease the stability of interleukin 1$\beta$ mRNA. *Proc. Nat. Acad. Sci. USA*, **85**, 1204–8.

Lemaire, I. (1988). Neurotensin enhances IL-1 production by activated alveolar macrophages. *J. Immunol.*, **140**, 2983–8.
Lephart, E. D., Baxter, C. B. & Parker, R. (1987). Effect of burn trauma on adrenal and testicular steroid hormone production. *J. Clin. Endocrinol. Metab.*, **64**, 842–8.
Leshin, L. S. & Malven, P. V. (1984). Bacteremia-induced changes in pituitary hormone release and effect of naloxone. *Am. J. Physiol.*, **247**, E585–91.
Levi-Montalcini, R., Aloe, L. & Alleva, E. (1990). A role for nerve growth factor in nervous, endocrine and immune systems. *Prog. Neuroendocrinimmunol.*, **3**, 1–10.
Lin, M.-T., Uang, W.-N. & Ho, L.-T. (1989). Hypothalamic somatostatin may mediate endotoxin-induced fever in the rat. *Naunyn. Schmeid. Arch. Pharmacol.*, **339**, 608–12.
Lindh, A., Carlstrom, K., Eklund, J. & Wilking, N. (1992). Serum steroids and prolactin during and after major surgical trauma. *Acta Anaesthesiol. Scand.*, **36**, 119–24.
Lissoni, P., Barni, S., Archili, C., Cattaneo, G., Rovelli, F., Conti, A., Maestroni, G. J. & Tancini, G. (1990). Endocrine effects on a 24-hour intravenous infusion of interleukin-2 in the immunotherapy of cancer. *Anticancer Res.*, **10**, 753–8.
Lotz, M., Vaughan, J. H. & Carson, D. A. (1988). Effect of neuropeptides on production of inflammatory cytokines by human monocytes. *Science*, **241**, 1218–21.
Lyson, K., Milenkovic, L. & McCann, S. M. (1991). The stimulatory effect of interleukin 6 on corticotropin-releasing hormone and thyrotropin-releasing hormone release *in vitro*. *Prog. Neuroendocrinimmunol.*, **4**, 161–5.
Malarkey, W. B. & Zvara, B. J. (1989). Interleukin-1-beta and other cytokines stimulate adrenocorticotropin release from cultured pituitary cells of patients with Cushing's disease. *J. Clin. Endocrinol. Metab.*, **69**, 196–9.
Malec, P. & Nowak, Z. (1988). Propranolol enhances *in vitro* interleukin 2 receptor expression on human lymphocytes. *Immunol. Lett.*, **17**, 319–22.
Malone, D. G., Pierce, J. H., Falko, J. P. & Metcalfe, D. D. (1988). Production of granulocyte–macrophage colony-stimulating factor by primary cultures of unstimulated rat microvascular endothelial cells. *Blood*, **71**, 684–9.
Marano, M. A., Moldawer, L. L., Fong, Y., Wei, H., Minei, J., Yurt, R., Cerami, A. & Lowry, S. F. (1988). Cachectin/TNF production in experimental burns and *Pseudomonas* infection. *Arch. Surg.*, **123**, 1383–8.
Markowe, H. L. J., Marmot, M. G., Shipley, M. J., Bulpitt, C. J., Meade, T. W., Stirling, Y., Vickers, M. V. & Semmence, A. (1985). Fibrinogen: a possible link between social class and coronary heart disease. *Br. Med. J.*, **291**, 1312–14.
Marks, J. D., Marks, C. B., Luce, J. M., Montgomery, A. B., Turner, J., Metz, C. A. & Murray, J. F. (1990). Plasma tumor necrosis factor in patients with septic shock. Mortality rate, incidence of adult respiratory distress syndrome, and effects of methylprednisolone administration. *Am. Rev. Respir. Dis.*, **141**, 94–7.
Marshall, J. S., Stead, R. H., McSharry, C., Nielsen, L. & Bienenstock, J. (1990). The role of mast cell deregulation products in mast cell hyperplasia. I. Mechanism of action of nerve growth factor. *J. Immunol.*, **144**, 1886–92.
Martin, L. W. & Lipton, J. M. (1990). Acute phase response to endotoxin – rise in plasma α-MSH and effects of α-MSH injection. *Am. J. Physiol.*, **259**, R768–72.
Masana, M. I., Heyes, M. P. & Mefford, I. N. (1990). Indomethacin prevents

increased catecholamine turnover in rat brain following systemic endotoxin challenge. *Prog. Neuro-Psych. Biol. Psych.*, **14**, 609–21.

Mathison, R., Hoogan, A., Helmer, D., Bauce, L., Woolner, J., Davison, J. S., Schultz, G. & Befus, D. (1992). Role for the submandibular gland in modulating pulmonary inflammation following induction of systemic anaphylaxis. *Brain Behav. Immun.*, **6**, 117–29.

Merrill, G. A. & Anderson, Jr, J. H. (1987). Involvement of endogenous opiates in glucose-stimulated hyperinsulinism of canine endotoxin shock: inhibition by naloxone. *Diabetes*, **36**, 585–91.

Metcalf, D. (1991). Control of granulocytes and macrophages: molecular, cellular, and clinical aspects. *Science*, **254**, 529–33.

Mier, J. W., Vachino, G., Klempner, M. S., Aronson, F. R., Noring, R., Smith, S., Brandon, E. P., Laird, W. & Atkins, M. B. (1990). Inhibition of interleukin-2-induced tumor necrosis factor release by dexamethasone – prevention of an acquired neutrophil chemotaxis defect and differential suppression of interleukin-2-associated side effects. *Blood*, **76**, 1933–40.

Mio, M., Izushi, K. & Tasaka, K. (1991). Substance-P-induced histamine release from rat peritoneal mast cells and its inhibition by antiallergic agents and calmodulin inhibitors. *Immunopharmacology*, **22**, 59–66.

Mochizuki, H., Trocki, O., Dominioni, L., Brackett, K. A., Joffe, S. N. & Alexander, J. W. (1984). Mechanism of prevention of postburn hypermetabolism and catabolism by early enteral feeding. *Ann. Surg.*, **200**, 297–310.

Mohammad, S. F., Mason, R. G., Eichwald, E. J. & Shively, J. A. (1984). Healthy and impaired vascular endothelium. In *Blood Platelet Function and Medical Chemistry*, ed. E. Lasslo, pp. 129–73. New York, Amsterdam, Oxford: Elsevier.

Morganelli, P. M. & Guyre, P. M. (1988). IFN-$\gamma$ plus glucocorticoids stimulate the expression of a newly identified human mononuclear phagocyte-specific antigen. *J. Immunol.*, **140**, 2296–304.

Morimoto, A., Nakamori, T., Watanabe, T., Ono, T. & Murakami, N. (1988). Pattern differences in experimental fevers induced by endotoxin, endogenous pyrogen, and prostaglandins. *Am. J. Physiol.*, **254**, R633–40.

Moss, F. M., Knight, J. & Lamb, J. R. (1984). The differential effects of hydrocortisone on activation and tolerance induction in human T lymphocyte clones. *Hum. Immunol.*, **11**, 259–70.

Mukherjee, P., Mastro, A. M. & Hymer, W. C. (1990). Prolactin induction of interleukin-2 receptors on rat splenic lymphocytes. *Endocrinology*, **126**, 88–94.

Müller-Eberhard, H. J. (1975). Complement. *Ann. Rev. Biochem.*, **44**, 697–724.

Murata, T. & Ying, S. Y. (1991). Transforming growth factor-$\beta$ and activin inhibit basal secretion of prolactin in a pituitary monolayer culture system. *Proc. Soc. Exp. Biol. Med.*, **198**, 599–605.

Murphy, M. T., Richards, D. B. & Lipton, J. M. (1983). Antipyretic potency of centrally administered alpha-melanocyte stimulating hormone. *Science*, **221**, 192–3.

Muscettola, M. & Grasso, G. (1990). Somatostatin and vasoactive intestinal peptide reduce interferon gamma production by human peripheral blood mononuclear cells. *Immunobiology*, **180**, 419–30.

Myers, A. K., Robey, J. W. & Price, R. M. (1990). Relationships between tumour necrosis factor, eicosanoids and platelet-activating factor as mediators of endotoxin-induced shock in mice. *Br. J. Pharmacol.*, **99**, 499–502.

Nagy, E. & Berczi, I. (1989). Pituitary dependence of bone marrow function. *Br. J. Haematol.*, **71**, 457–62.
Nagy, E. & Berczi, I. (1991). Hypophysectomized rats depend on residual prolactin for survival. *Endocrinology*, **146**, 2776–84.
Nagy, E., Berczi, I. & Sabbadini, E. (1992). Endocrine control of the immunosuppressive activity of the submandibular gland. *Brain Behav. Immun.*, **6**, 418–28.
Nagy, S. U. & Bertok, L. (1990). Influence of experimentally induced endotoxemias on the thyroid function of rats. *Acta Physiol. Hung.*, **76**, 137–41.
Nagy, Z., Berczi, I. & Bertok, L. (1968). Experimental data on the pathogenesis of edema disease of swine. Clinical picture, gross and microscopic lesions related to endotoxic shock. *Zbl. Vet. Med. Reihe B.*, **15**, 504–11.
Nelson, J. L. & Steinberg, A. D. (1987). Sex steroids, autoimmunity and autoimmune disease. In *Hormones and Immunity*, ed. I. Berczi & K. Kovacs, pp. 93–119. London: MTP Press.
Neta, R., Perlstein, R., Vogel, S. N., Ledney, G. D. & Abrams, J. (1992). Role of interleukin-6 (IL-6) in protection from lethal irradiation and in endocrine responses to IL-1 and tumor necrosis factor. *J. Exp. Med.*, **175**, 689–94.
Newsome, H. H. & Rose, J. C. (1971). The response of human adrenocorticotrophic hormone and growth hormone to surgical stress. *J. Clin. Endocrinol.*, **33**, 481–7.
Nieto, M. A. & Lopez-Rivas, A. (1989). IL-2 protects T lymphocytes from glucocorticoid-induced DNA fragmentation and cell death. *J. Immunol.*, **143**, 4166–70.
Ninneman, J. L. (1989). The immune consequences of trauma: an overview. In *Immune Consequences of Trauma, Shock and Sepsis. Mechanisms and Therapeutic Approaches*, ed. E. Faist, J. Ninneman & D. Green, pp. 1–8. Berlin, New York: Springer-Verlag.
Noel, G. L., Suh, H. K., Stone, G. J. & Frantz, A. G. (1971). Human prolactin and growth hormone release during surgery and other conditions of stress. *J. Clin. Endocrinol. Metab.*, **35**, 840–51.
Nong, Y.-H., Titus, R. G., Ribeiro, J. M. C. & Remold, H. G. (1989). Peptides encoded by the calcitonin gene inhibit macrophage function. *J. Immunol.*, **145**, 45–9.
North, R. J. & Havell, E. A. (1989). Glucocorticoid-mediated inhibition of endotoxin-induced intratumor necrosis factor production and tumor hemorrhagic necrosis and regression. *J. Exp. Med.*, **170**, 703–10.
Nuytinck, J. K. S., Goris, R. J. A., Redl, H., Schlag, G. & van Munster, P. J. J. (1986). Posttraumatic complications and inflammatory mediators. *Arch. Surg.*, **121**, 886–90.
Ohalloran, D. J., Jones, P. M. & Bloom, S. R. (1991). Neuropeptides synthesized in the anterior pituitary – possible paracrine role. *Mol. Cell. Endocrinol.*, **75**, C7–12.
Ohlsson, K., Bjork, P., Bergenfeldt, M. Hageman, R. & Thompson, R. C. (1990). Interleukin-1 receptor antagonist reduces mortality from endotoxin shock. *Nature*, **348**, 550–2.
Oppenheim, J. J., Zachariae, C. O. C., Mukaida, N. & Matsushima, K. (1991). Properties of the novel proinflammatory supergene 'intercrine' cytokine family. *Ann. Rev. Immunol.*, **9**, 617–48.
Ottaway, C. A. (1987). Selective effects of vasoactive intestinal peptide on the mitogenic response of murine T-cells. *Immunology*, **62**, 291–7.
Packham, M. A. & Mustard, J. F. (1984). Normal and abnormal platelet activity.

In *Blood Platelet Function and Medical Chemistry*, ed. E. Lasslo, pp. 61–128. New York, Amsterdam, Oxford: Elsevier.
Pang, X.-P., Hershman, J. M., Mirell, C. J. & Pekary, A. E. (1989). Impairment of hypothalamic–pituitary–thyroid function in rats treated with human recombinant tumor necrosis factor-α (cachectin). *Endocrinology*, **125**, 76–84.
Parant, M., Lecontel, C., Parant, F. & Chedid, L. (1991). Influence of endogenous glucocorticoid on endotoxin-induced production of circulating TNF-α. *Lymphokine Cytokine Res.*, **10**, 265–71.
Paul, W. E. (1989). The immune system: an introduction. In *Fundamental Immunology*, 2nd edn, ed. W. E. Paul, pp. 3–19. New York: Raven Press.
Pearce, F. L., Kassessinoff, T. A. & Liu, W. L. (1989). Characteristics of histamine secretion induced by neuropeptides: implications for the relevance of peptide–mast cell interactions in allergy and inflammation. *Int. Arch. Allergy Appl. Immunol.*, **88**, 129–31.
Perretti, M., Mugridge, K. G., Becherucci, C. & Parente, L. (1991). Evidence that interleukin-1 and lipoxygenase metabolites mediate the lethal effect of complete Freund's adjuvant in adrenalectomized rats. *Lymphokine Cytokine Res.*, **10**, 239–43.
Pullicino, E. A., Carli, F., Poole, S., Rafferty, B., Malik, S. T. A. & Elia, M. (1990). The relationship between the circulating concentrations of interleukin (IL-6), tumor necrosis factor (TNF) and the acute phase response to elective surgery and accidental injury. *Lymphokine Res.*, **9**, 231–8.
Quesenberry, P., Morley, A., Stohlman Jr, F., Richard, K., Howard, D. & Smith, M. (1972). Effect of endotoxin on granulopoiesis and colony-stimulating factor. *N. Engl. J. Med.*, **286**, 227–32.
Raetz, C. R. H., Ulevitch, R. J., Wright, S. D., Sibley, C. H., Ding, A. & Nathan, C. F. (1991). Gram-negative endotoxin: an extraordinary lipid with profound effects on eukaryotic signal transduction. *Fed. Am. Soc. Exp. Biol. J.*, **5**, 2652–60.
Ramachandra, R. N., Berczi, A., Sehon, A. H. & Berczi, I. (1993). Inhibition of lipid A- and lipopolysaccharide-induced cytokine secretion, B cell mitogenesis, and lethal shock by lipid A-specific monoclonal antibodies. *J. Infect. Dis.*, **167**, 1151–9.
Ramachandra, R. N., Sehon, A. H. & Berczi, I. (1992). Neuro-hormonal host defence in endotoxin shock. *Brain Behav. Immun.*, **6**, 157–69.
Rameshwar, P., Gascon, P. & Ganea, D. (1992). Immunoregulatory effects of neuropeptides. Stimulation of interleukin-2 production by substance-P. *J. Neuroimmunol.*, **37**, 65–74.
Raveche, E. S. & Steinberg, A. D. (1986). Sex hormones in autoimmunity. In *Pituitary Function and Immunity*, ed. I. Berczi, pp. 283–301. Boca Raton, FL: CRC Press.
Richard, A., McColl, S. R. & Pelletier, G. (1992). Interleukin-4 and nerve growth factor can act as cofactors for interleukin-3-induced histamine production in human umbilical cord blood cells in serum-free culture. *Br. J. Haematol.*, **81**, 6–11.
Richardson, R. P., Rhyne, C. D., Fong, Y., Hesse, D. G., Tracey, K. J., Marano, M. A., Lowry, S. F., Antonacci, A. C. & Calvano, S. E. (1989). Peripheral blood leukocyte kinetics following *in vivo* lipopolysaccharide (LPS) administration to normal human subjects: influence of elicited hormones and cytokines. *Ann. Surg.*, **210**, 239–45.
Rivier, C., Chizzonite, R. & Vale, W. (1989). In the mouse, the activation of the

hypothalamic–pituitary–adrenal axis by a lipopolysaccharide (endotoxin) is mediated through interleukin-1. *Endocrinology*, **125**, 2800–5.

Rivier, C. & Vale, W. (1989). In the rat, interleukin-1-alpha acts at the level of the brain and the gonads to interfere with gonadotropin and sex steroid secretion. *Endocrinology*, **124**, 2105–9.

Robertson, B., Dostal, K. & Daynes, R. A. (1988). Neuropeptide regulation of inflammatory and immunologic responses. The capacity of $\alpha$-melanocyte-stimulating hormone to inhibit tumor necrosis factor and IL-1-inducible biologic responses. *J. Immunol.*, **140**, 4300–7.

Robertson, B., Gahring, L., Newton, R. & Daynes, R. A. (1987). *In vivo* administration of IL-1 to normal mice decreases their capacity to elicit contact hypersensitivity responses: Prostaglandins are involved in this modification of the immune response. *J. Invest. Dermatol.*, **88**, 380–7.

Robin, J. L., Seldin, D. C., Austen, K. F. & Lewis, R. A. (1985). Regulation of mediator release from mouse bone marrow-derived mast cells by glucocorticoids. *J. Immunol.*, **135**, 2719–26.

Rook, G. (1989). Immunity to viruses, bacteria and fungi. In *Immunology*, 2nd edn, ed. I. Roit, J. Brostoff & E. Male, pp. 16.1–16.16. London: Gower Medical.

Rothwell, N. J. (1989). CRF is involved in the pyrogenic and thermogenic effects of interleukin-1$\beta$ in the rat. *Am. J. Physiol.*, **256**, E111–15.

Rothwell, N. J. (1991). The endocrine significance of cytokines. *J. Endocrinol.*, **128**, 171–3.

Rougeot, C., Junier, M. P., Minary, P., Weidenfeld, J., Braquet, P. & Dray, F. (1990). Intracerebroventricular injection of platelet-activating factor induces secretion of adrenocorticotropin, beta-endorphin and corticosterone in conscious rats: a possible link between the immune and nervous systems. *Neuroendocrinology*, **51**, 267–75.

Rovensky, J., Ferencikova, J., Vigas, M. & Lukac, P. (1985). Effect of growth hormone on the activity of some lysosomal enzymes in neutrophilic polymorphonuclear leukocytes of hypopituitary dwarfs. *Int. J. Tissue React.*, **7**, 153–9.

Said, S. I. (1990). Neuropeptides as modulators of injury and inflammation. *Life Sci.*, **47**, PL19–21.

Salkowski, C. A. & Vogel, S. N. (1992). IFN-$\gamma$ mediates increased glucocorticoid receptor expression in murine macrophages. *J. Immunol.*, **148**, 2770–7.

Sanchez-Cantu, L., Rode, H. N., Yun, T. J. & Christou, N. V. (1991). Tumor necrosis factor alone does not explain the lethal effect of lipopolysaccharide. *Arch. Surg.*, **126**, 231–5.

Sanders, V. M. & Munson, A. E. (1985). Norepinephrine and the antibody response. *Pharmacol. Rev.*, **37**, 229–48.

Schimpff, R.-M. & Repellin, A.-M. (1990). Production of interleukin-1-alpha and interleukin-2 by mononuclear cells in healthy adults in relation to different experimental conditions and to the presence of growth hormone. *Hormone Res.*, **33**, 171–6.

Schluter, B., Konig, B., Bergmann, U., Muller, F. E. & Konig, W. (1991). Interleukin 6 – a potential mediator of lethal sepsis after major thermal trauma: evidence for increased IL-6 production by peripheral blood mononuclear cells. *J. Trauma*, **31**, 1663–70.

Schooltink, H., Stoyan, T., Roeb, E., Heinrich, P. C. & Rose-John, S. (1992). Ciliary neurotropic factor induces acute-phase protein expression in hepatocytes. *FEBS Lett.*, **314**, 280–4.

Schwartz, R. A. (1990). A cell culture model for T lymphocyte clonal anergy. *Science*, **248**, 1349–56.

Schwarz, T., Urbanska, A., Gschnait, F. & Luger, T. A. (1986). Inhibition of the induction of contact hypersensitivity by a UV-mediated epidermal cytokine. *J. Invest. Dermatol.*, **87**, 289–91.

Schwarz, T., Urbanska, A., Gschnait, F. & Luger, T. A. (1987). UV-irradiated epidermal cells produce a specific inhibitor of IL-1 activity. *J. Immunol.*, **138**, 1457–63.

Selye, H. (1936*a*). A syndrome produced by diverse nocuous agents. *Nature*, **138**, 32.

Selye, H. (1936*b*). Thymus and the adrenals in response of the organism to injuries and intoxications. *Br. J. Exp. Pathol.*, **17**, 234–48.

Selye, H. (1943). Morphological changes in the fowl following chronic overdosage with various steroids. *J. Morphol.*, **73**, 401–21.

Selye, H. (1946). The general adaptation syndrome and the diseases of adaptation. *J. Clin. Endocrinol.*, **6**, 117–230.

Selye, H. (1949). Effect of ACTH and cortisone upon an 'anaphylactoid reaction'. *Can. Med. Assoc. J.*, **61**, 553–6.

Selye, H. (1955). Stress and disease. *Science*, **122**, 625.

Serra, M. C., Bazzoni, F., Della Bianca, V., Greskowiak, M. & Rossi, F. (1988). Activation of human neutrophils by substance P. Effect on oxidative metabolism, exocytosis, cytosolic $Ca^{2+}$ concentration and inositol phosphate formation. *J. Immunol.*, **141**, 2118–24.

Severn, A., Rapson, N. T., Hunter, C. A. & Liew, F. Y. (1992). Regulation of tumor necrosis factor production by adrenaline and $\beta$-adrenergic agonists. *J. Immunol.*, **148**, 3441–5.

Shanahan, F., Lee, T. D. G., Bienenstock, J. & Befus, A. D. (1986). Mast cell heterogeneity: effect of anti-allergic compounds on neuropeptide-induced histamine release. *Int. Arch. Allergy Appl. Immunol.*, **80**, 424–6.

Sharkey, K. A. (1992). Substance P and calcitonin gene-related peptide (CGRP) in gastrointestinal inflammation. *Ann. NY Acad. Sci.*, **664**, 425–42.

Sharp, B. M., Matta, S. G., Peterson, P. K., Newton, R., Chao, C. & McAllen, K. (1989). Tumor necrosis factor-alpha is a potent ACTH secretagogue: comparison to interleukin-1. *Endocrinology*, **124**, 3131–3.

Shavit, Y. (1991). Stress-induced immune modulation in animals: opiates and endogenous opioid peptides. In *Psychoneuroimmunology*, 2nd edn, ed. R. Ader, D. L. Felten & N. Cohen, pp. 789–806. San Diego: Academic Press.

Shenep, J. L., Flynn, P. M., Barette, F. F., Stidham, G. L. & Westenkirchner, D. F. (1988). Serial quantitation of endotoxemia and bacteremia during therapy for Gram-negative bacterial sepsis. *J. Infect. Dis.*, **157**, 565–8.

Sheppard, B. C., Fraker, D. L. & Norton, J. A. (1989). Prevention and treatment of endotoxin and sepsis lethality with recombinant human tumor necrosis factor. *Surgery*, **106**, 156–61.

Sibbald, W. J., Short, A., Chohen, M. P. & Wilson, R. F. (1977). Variations in adrenocortical responsiveness during severe bacterial infections. Unrecognized adrenocortical insufficiency in severe bacterial infections. *Ann. Surg.*, **186**, 29–33.

Singh, V. K. (1989). Stimulatory effect of corticotropin-releasing neurohormone on human lymphocyte proliferation and interleukin-2 receptor expression. *J. Neuroimmunol.*, **23**, 257–62.

Sinha, A. A., Lopez, M. T. & McDevitt, H. O. (1990). Autoimmune disease. The failure of self tolerance. *Science*, **248**, 1380–8.

Smith, B. B. & Wagner, W. C. (1984). Suppression of prolactin in pigs by *Escherichia coli* endotoxin. *Science*, **224**, 605–7.
Smith, B. B. & Wagner, W. C. (1985). Effect of *Escherichia coli* endotoxin and thyrotropin-releasing hormone on prolactin in lactating sows. *Am. J. Vet. Res.*, **46**, 175–80.
Smith, L. R., Brown, S. L. & Blalock, J. E. (1989). Interleukin-2 induction of ACTH secretion: presence of an interleukin-2 receptor alpha-chain-like molecule on pituitary cells. *J. Neuroimmunol.*, **21**, 249–54.
Smolen, J. E. & Boxer, L. A. (1990). Function of neutrophils. In *Hematology*, 4th edn, ed. W. W. Williams, E. Beutler, A. J. Erslev & M. A. Lichtman, pp. 780–94. New York: McGraw-Hill.
Snyers, L., De Wit, L. & Content, J. (1990). Glucocorticoid up-regulation of high-affinity interleukin 6 receptors on human epithelial cells. *Proc. Natl. Acad. Sci. USA*, **87**, 2838–42.
Spadoni, G. L., Spagnoli, A., Cianfarani, S., Del Principe, D., Menicheli, A., Di Giulio, S. & Boscherini, B. (1990). Enhancement by growth hormone of phorbol diester-stimulated respiratory burst in human polymorphonuclear leukocytes. *Acta Endocrinol.*, **124**, 589–94.
Spangelo, B. L. & MacLeod, R. M. (1990). Regulation of the acute phase response and neuroendocrine function by interleukin 6. *Prog. Neuroendocrinimmunol.*, **3**, 167–75.
Spengler, R. N., Allen, R. M., Remick, D. G., Strieter, R. M. & Kunkel, S. L. (1990). Stimulation of α-adrenergic receptor augments the production of macrophage-derived tumor necrosis factor. *J. Immunol.*, **145**, 1430–4.
Sprung, C. L., Caralis, P. V., Marcial, E. H., Pierce, M., Gelbard, M. A., Long, W. M., Duncan, R. C., Tendler, M. D. & Karpf, M. (1984). The effects of high-dose corticosteroids in patients with septic shock: a prospective, controlled study. *N. Engl. J. Med.*, **311**, 1137–43.
Stead, R. H. (1992). Nerve remodelling during intestinal inflammation. *Ann. NY Acad. Sci.*, **664**, 443–55.
Stern, R. S. (1989). PUVA and the induction of skin cancer. In *Carcinogenesis – A Comprehensive Survey*, vol. 11, ed. C. J. Conti, T. J. Slaga & A. J. P. Klein-Szanto, pp. 85–101. New York: Raven Press.
Stimson, W. H. (1987). Sex steroids, steroid receptors and immunity. In *Hormones and Immunity*, ed. I. Berczi & K. Kovacs, pp. 43–53. Lancaster, UK: MTP Press.
Strickland, R. W., Wahl, L. M. & Finbloom, D. S. (1986). Corticosteroids enhance the binding of recombinant interferon-γ to cultured human monocytes. *J. Immunol.*, **137**, 1577–80.
Sullivan, N. J. & Tashjian Jr, A. H. (1983). Platelet-derived growth factor selectively decreases prolactin production in pituitary cells in culture. *Endocrinology*, **113**, 639–45.
Sundar, S. K., Becker, K. J., Cierpial, M. A., Carpenter, M. D., Rankin, L. A., Fleener, S. L., Ritchie, J. C., Simson, P. E. & Weiss, J. M. (1989). Intracerebro-ventricular infusion of interleukin 1 rapidly decreases peripheral cellular immune responses. *Proc. Natl. Acad. Sci. USA*, **86**, 6398–402.
Suzuki, S., Oh, C. & Nakano, K. (1986). Pituitary-dependent and -independent secretion of CS caused by bacterial endotoxin in rats. *Am. J. Physiol.*, **250**, E470–4.
Sydbom, A. (1988). Effects of β-endorphin on rat mast cells. *Agent. Action*, **23**, 204–6.

Szabo, G., Kodys, K. & Miller-Graziano, C. L. (1991*a*). Elevated monocyte interleukin-6 (IL-6) production in immunosuppressed trauma patients. 1. Role of Fc-γ-RI crosslinking stimulation. *J. Clin. Immunol.*, **11**, 326–35.

Szabo, G., Kodys, K. & Miller-Graziano, C. L. (1991*b*). Elevated monocyte interleukin-6 (IL-6) production in immunosuppressed trauma patients. 2. Downregulation by IL-4. *J. Clin. Immunol.*, **11**, 336–44.

Tache, Y. & Saperas, E. (1992). Potent inhibition of gastric acid secretion and ulcer formation by centrally and peripherally administered interleukin-1. *Ann. NY Acad. Sci.*, **664**, 353–68.

Takayama, T. K., Miller, C. & Czabo, G. (1990). Elevated tumor necrosis factor α production concomitant to elevated E2 production by trauma patients' monocytes. *Arch. Surg.*, **125**, 29–35.

Talal, N. (ed.) (1977). *Autoimmunity. Genetic, Immunologic, Virologic and Clinical Aspects.* New York, San Francisco, London: Academic Press.

Taverne, J. (1989). Immunity to protozoa and worms. In *Immunology*, 2nd edn, ed. I. Roitt, J. Brostoff & D. Male, pp. 17.1–17.21. London: Gower Medical.

Teodorczyk-Injeyan, J. A., Sparkes, B. G., Mills, G. B. & Peters, W. J. (1991). Soluble interleukin 2-receptor α secretion is related to altered interleukin 2 production in thermally injured patients. *Burns*, **17**, 290–5.

Teodorczyk-Injeyan, J. A., Sparkes, B. G. & Peters, W. J. (1989). Serum interleukin-2 receptor as a possible mediator of immunosuppression after burn injury. *J. Burn Care Rehab.*, **10**, 112–18.

Tobler, A., Meier, R., Seitz, M., Dewald, B., Baggiolini, M. & Fey, M. F. (1992). Glucocorticoids downregulate gene expression of GM-CSF, NAP-1/IL-8, and IL-6, but not of M-CSF in human fibroblasts. *Blood*, **79**, 45–51.

Tomioka, M., Stead, R. H., Nielsen, L., Coughlin, M. D. & Bienenstock, J. (1988). Nerve growth factor enhances antigen and other secretagogue-induced histamine release from rat peritoneal mast cells in the absence of phosphatidylserine. *J. Allergy Clin. Immunol.*, **82**, 599–607.

Tracey, K. J., Fong, Y., Hesse, D. G., Manogue, K. R., Lee, A. T., Kuo, G. C., Lowry, S. F. & Cerami, A. (1987). Anti-cachectin/TNF monoclonal antibodies prevent septic shock during lethal bacteremia. *Nature*, **330**, 662–4.

Ullrich, S. E., Alcalay, J., Applegate, L. A. & Kripke, M. L. (1989). Immunosuppression in phototherapy. *Ciba Found. Symp.*, **146**, 131–47.

Urbaschek, B. & Urbaschek, R. (1987). Tumor necrosis factor and interleukin-1 as mediators of endotoxin-induced beneficial effects. *Rev. Infect. Dis.*, **9**, S607–15.

Van Dam, A. M., Brouns, M., Louisse, S. & Berkenbosch, F. (1992). Appearance of interleukin-1 in macrophages and in ramified microglia in the brain of endotoxin-treated rats: a pathway for the induction of non-specific symptoms of sickness? *Brain Res.*, **588**, 291–6.

Van Dijk, H. & Rademaker, P. M. (1985). Infectious disease, fever and the immune response. *Immunol. Today*, **6**, 318.

Van Gool, J., Boers, W., Sala, M. & Ladiges, N. C. J. J. (1984). Glucocorticoids and catecholamines as mediators of acute-phase proteins, especially rat α-macrofoetoprotein. *Biochem. J.*, **220**, 125–32.

Van Gool, J., Van Vugt, H., Helle, M. & Aarden, L. A. (1990). The relation among stress, adrenalin, interleukin 6, and acute phase proteins in the rat. *Clin. Immunol. Immunopathol.*, **57**, 200–10.

Vankelecom, H., Carmeliet, P., Heremans, H., Van Damme, J., Dijkamans, A. , Billiau, A. & Denef, C. (1990). Interferon-γ inhibits stimulated adrenocortico-tropin, prolactin, and growth hormone secretion in normal rat anterior pituitary cell cultures. *Endocrinology*, **126**, 2919–26.

Vemulapalli, S., Chiu, P. J. S., Rivelli, M., Foster, C. J. & Sybertz, E. J. (1991). Modulation of circulating endothelin levels in hypertension and endotoxemia in rats. *J. Cardiovasc. Pharmacol*, **18**, 895–903.

Veterans Administration Systemic Sepsis Cooperative Study Group (1987). Effect of high-dose glucocorticoid therapy on mortality in patients with clinical signs of systemic sepsis. *N. Engl. J. Med.*, **317**, 659–65.

Waage, A. (1987). Production and clearance of tumor necrosis factor in rats exposed to endotoxin and dexamethasone. *Clin. Immunol. Immunopathol.*, **43**, 348–55.

Wahl, S. M. (1992). Transforming growth factor beta (TGF-$\beta$) in inflammation – a cause and a cure. *J. Clin. Immunol.*, **12**, 61–74.

Wallace, D. J. (1987). The role of stress and trauma in rheumatoid arthritis and systemic lupus erythematosus. *Sem. Arthritis Rheum.*, **16**, 153–7.

Wannemacher Jr, R. W., Pekarek, R. S., Thompson, W. L., Curnow, R. T., Beall, F. A., Zenser, T. V., deRubertis, R. F. & Beisel, W. R. (1975). A protein from polymorphonuclear leukocytes (LEM) which affects the rate of hepatic amino acid transport and synthesis of acute-phase globulins. *Endocrinology*, **96**, 651–61.

Waris, T. & Kyösala, K. (1982). Cold injury of the rat skin. *Scand. J. Plast. Reconstr. Surg.*, **16**, 1–9.

Wei, E. T., Wong, J. C. & Kiang, J. C. (1990). Decreased inflammatory responsiveness of hypophysectomized rats to heat is reversed by a corticotropin-releasing factor (CRF) antagonist. *Regul. Peptides*, **27**, 317–23.

Wells, M. T., Gaffin, S. L., Wessels, B. C., Brock-Utne, J. G., Jordaan, J. P. & VanDenEnde, J. (1990). Anti-LPS antibodies reduce endotoxemia in whole body $^{60}$Co irradiated primates: a preliminary report. *Aviat. Space Environ. Med.*, **61**, 802–6.

Wexler, B. C., Dolgin, A. E. & Tryczynski, E. W. (1957). Effects of bacterial polysaccharide (Piromen) on the pituitary–adrenal axis: adrenal ascorbic acid, cholesterol and histological alterations. *Endocrinology*, **61**, 300–8.

Whitehouse, B. J. (1989). Commentary: lipocortins, mediators of the anti-inflammatory actions of corticosteroids? *J. Endocrinol.*, **123**, 363–6.

Wiedermann, C. J., Niedermuhlbichler, M., Beimpold, H. & Braunsteiner, H. (1991*a*). *In vitro* activation of neutrophils of the aged by recombinant human growth hormone. *J. Infect. Dis.*, **164**, 1017–20.

Wiedermann, C. J., Niedermuhlbichler, M., Geissler, D., Beimpold, H. & Braunsteiner, H. (1991*b*). Priming of normal human neutrophils by recombinant human growth hormone. *Br. J. Haematol.*, **78**, 19–22.

Wieser, M., Bonifer, R., Oster, W., Lindemann, A., Mertelsmann, R. & Herrmann, F. (1989). Interleukin-4 induces secretion of CSF for granulocytes and CSF for macrophages by peripheral blood monocytes. *Blood*, **73**, 1105–8.

Wira, C. R. & Rossoll, R. M. (1991). Glucocorticoid regulation of the humoral immune system. Dexamethasone stimulation of secretory component in serum, saliva, and bile. *Endocrinology*, **128**, 835–42.

Wodnar-Filipowicz, A., Heusser, C. H. & Moroni, C. (1989). Production of the haemopoietic growth factors GM-CSF and interleukin-3 by mast cells in response to IgE receptor-mediated activation. *Nature*, **339**, 150–2.

Woloski, B. M. R. N. J., Smith, E. M., Meyer III, W. J., Fuller, G. M. &

Blalock, J. E. (1985). Corticotropin-releasing activity of monokines. *Science*, **230**, 1035–7.

Wood, J. D. (1992). Histamine signals in enteric neuroimmune interactions. *Ann. NY Acad. Sci.*, **664**, 275–83.

Yamaguchi, M., Matsuzaki, N., Hirota, K., Miyake, A. & Tanizawa, O. (1990*a*). Interleukin-6 possibly induced by interleukin 1-beta in the pituitary gland stimulates the release of gonadotropins and prolactin. *Acta Endocrinol.*, **122**, 201–5.

Yamaguchi, M., Sakata, M., Matsuzaki, N., Koike, K., Miyake, A. & Tanizawa, O. (1990*b*). Induction by tumor necrosis factor-alpha of rapid release of immunoreactive and bioactive luteinizing hormone from rat pituitary cell *in vitro*. *Neuroendocrinology*, **52**, 468–72.

Yamashita, S., Kimura, H., Ashizawa, K., Nagayama, Y., Hirayu, H., Izumi, M. & Nagataki, S. (1989). Interleukin-1 inhibits thyrotrophin-induced human thyroglobulin gene expression. *J. Endocrinol.*, **122**, 177–83.

Yasumoto, S., Hayashi, Y. & Aurelian, L. (1987). Immunity to herpes simplex virus type 2: suppression of virus-induced immune responses in ultraviolet B-irradiated mice. *J. Immunol.*, **139**, 2788–93.

Yelich, M. R. (1990). *In vivo* endotoxin and IL-1 potentiate insulin secretion in pancreatic islets. *Am. J. Physiol.*, **258**, R1070–7.

Yelich, M. R., Havdala, H. S. & Filkins, J. P. (1987). Dexamethasone alters glucose, lactate, and insulin dyshomeostasis during endotoxicosis in the rat. *Circ. Shock*, **22**, 155–71.

Yelich, M. R., Umporowicz, D. M., Qi, M. & Jones, S. B. (1991). Insulin-inhibiting effects of epinephrine are blunted during endotoxicosis in the rat. *Circ. Shock.*, **35**, 129–38.

Yurt, R. W. & Lowry, S. F. (1990). Role of macrophage and endogenous mediators in multiple organ failure. In *Multiple Organ Failure. Pathophysiology and Basic Concepts of Therapy*, ed. E. A. Deitch, pp. 60–71. New York: Thieme Medical.

Zanetti, G., Heumann, D., Kohler, J., Abbet, P., Barras, C., Lucas, R., Glauser, M.-P. & Baumgartner, J.-D. (1992). Cytokine production after intravenous or peritoneal gram-negative bacterial challenge in mice. Comparative protective efficacy of antibodies to tumor necrosis factor-α and to lipopolysaccharide. *J. Immunol.*, **148**, 1890–7.

Zanker, B., Walz, G., Wieder, K. J. & Strom, T. B. (1990). Evidence that glucocorticosteroids block transcription of human interleukin-6 gene by accessory cells. *Transplantation*, **49**, 183–5.

Ziegler, E. J., Fisher, C. J., Sprung, C. L., Straube, R. C., Sadoff, J. C., Foulke, G. E., Wortel, C. H., Mitchell, P. F., Dellinger, R. P., Teng, N. N. H., Allen, I. E., Berger, H. J., Knatterud, G. L., LoBuglio, A. F., Smith, C. R., the HA-1A Sepsis Study Group (1991). Treatment of gram-negative bacteremia and septic shock with HA-1A human monoclonal antibody against endotoxin. A randomized double-blind, placebo-controlled trial. *N. Engl. J. Med.*, **324**, 429–36.

# 5

# Brain regions involved in modulation of immune responses

BRIGITTE DELEPLANQUE and PIERRE J. NEVEU

From the experimental and clinical evidence of brain–immune relationships (Blalock, 1989; O'Leary, 1990; Khansari *et al.*, 1990) two main questions arise: what are the central nervous structures involved in neuroimmunomodulation? and how do the brain and the immune system communicate?

In order to answer the first question, the most useful approach is to study the immune effects of lesioning different areas of the central nervous system. Even though this approach contains some inbuilt methodological problems related to the plasticity of the immune and central nervous systems, the data now available permit us to answer this question, at least partly, and also suggest the existence of functional brain networks in neuroimmunomodulation.

## Effects of brain lesions on immune reactivity

### *Hypothalamic and brainstem lesions*

Bilateral lesions of the hypothalamus have been consistently shown to induce changes in immunity. Early works showed that local lesions of the hypothalamus protected guinea pigs (Filipp & Szentivanyi, 1958; Szentivanyi & Filipp, 1958) and rats (Luparello *et al.*, 1964) from lethal anaphylactic shock. Moreover, these protective effects of hypothalamic lesions were not necessarily associated with lower titres of antibodies as measured by passive cutaneous anaphylaxis (Stein *et al.*, 1976). Later, it was demonstrated that rats showed profound alterations in the architecture of lymphoid organs 32 days after electrolytic lesions of the hypothalamus. In the thymus, there was a profound depletion of lymphocytes, a reduction of the cortex and a disappearance of the corticomedullary junction. In spleen and lymph nodes, there was a decrease in the number of lymphocytes and plasma cells, as well as an absence of germinal centres (Isakovic & Jankovic, 1973). The same electrolytic lesions, performed 24 h before immunization against bovine serum albumin, lowered serum antibody levels and reduced the intensity of Arthus and delayed hypersensitivity reactions as late as 30 days after the first antigen challenge (Jankovic & Isakovic, 1973). More recently, Keller *et al.* (1980) reported that, in guinea pigs, electrolytic lesions of the anterior hypothalamic area suppressed delayed hypersensitivity to tuberculin. These lesions also depressed mitogenesis induced by phytohaemagglutinin (PHA) when using whole blood but not when using purified lymphocytes. Similarly, the depression of spleen lymphocyte mitogenesis observed after electrolytic lesions of preoptic and anterior areas has been reversed by removing macrophages from spleen cells (Roszman *et al.*, 1982). Furthermore, macrophages taken from lesioned animals suppressed mitogen-induced proliferation of normal lymphocytes. Therefore, lesions of the preoptic and anterior areas of the hypothalamus may stimulate the suppressive function of macrophages. The hypothalamus may also be involved in modulation of other macrophage functions, as suggested by the fact that electrical stimulation of the ventromedial area transiently decreased phagocytic activity of the reticuloendothelial system, as measured by carbon clearance (Lambert *et al.*, 1981).

Finally, lesions of the preoptic anterior areas of the hypothalamus have been shown to suppress natural killer (NK) cell activity transiently in the spleen (Cross *et al.*, 1984). However, a persistent abrogation of NK cell activity has been observed after lesions of the hypothalamus, including the ventromedial, dorsomedial and arcuate nucleus. This depression was demonstrated to be due to a block of NK lineage maturation (Forni *et al.*, 1983).

The mechanisms involved in hypothalamus-mediated immunomodulation remain unclear, and the role of the pituitary–adrenal axis is particularly controversial. Inhibition of mitogenesis induced by anterior lesions was not observed in hypophysectomized animals (Cross *et al.*, 1982). These results are in agreement with those reported by Kato *et al.* (1986), in which chemical lesions of the preoptic and arcuate nuclei depressed the delayed hypersensitivity to bacillus Calmette–Guérin (BCG) and *Listeria* in suckling mice. Interestingly, this depression was accompanied by an increase of plasma adrenocorticotropic hormone (ACTH) (Kato *et al.*, 1986). However, the pituitary axis may not be involved in hypothalamic regulation of immune reactivity. In the study of the effects of tuberal hypothalamic lesions on graft rejection in normal and hypophysectomized rats, it was shown that hypothalamic lesions depressed graft rejection and that the mechanism governing this response involved a direct neural pathway that bypassed the hypothalamic–pituitary–adrenal axis (Dann *et al.*, 1979).

The first described immunological effects of electrolytic lesions of the reticular formation were quite similar to those reported in the hypothalamus. Cellular architecture of the thymus, but not that of the spleen and lymph nodes, was equally altered after both types of lesion (Isakovic & Jankovic, 1973). Likewise, in rats with lesions of the reticular formation, the levels of serum antibody were depressed and the intensity of Arthus and delayed hypersensitivity reactions was reduced (Jankovic & Isakovic, 1973). In fact, the immunological effects of electrolytic lesions of the reticular formation appeared to depend on their rostrocaudal location. Rostral lesions, performed 1 week before immunization against bovine serum albumin, potentiated early and delayed hypersensitivity as well as the development of adjuvant arthritis. In contrast, caudal lesions, including those of the pons and medulla oblongata, were shown to impair these reactions (Masek *et al.*, 1983). The brainstem probably modulates the immune response via the autonomic nervous sytem, which innervates the immune tissues, but the mechanisms involved in such a modulation are still unknown.

### *Lesion of limbic structures*

In rats, lesions of the limbic structures, hippocampus and amygdala appeared to act in an opposite way to hypothalamic lesions. Indeed, an enhancement of the number of splenic and thymic cells, as well as an increase in T-cell mitogenesis, were observed in these two organs after bilateral lesions of the dorsal part of the hippocampus. These effects, which were maximal 4 to 7 days after surgery, were reversed by hypophysectomy (Cross *et al.*, 1982). Furthermore, lesions in the hippocampus were shown to increase IgG and IgM antibody production and to reduce IgA after immunization against ovalbumin. These results suggest that the hippocampus may have selective effects on certain components of the immune system (Nance *et al.*, 1987). Lesions of the amygdala induced an enhancement of T-cell mitogenesis similar to that observed after a lesion of the hippocampus, but did not modify the number of splenic or thymic cells. Similarly, the enhanced mitogenesis was reversed by hypophysectomy (Cross *et al.*, 1982).

### *Lesions of cortical and other subcortical structures*

Several other subcortical and cortical structures have been lesioned in order to investigate their possible immunoregulatory roles. Kainic acid lesions of the lateral septum significantly reduced production of antibodies of the IgG, IgA and IgM isotypes (Nance *et al.*, 1987). We have also observed that septal lesions may slightly depress the mitogen-induced proliferation of spleen lymphocytes (unpublished observations). In contrast, bilateral electrolytic lesions of the thalamus or superior colliculus did not modify cellular or humoral responsiveness to bovine serum albumin (Jankovic and Isakovic, 1973). Likewise, small striatal lesions in mice did not modify lymphocyte proliferation or NK cell activity (unpublished observations). However, profound unilateral depletion of striatal dopamine (over 90% when compared to the non-operated side), induced by injection of the toxin 6-hydroxydopamine in the substantia nigra, modified immune reactivity (Neveu *et al.*, 1992; Deleplanque *et al.*, 1992). Indeed, proliferation of T lymphocytes, but not B cells, was depressed 2 weeks after right or left lesions. Four weeks postoperatively, T-cell mitogenesis of left-lesioned mice returned to control levels, while that of right-lesioned animals was slightly potentiated 4 and 6 weeks after surgery. These dopaminergic lesions did not modify NK-cell activity. On the other hand, bilateral excitotoxic lesions of the nucleus basalis magnocellularis strongly enhanced T-cell mitogenesis and NK-cell activity when tested 3 weeks later. B-cell mitogenesis as well as blood T-cell subsets remained unchanged (Cherkaoui *et al.*, 1990).

The brain cortex has also been shown to have immunomodulatory functions. As a number of cerebral functions are lateralized, cortical lesions were mainly performed unilaterally. First, Renoux *et al.* (1983) showed that both mitogen-induced T-cell proliferation and production of antibodies of the IgG isotype were depressed after neocortical ablation of the left hemisphere, but enhanced after right hemisphere ablation. Additionally, NK cell activity was impaired after left hemisphere cortical ablation (Bardos *et al.*, 1981). B-lymphocyte and macrophage functions were claimed to be unaffected by cortical lesions. We replicated the effects of left vs right hemisphere cortical ablation on mitogen-induced proliferation of spleen T cells (Neveu *et al.*, 1986). Mitogenesis was decreased 6 to 10 weeks after ablation of the left fronto–parieto–occipital cortex. Differences were statistically significant only when left-hemisphere and right-hemisphere groups were compared. Neither of these groups differed from the unoperated controls. These modifications in T-cell proliferation have been shown to parallel those of interleukin-2 production (Neveu *et al.*, 1989*b*). Cortical lesions also modified, but only slightly, the mitogen-induced proliferation of B cells ($p = 0.05–0.1$). In further studies, we have found that the brain asymmetrically modulates macrophage activation (Neveu *et al.*, 1989*a*). The intraperitoneal injection of BCG is known to induce an accumulation of activated macrophages in the peritoneum. This accumulation was impaired by cortical lesions, especially in the left hemisphere. Moreover, oxidative metabolism was decreased in left-lesioned mice as compared to right-lesioned animals or controls. The function of non-activated resident macrophages was not affected by damaging the cortex. Although we have shown that the neocortex modulates the activity of both lymphocytes (T and B) and macrophages, the cellular target of brain cortex immunomodulation is not yet known. Cortical lesions do not induce a lymphocyte redistribution similar to that observed during stress. Furthermore, cortical lesions modulate concanavalin A-induced proliferation of lymphocytes of both lymph node and spleen in a similar way (Barnéoud *et al.*, 1990*b*). It is possible that the brain neocortex acts on a haematopoietic stem cell at the bone-marrow level as previously postulated (Neveu *et al.*, 1989*a*). On the other hand, the neocortex may first act on T lymphocytes and only secondarily modulate B-cell and macrophage functions through the lymphokines produced by T lymphocytes. In fact, it has been shown that left cortical lesions decreased production and/or release of serum factor(s) involved in T-cell maturation (Renoux *et al.*, 1983).

It is not known how brain structures produce asymmetrical modulation of the immune system. Renoux & Bizière (1986) have postulated that the right hemicortex modulates the activity of the left, which in turn controls the immune system. According to this hypothesis, the effects of bilateral cortical ablation should be similar to those of a left lesion alone. Indeed, they have shown that both bilateral and left lesions decreased NK-cell activity to the same extent. However, in our experiments, bilateral lesions (two unilateral lesions performed within a time interval of 3 weeks to avoid the high mortality rates of one-stage bilateral damage) did not modify mitogen-induced lymphoproliferation (Neveu *et al.*, 1988). Suppression of the asymmetrical immunomodulatory effects with bilateral lesions suggests that each hemicortex may be active on the immune system in an opposing fashion. That is, the left hemisphere may increase T-cell functions and the right hemisphere may decrease T-cell functions. Furthermore, cortical areas appeared to be differently involved in the modulation of immune responses.

Frontal cortex lesions, performed bilaterally (Cross *et al.*, 1982) or unilaterally (unpublished data) had no immunological effect. However, unilateral cortical lesions restricted to the parietooccipital areas had immunoregulatory functions, but the effects of these lesions were different from those observed after lesions involving all of the fronto–parieto–occipital cortex (Barnéoud *et al.*, 1987). In contrast to large neocortical ablations, small left posterior cortical lesions had no effect, while symmetrical right lesions altered only some of the immune parameters studied. These results suggest that each hemisphere may contain both activating and suppressing zones that interact within a hemisphere and between hemispheres. The effects of cortical lesions on T-cell mitogenesis, first described in female mice, were replicated with both small (Lahoste *et al.*, 1989) and large (Barnéoud *et al.*, 1988*a*) lesions in female and male rats. Furthermore, asymmetrical brain immunomodulation may occur in humans, as different perturbations of blood lymphocyte subsets have been reported 3 weeks after right- or left-sided stroke (Czlonkowska *et al.*, 1987).

## Specification of immune parameters susceptible to modulation by the brain

Taken together, the findings summarized above suggest that lesions of several distinct brain areas may change immune responsiveness. One could ask whether it is possible to characterize the general effects of brain lesions. Several methodological problems make it difficult to answer such a question. From an immunological point of view, none of these workers systematically studied the functions of each population of immune cells. Furthermore, immunological determinations were usually made only in spleen or blood, and rarely in several lymphoid organs from the same lesioned animal. In recent reports, lymphocytes and NK cells in the spleen were usually studied, but macrophage functions were not systematically investigated. The number and mitogenesis of B cells appeared not to be modified by brain lesions. Modifications of antibody production, observed after lesioning of the hypothalamus (Jankovic & Isakovic, 1973), hippocampus (Nance *et al.*, 1987) or neocortex (Renoux *et al.*, 1983) may reflect the activity of the helper T cells rather than B cells, as T-dependent antigens were usually used for immunization. Spleen T-lymphocyte mitogenesis and NK activity sometimes demonstrated parallel changes after lesions of the hypothalamus (Cross *et al.*, 1984) or of the nucleus basalis magnocellularis (Cherkaoui *et al.*, 1990). In other experiments,

T-cell mitogenesis was modified, while no alteration of NK-cell activity was observed, after lesion of the substantia nigra (Deleplanque *et al.*, 1992; Neveu *et al.*, 1992) or the right neocortex (Bardos *et al.*, 1981; Betancur *et al.*, 1991). Taken together, these results suggest that the various components of the immune system are specifically modulated by different brain structures.

Usually, immune modifications induced by brain lesions are studied in only one or two lymphoid organs, never in more. In some experiments, the functions of lymphocytes from two different lymphoid organs were equally altered. For example, modulation of T-cell mitogenesis induced by unilateral neocortex ablation was similarly observed in the spleen and lymph nodes (Barnéoud *et al.*, 1990*b*). In contrast, in other experiments, brain lesions may have induced changes selectively in one location. Indeed, T-cell mitogenesis in the spleen but not in the thymus was shown to be affected by hypothalamic lesions of the preoptic area (Cross *et al.*, 1982).

Another methodological problem makes it difficult to interpret immunological effects induced by various brain structures. Most of the immune alterations induced by lesioning various brain structures, including the hypothalamus, hippocampus or amygdala, were observed only a short time (less than 1 week) after lesioning. A single study reported a long-lasting depression of NK cell activity after destruction of the tuberoinfindibular region of the hypothalamus (Forni *et al.*, 1983). However, immune modifications induced by brain lesions may change with time, possibly because of the plasticity of both the immune and central nervous sytems. In fact, when studying the immunological effects of unilateral lesions of the neocortex (Neveu, 1992) or the substantia nigra (Deleplanque *et al.*, 1992; Neveu *et al.*, 1992), it was clearly shown that the effects observed 2 weeks after lesioning were quite different from those observed 6 to 10 weeks after surgery. Some immunological changes may even be reversed with time. To gain a better understanding of the role of brain areas in neuroimmunomodulation, the kinetic analysis of immunological effects of brain lesions should be more extensively studied. Furthermore, even though immune parameters studied in a steady state may appear to be normal after a certain interval of time, it is possible that the immune system is in an unstable equilibrium, which may be broken by immunization or stress.

Finally, the lesion model contains another inbuilt methodological problem. The immune system is known to send information to the central nervous system. For example, interleukin-1, produced by activated macrophages, has been shown to stimulate the corticotrophic axis at the hypothalamic (Berkenbosch *et al.*, 1987) and/or pituitary level (Bernton *et al.*, 1987). Changes in the firing rate of hypothalamic neurones, as well as in monoamine turnover in various limbic structures, were shown to occur after antigenic stimulation (Besedovsky *et al.*, 1977, 1983; Carlson *et al.*, 1987). Likewise, an increase of norepinephrine was observed 13 days after stimulation of the immune system by BCG in the right hemisphere, and this increase was correlated with lymphoproliferation (Barnéoud, *et al.*, 1988*b*). Even 8 weeks after BCG injection, variations of neurotransmitter concentrations were observed in various brain areas (Deleplanque *et al.*, 1993). These feedback mechanisms could interfere with the immunological effects of brain lesioning.

**Brain structures involved in neuroimmunomodulation**

Depending on their location, cerebral lesions may enhance or depress the immune parameters studied. For example, there was a clear-cut opposition between the effects of anterior hypothalamic and limbic lesions in the number and function of splenic and thymic T cells. (Cross *et al.*, 1982) or between lesions of the hippocampus and lateral septum on antibody production (Nance *et al.*, 1987). Therefore, it appears that some specificity may exist in the immunoregulatory effects of different brain lesions. In some circumstances, a specificity has not been found. For example, destruction of the hypothalamus (Forni *et al.*, 1983; Cross *et al.*, 1984) or ablation of the left neocortex (Renoux *et al.*, 1983; Betancur *et al.*, 1991) depresses spleen lymphocyte mitogenesis and NK-cell activity. However, the mechanisms involved in modulation of the same immune parameters by different brain lesions may be different. Such a hypothesis has not yet been tested. Keeping in mind that known mediators of brain–immune relationships are the hypothalamic–pituitary–adrenal axis and the autonomic nervous system (Bateman *et al.*, 1989; Ader *et al.*, 1990), it is not surprising to observe a modulation of immune responsiveness after hypothalamic or brainstem lesions. Hypothalamic nuclei are involved in neurosecretion, via the control of pituitary hormonal outflow. In fact, it was demonstrated that some of the effects of hypothalamic lesions were abolished by hypophysectomy (Cross *et al.*, 1982). However, plasma levels of ACTH, corticosterone or prolactin, which also have immunoregulatory functions (Cross & Roszman, 1989), were not usually determined. On the other hand, the hypothalamic paraventricular nuclei send descending projections to sympathetic and parasympathetic formations of the brainstem as well as to the intermediolateralis column of the spinal cord (Smith

& De Vito, 1984; Swanson & Sawchenko, 1983). Therefore, the hypothalamus and brainstem may be involved in the preganglionic control of the autonomic innervation of lymphoid organs. Unfortunately, the immunological effects of lesioning these two structures have never been linked to a possible modification of peripheral neurotransmission in the lymphoid organs. The reticular formation of the brainstem and the hypothalamus are certainly implicated in brain modulation of the immune system, but these regions may be considered only as effectors under the control of higher structures of the central nervous system.

Limbic structures may effectively modulate the immune response via the hypothalamus. The hippocampus and amygdala have anatomical and functional connections with the hypothalamus (Bjorklund & Lindvall, 1984; Feldman, 1985; Herman *et al.*, 1989). It was shown that lesion or stimulation of the hippocampus induced changes in the activity of the corticotropic axis (Dunn & Orr, 1984; De Kloet *et al.*, 1988; Herman *et al.*, 1989) but other hormones and neuropeptides may also be involved. Interestingly, hypophysectomy abolished the immune effects of hippocampal lesions (Cross *et al.*, 1982). However, some of the hormonal changes observed after limbic stimulation appear to depend on the site, ventral or dorsal, of stimulation (Dunn & Whitener, 1986). The amygdala–hippocampal complex may be considered as neuroimmunomodulatory structures. These areas are involved in the behavioural and neuroendocrine responses to stressful events (De Kloet *et al.*, 1988), known to alter immune functions, and are connected with effector structures. The possibility that different pathways involved in the control of neurosecretion by the various limbic areas may be reflected at the level of the immune system could represent the basis for a possible specific brain modulation of the immune response. More difficult to explain are the immune changes induced by other subcortical or cortical lesions. First, it must be noted that such lesions usually have to be extensive or to induce profound functional alterations. Indeed, only large, unilateral fronto–parieto–occipital or parieto–occipital decortications (Neveu, 1992) or drastic dopamine depletion (Neveu *et al.*, 1992; Deleplanque *et al.*, 1992) induce changes in immune reactivity. The involvement of the hypothalamus or brainstem in the immune effects of such lesions is still debated. There are no available data on the turnover of peripheral transmitters after lesioning. On the other hand, plasma levels of ACTH, corticosterone or prolactin were normal 7 weeks after unilateral lesion of the frontal–parietal–occipital cortex in rats at the time that immunological effects were studied (Barnéoud *et al.*, 1988*a*). Enhanced plasma levels of prolactin have been reported only when unilateral or bilateral cortex lesions were restricted to the parieto–occipital areas (Lahoste *et al.*, 1989). However, no kinetic studies of hormonal activity of the hypothalamic–pituitary–adrenal axis have yet been performed after such lesioning, and it may be that hormonal modifications were not concomitant but preceded the observed immune alterations. Furthermore, the role of corticotropin-releasing factor (CRF) which is known to have immunoregulatory functions (Jain *et al.*, 1991), has never been determined. The brain neocortex and substantia nigra, which have been shown to modulate immune functions asymmetrically (Neveu *et al.*, 1992; Deleplanque *et al.*, 1992), may also implicate the hypothalamus, as hypothalamic regulation of some neuroendocrine pathways was demonstrated to be lateralized (Gerendai, 1984). Furthermore, some experimental data suggest that the autonomic nervous system may also function asymmetrically (Bereiter, 1989; Shannahoff-Khalsa, 1991; Zamrini *et al.*, 1990). Brain areas other than those already studied are possibly involved in neuroimmunomodulation. The prefrontal cortex, now considered a limbic structure, may have anatomical connections with the hypothalamus and brainstem. Moreover, prefrontal cortex and nucleus accumbens are functionally interconnected (Jaskin *et al.*, 1990), are involved in various types of stress (Thierry *et al.*, 1976) and appear to function asymmetrically (Carlson *et al.*, 1991). The immunological effects of lesioning these structures are currently under investigation.

Even though one of the most useful approaches to study the influence of different brain structures on immune reactivity appears to be lesioning nervous tissue, it is difficult to conclude whether the lesioned area, or other functionally related structures that are secondarily altered by post-operative brain reorganization, are directly involved in neuroimmunomodulation. In order to overcome the difficulties of interpretation encountered in lesion models, some other experimental paradigms have also been set up. These paradigms are attempts to establish correlations between brain organization related to behaviour, and immune reactivity. For example, immune reactivity was shown to differ in two lines of rats (Roman low- and high-avoidance rats) that were genetically selected on the basis of their active avoidance behaviour; lymphocytes of the high-avoidance line were less reactive (Sandi *et al.*, 1991). Even though adult Roman rats differ in their basal and stimulated hypothalamus–pituitary–adrenocortical reactivity (Walker *et al.*, 1989) and in stress-induced changes of central monoamine metabolism (D'Angio *et al.*, 1988), it is not yet possible to link these patterns of brain organization to immune responsiveness. Furthermore, in this model, differences in immune reactivity may be related to genetic factors that are not necessarily involved in behaviour. The possible genetic bias has been obviated using another experimental approach, in which inbred mice were selected for paw preference. Left- and right-handed mice differed in their immune reactivity, including T-cell mitogenesis, NK-cell activity and autoantibody production (Neveu, 1992). Likewise, they exhibited differences in the distribution of brain monoamines (Barnéoud *et al.*, 1990*a*; Deleplanque *et al.*, 1993). However, it is still not possible to correlate immune response with the activity of given brain structures. In other, experimental designs it was possible to establish some correlations between stress-induced changes in catecholamine turnover in prefrontal areas and variations of NK-cell activity (Zalcman *et al.*, 1990).

These non-lesional models, which avoid the role of neural plasticity in the interpretation of brain–immune relationships, are not able to give us definitive conclusions about the brain structures involved in neuroimmunomodulation. We hope that they can be improved in the near future, in order to clarify the mechanisms involved in brain–immune interactions.

## Conclusion

From the present data in the literature, it can be concluded that various anatomically and functionally distinct regions may be involved in neuroimmunomodulation.

The hypothalamus and brainstem may be considered as effector structures in neuroimmunomodulation, as they control neuroendocrine pathways and autonomic nervous system activity, which are directly involved in modulation of immune reactivity.

Limbic structures, such as the hippocampus, amygdala or possibly the prefrontal cortex, may be considered as higher brain regions which are anatomically and functionally connected to the effector structures, and are implicated during stressful situations known to alter the immune response. It is more difficult to explain the mechanisms whereby the substantia nigra and neocortex (the latter being in charge of higher integrative functions) asymmetrically modulate immune responsiveness.

All these important data come from experimental lesion models, even though these models contain inbuilt methodological problems related to postlesional plasticity of the central nervous system and possibly of the immune system as well. Chemical lesioning of precise neurotransmitter pathways, as well as kinetic studies of immune reactivity in various lymphoid organs, would be useful in the future to delineate the mechanisms whereby different brain structures modulate the activity of the various components of the immune system.

## References

Ader, R., Felten, D. & Cohen, N. (1990). Interactions between the brain and the immune system. *Ann. Rev. Pharmacol. Toxicol.*, **30**, 561–602.

Bardos, P., Degenne, D., Lebranchu, Y., Biziere, K. & Renoux, G. (1981). Neocortical lateralization of NK activity in mice. *Scand. J. Immunol.*, **13**, 609–11.

Barnéoud, P., Le Moal, M. & Neveu, P. J. (1990*a*). Asymmetric distribution of brain monoamines in left- and right-handed mice. *Brain Res.*, **520**, 317–21.

Barnéoud, P., Neveu, P. J., Vitiello, S. & Le Moal, M. (1987). Functional heterogeneity of the right and left cerebral neocortex in the modulation of the immune system. *Physiol. Behav.*, **41**, 525–30.

Barnéoud, P., Neveu, P. J., Vitiello, S. & Le Moal, M. (1988*a*) Brain neocortex immunomodulation in rats. *Brain Res.*, **474**, 394–8.

Barnéoud, P., Neveu, P. J., Vitiello, S. & Le Moal, (1990*b*). Lymphocyte homing after left or right brain neocortex ablation. *Immunol. Lett.*, **24**, 31–6.

Barnéoud, P., Rivet, J. M., Vitiello, S., Le Moal, M. & Neveu, P. J. (1988*b*). Brain norepinephrine levels after BCG-stimulation of the immune system. *Immunol. Lett.*, **18**, 201–4.

Bateman, A., Singh, A., Kral, T. & Solomon, S. (1989). The immune hypothalamic pituitary–adrenal axis. *Endocrine Rev.*, **10**, 92–112.

Bereiter, D. A. (1989). Partial transection of the ipsilateral cervical spinal cord evokes a sustained increase in the adrenal secretion of catecholamines in the cat. *J. Autonomic Nerv. Syst.*, **27**, 181–92.

Berkenbosch, F., Van Oers, J., Del Rey, A., Tilders, F. & Besedovsky, H. (1987). Corticotropin-releasing factor – producing neurons in the rat activated by interleukin-I. *Science*, **238**, 524–6.

Bernton, E. W., Beach, J. F., Holaday, J. W., Smallridge, R. C. & Fein, H. G. (1987). Release of multiple hormones by a direct action of interleukin 1 on pituitary cells. *Science*, **238**, 519–21.

Besedovsky, H. O., Del Rey, A., Sorkin, E., Da Prada, M., Burri, R. & Honegger, C. (1983). The immune response evokes changes in brain noradrenergic neurons. *Science*, **221**, 564–6.

Besedovsky, H. O., Sorkin, E., Felix, D. & Haas, H. (1977). Hypothalamic changes during the immune response. *Eur. J. Immunol.*, **7**, 323–25.

Betancur, C., Neveu, P. J., Vitiello, S. & Le Moal, M. (1991). Natural killer cell activity is associated with brain asymmetry in male mice. *Brain Behav. Immun.*, **5**, 162–9.

Bjorklund, A. & Lindvall, O. (1984). Dopamine-containing system in the CNS. In *Handbook of Chemical Neuroanatomy. Classical Neurotransmitters in the CNS*, vol. 2, ed. A. Bjorklund & T. Holkfelt, pp. 55–122. Amsterdam: Elsevier.

Blalock, J. E. (1989). A molecular basis for bidirectional communication between the immune and neuroendocrine systems. *Physiol. Rev.*, **69**, 1–32.

Carlson, J. N., Fitzgerald, L. W., Keller, R. W. & Glick, S. D. (1991). Side and region dependent charges in dopamine activation with various durations of restraint stress. *Brain Res.*, **550**, 313–18.

Carlson, S. L., Felten, D. L., Livnat, S. & Felten, S. Y. (1987). Alterations of monoamines in specific central autonomic nuclei following immunization in mice. *Brain Behav. Immun.*, **1**, 52–63.

Cherkaoui, J., Mayo, W., Neveu, P. J., Kelley, K. W., Vitiello, S., Le Moal, M. & Simon, H. (1990). The nucleus basalis is involved in brain modulation of the immune system in rats. *Brain Res.*, **516**, 345–8.

Cross, R. J., Brooks, W. H., Roszman, T. L. & Markesbery, W. R. (1982). Hypothalamic–immune interactions: effect of hypophysectomy on neuroimmunomodulation. *J. Neurol. Sci.*, **53**, 557–66.

Cross, R. J., Markesbery, W. R., Brooks, W. H. & Roszman, T. L. (1984). Hypothalamic–immune interactions: neuromodulation of natural killer activity by lesioning of the anterior hypothalamus. *Immunology*, **51**, 399–406.

Cross, R. J. and Roszman, T. L. (1989). Neuroendocrine modulation of immune function: the role of prolactin. *Prog. Neuroendocr. Immunol.*, **2**, 17–20.

Czlonkowska, A., Korlak, J. & Kuczynska-Zardzewialy, A. (1987). Lymphocyte subsets after stroke. *J. Neuroimmunol.*, **16**, 40 (abstract).

D'Angio, M., Serrano, A., Driscoll, P. & Scatton, B. (1988). Stressful environmental stimuli increase extracellular DOPAC levels in the prefrontal cortex of hypoemotional (Roman high-avoidance) but not hyperemotional (Roman low-avoidance) rats. An *in vivo* voltametric study. *Brain Res.*, **451**, 237–47.

Dann, J. A., Wachtel, S. S. & Rubin, A. L. (1979). Possible involvement of the central nervous system in graft rejection. *Transplantation*, **27**, 223–6.

Deleplanque, B., Delrue, C., Vitiello, S. & Neveu, P. J. (1993). Effects of BCG-stimulation of the immune system on distribution of brain monoamines in left- and right-handed mice. *Int. J. Neurosci.*, in press.

Deleplanque, B., Neveu, P., Vitiello, S. & Le Moal, M. (1992). Early effects of unilateral lesions of substantia nigra on immune reactivity. *Neurosci. Lett.*, **135**, 205–9.

De Kloet, E. R., De Kock, S., Schild, V. & Veldhuis, H. D. (1988). Antiglucocorticoid RU 38486 attenuates retention of a behavior and disinhibits the hypothalamic–pituitary–adrenal axis at different brain sites. *Neuroendocrinology*, **47**, 109–15.

Dunn, J. D. & Orr, S. E. (1984). Differential plasma corticosterone to hippocampal stimulation. *Exp. Brain Res.*, **54**, 1–6.

Dunn, J. D. & Whitener, J. (1986). Plasma corticosterone response to electrical stimulation of the amygdaloid complex: cytoarchitectural specificity. *Neuroendocrinology*, **42**, 211–17.

Feldman, S. (1985). Neural pathways mediating adrenocortical responses. *Fed. Proc.*, **44**, 169–75.

Filipp, G. & Szentivanyi, A. (1958). Anaphylaxis and the immune system. Part III. *Ann. Allergy*, **16**, 306–11.

Forni, G., Bindoni, M., Santoni, A., Belluardo, N., Marchese, A. E. & Giovarelli, M. (1983). Radiofrequency destruction of the tubero-infundibular region of hypothalamus permanently abrogates NK cell activity in mice. *Nature*, **306**, 181–3.

Gerendai, I. (1984). Lateralization of neuroendocrine control. In *Cerebral Dominance: the Biological Foundations*, ed. N. Geschwind & A. M. Galaburda, pp. 167–78. London: Harvard University Press.

Herman, J. P., Shafer, M. K. H., Young, E., Thompson, R., Douglass, J., Akil, H. & Watson, S. J. (1989). Evidence for hippocampal regulation of the hypothalamo–pituitary–adrenal axis. *J. Neurosci.*, **9**, 3072–82.

Isakovic, K. & Jankovic, B. D. (1973). Neuro-endocrine correlates of immune response. II Changes in the lymphatic organs of brain-lesioned rats. *Int. Arch. Allergy*, **45**, 373–84.

Jain, R., Zwickler, D., Hollander, C. S., Brand, H., Saperstein, A., Hutchinson, B., Brown, C. & Audhya, T. (1991). Corticotropin-releasing factor modulates the immune response to stress in the rat. *Endocrinology*, **128**, 1329–36.

Jankovic, B. D. & Isakovic, K. (1973). Neuroendocrine correlate of immune response. Effects of brain lesions on antibody production, Arthus reactivity and delayed hypersensitivity in the rat. *Int. Arch. Allergy*, **45**, 360–72.

Jaskin, G. E., Karoum, F. K. & Weinberger, D. R. (1990). Persistent elevations in dopamine and its metabolites in the nucleus accumbens after mild subchronic stress in rats with ibotenic lesions of the medial prefrontal cortex. *Brain Res.*, **534**, 321–3.

Kato, K., Hamada, N., Mizukoshi, N., Yamamoto, K. I., Kimura, T., Ishihara, C., Fujioka, Y., Kato, T., Fujieda, K. & Matsuura, N. (1986). Depression of delayed-type hypersensitivity in mice with hypothalamic lesion induced by monosodium glutamate. Involvement of neuroendocrine system in immunomodulation. *Immunology*, **58**, 389–95.

Keller, S. E., Stein, M., Camerino, M. S., Schleifer, S. J. & Sherman, J. (1980). Suppression of lymphocyte stimulation by anterior hypothalamic lesions in guinea pigs. *Cell Immunol.*, **52**, 334–40.

Khansari, D. N., Murgo, A. J. & Faith, R. E. (1990). Effects of stress on the immune system. *Immunol. Today*, **11**, 170–5.

Lahoste, G., Neveu, P. J., Mormede, P. & Le Moal, M. (1989). Hemispheric asymmetry in the effects of cerebral cortical ablation on mitogen-induced lymphoproliferation and plasma prolactin levels in female rats. *Brain Res.*, **483**, 123–9.

Lambert, P. L., Harrell, E. H. & Achterberg, J. (1981). Medial hypothalamic stimulation decreases the phagocytic activity of the reticuloendothelial system. *Physiol. Psychol.*, **9**, 193–6.

Luparello, T. J., Stein, M. & Park, D. C. (1964). Effect of hypothalamic lesions on rat anaphylaxis. *Am. J. Physiol.*, **207**, 911–14.

Masek, K., Kadlecov, O. & Petrovicky, A. P. (1983). The effect of brain stem lesions on the immune response. In *Advances in Immunopharmacology*, 2nd edn, ed. J. W. Hadden, L. Cheldid, P. Dukor, F. Spereafico & D. Willoughby, pp. 443–50. Oxford: Pergamon Press.

Nance, D. M., Rayson, D. & Carr, R. I. (1987). The effects of lesions in the septal and hippocampal areas on the humoral immune response of adult female rats. *Brain Behav. Immun.*, **1**, 292–305.

Neveu, P. J. (1992). Asymmetrical brain modulation of the immune response. *Brain Res. Rev.*, **17**, 101–7.

Neveu, P. J., Barnéoud, P., Georgiades, O., Vitiello, S., Vincendeau, P. & Le Moal, M. (1989*a*). Brain neocortex influence on the mononuclear phagocytic system. *J. Neurol. Sci.*, **22**, 188–93.

Neveu, P. J., Barnéoud, P., Vitiello, S., Kelley, K. W. & Le Moal, M. (1989*b*). Brain neocortex modulation of mitogen-induced interleukin-2, but not interleukin-1, production. *Immunol. Lett.*, **21**, 307–10.

Neveu, P. J., Barnéoud, P., Vitiello, S. & Le Moal, M. (1988). Immune functions after bilateral neocortex ablation in mice. *Neurosci. Res. Commun.*, **3**, 183–90.

Neveu, P. J., Deleplanque, B., Vitiello, S., Rouge-Pont, F. & Le Moal, M.

(1992). Hemispheric asymmetry in the effects of substantia nigra lesioning on lymphocyte reactivity in mice. *Int. J. Neurosci.*, **64**, 267–73.

Neveu, P. J., Taghzouti, K., Dantzer, R., Simon, H. & Le Moal, M. (1986). Modulation of mitogen-induced lymphoproliferation by cerebral neocortex. *Life Sci.*, **38**, 1907–13.

O'Leary, A. (1990). Stress, emotion and human immune function. *Psychol. Bull.*, **108**, 363–82.

Renoux, G. & Bizière, K. (1986). Brain neocortex lateralized control of immune recognition. *Integr. Psychiatry*, **4**, 32–40.

Renoux, G., Bizière, K., Renoux, M., Guillaumin, J. M. & Degenne, D. J. (1983). A balanced brain asymmetry modulates T cell mediated events. *J. Neuroimmunol.*, **5**, 227–38.

Roszman, T. L., Cross, R. J., Brooks, W. H. & Markesbery, W. R. (1982). Hypothalamic-immune interactions II. The effect of hypothalamic lesions on the ability of adherent spleen cells to limit lymphocyte blastogenesis. *Immunology*, **45**, 737–43.

Sandi, C., Castanon, N., Vitiello, S., Neveu, P. J. & Mormede, P. (1991). Different responsiveness of spleen lymphocytes from two lines of psychogenetically selected rat (Roman high and low avoidance). *J. Neuroimmunol.*, **31**, 27–33.

Shannahoff-Khalsa, D. (1991). Lateralized rhythms of the central and autonomic nervous system. *Int. J. Psychophysiol.*, **11**, 225–51.

Smith, O. A. & De Vito, J. L. (1984). Central neural integration for the control of antonomic responses associated with emotion. *Ann. Rev. Neurosci.*, **7**, 43–65.

Stein, M., Schiavi, R. C. & Camerino, M. (1976). Influence of brain and behavior on the immune system. *Science*, **191**, 435–40.

Swanson, L. W. & Sawchenko, P. E. (1983). Hypothalamic integration: organisation of the paraventricular and supraoptic nuclei. *Ann. Rev. Neurosci.*, **6**, 269–324.

Szentivanyi, A. & Filipp, G. (1958). Anaphylaxis and the immune system part II. *Ann. Allergy.*, **16**, 143–51.

Thierry, A. M., Tassin, J. P., Blanc, G. & Glowinski, J. (1976). Selective activation of the mesocortical DA system by stress. *Nature*, **263**, 242–4.

Walker, C. D., Rivest, R. W., Meaney, M. J. & Aubert, M. L. (1989). Differential activation of the pituitary–adrenocortical axis after stress in the rat: use of two genetically selected lines (Roman low- and high-avoidance rats) as a model. *Endocrinology*, **123**, 477–85.

Zalcman, S., Irwin, J. & Anisman, H. (1990). Stressor-induced alterations of natural killer cell activity and central catecholamines in mice. *Biol. Biochem. Behav.*, **39**, 361–6.

Zamrini, E. Y., Meador, K. J., Loring, D. W., Nichols, F. T., Lee, G. P., Figueroa, R. E. & Thompson, W. O. (1990). Unilateral cerebral inactivation produces differential left/right heart rate responses, *Neurology*, **40**, 1408–11.

# 6

# Psychological and neurobiological consequences of trauma

BARBARA O. ROTHBAUM and
CHARLES B. NEMEROFF

## Introduction

Human reactions to trauma have been characterized for more than a century by various labels, including compensation neurosis (Rigler, 1879), hysteria (Putnam, 1881), nervous shock (Page, 1885), traumatophobia (Rado, 1942), and war neurosis (Grinker & Spiegel, 1943). More recently, a large cluster of these reactions has been subsumed under posttraumatic stress disorder (PTSD) (American Psychiatric Association, 1980), described as an anxiety disorder precipitated by an event 'outside the range of usual human experience' (p. 250) and characterized by symptoms of reexperiencing (e.g. nightmares, flashbacks), avoidance and numbing (e.g. avoidance of reminders, psychogenic amnesia), and arousal (e.g. difficulty sleeping, exaggerated startle) that persist longer than 1 month posttrauma. The fourth edition of the *Diagnostic and Statistical Manual of Mental Disorders* (DSM-IV) is expected to retain the symptoms described above, but modify the trauma criterion to include the individual's perception of threat rather than the rarity of the event. The duration criterion is likely to include the subtypes of 'acute' and 'chronic' to describe the course of the reaction.

PTSD was introduced into the third edition of the DSM (DSM-III) (American Psychiatric Association, 1980) primarily in response to the large number of Vietnam combat veterans who manifested the above symptoms, but the disorder has been evidenced following other traumas as well, including rape (Kilpatrick *et al.*, 1987; Rothbaum *et al.*, 1992), accidents (Muse, 1986; Burstein *et al.*, 1988), natural disasters such as volcanoes, fires, tornadoes, floods, and mudslides (Lindy *et al.*, 1983; Shore *et al.*, 1986; Smith *et al.*, 1986; Bravo *et al.*, 1990; Green *et al.*, 1990, 1991), and disasters such as the nuclear accident at Three Mile Island, fire, and collapse of dams and skywalks (Baum *et al.*, 1983; Wilkinson, 1983;

Bromet *et al.*, 1984; Green *et al.*, 1990, 1991). The duration of these reactions is quite variable: some individuals experience traumatic events with apparently no long-lasting adverse effects, whereas other victims seem to suffer permanent damage, with one study finding continuing negative effects after 14 years posttrauma (Green *et al.*, 1990). The percentage of people who develop PTSD following various traumas, and the course of their reactions, are addressed below.

In this chapter, we review some of the characteristic psychological and neurobiological consequences of trauma as experienced by humans. The animal literature is not reviewed here. A significant focus is given to PTSD symptoms and markers, as this syndrome succinctly describes the reactions of many individuals to threatening events. Neuroendocrine and neurochemical alterations in humans following trauma are examined, as well as psychophysiological, affective, and behavioral reactions. The course and duration of PTSD reactions following various traumas is also reviewed. A substantial emphasis is placed on studies of rape victims, as the nature of the trauma lends itself to the prospective examination of reactions beginning very soon after the trauma.

## Posttraumatic stress disorder

Some of the reactions to criminal victimization that have been noted include anxiety, depression, intrusive thoughts and images of the assault, and sleep disturbances such as nightmares and insomnia (Kilpatrick *et al.*, 1979; Ellis *et al.*, 1981; Calhoun *et al.*, 1982; Nadelson *et al.*, 1982; Frank & Stewart, 1984; Kilpatrick & Veronen, 1984; Resick, 1987). Rape victims have reported intrusive thoughts and images of the assault that they have actively attempted to avoid (Kilpatrick & Veronen, 1984; Resick, 1987). They have also reported more sleep disturbance, including nightmares and insomnia (Ellis *et al.*, 1981; Nadelson *et al.*, 1982), and more difficulty concentrating (Nadelson *et al.*, 1982) than non-victimized controls. Research indicates that the postassault psychopathology of rape victims may best be described as posttraumatic stress disorder. For example, Resick *et al.* (unpublished data) found that 76% of rape victims fulfilled the diagnostic criteria for PTSD at some point within a year after the assault.

### *Duration of symptoms*

It is important to differentiate between the duration of the normal response to trauma and a chronic pathological response. To do so, repeated assessments of PTSD symptoms are necessary over time, beginning soon after the trauma. Several studies using such prospective methodology are summarized below. Unfortunately, such studies of Vietnam veterans are not available, because PTSD was not included as a diagnostic entity until the DSM-III was published in 1980, long after the Vietnam War. By the time PTSD was studied in this population, most of the subjects were 'contaminated' by chronic hospitalizations, substance abuse, etc., due to the time lag. Therefore, the criterion of repeated assessments for PTSD beginning soon after the trauma was not fulfilled regarding Vietnam veterans. However, the results of two recent retrospective studies of the prevalence of PTSD in Vietnam veterans are included.

A prospective study of rape and crime victims was conducted by Foa and Rothbaum and colleagues (Rothbaum *et al.*, 1992). The following PTSD symptoms were assessed via a structured interview: reliving experiences, nightmares, flashbacks, avoidance of reminders and thoughts of the assault, impaired leisure activities, sense of detachment, blunted affect, disturbed sleep, memory and concentration difficulties, hyperalertness, increased startle response, feelings of guilt and increased fearfulness.

Rape victims ($N = 95$) were first interviewed within two weeks following their assault (mean = 12.64 days) and once weekly thereafter, for 12 weeks. Follow-up assessments were conducted 6 and 9 months following the assault ($N = 24$). The results indicated that at the initial interview, 94% of rape victims met symptomatic but not duration criteria for a PTSD diagnosis. At 1 month postassault (mean = 35 days), 65% met criteria for PTSD, decreasing to 52.5% by 2 months postassault and to 47% by 3 months postassault. At 6 months postassault, 41.7% were classified as PTSD, and at 9 months postassault, 47.1% fulfilled PTSD criteria. PTSD and related psychopathology decreased sharply between assessments 1 and 4 for all women. Women who did not meet criteria for PTSD 3 months postassault showed steady improvement over time. However, women whose PTSD persisted throughout the 3-month study did not show improvement after the fourth assessment. Thus, nearly all of the rape victims in this sample appeared to have PTSD immediately following the assault, but fewer than half continued to meet criteria for this disorder 3 months later. The incidence of PTSD did not change appreciably after the 3-month assessment.

The course of PTSD was similar for victims of non-sexual criminal assault (simple and aggravated assault and robbery) to that found for the rape victims. A majority of the crime victims responded with PTSD symptoms initially but the incidence of PTSD decreased over time (Foa & Rothbaum, unpublished data). Approximately 1 week following the assault, 64.7% ($N = 51$) fulfilled the requisite PTSD criteria, decreasing to 36.7% 1 month postassault, 25% 2 months postassault, 14.6% 3 months postassault, and 11.5% 6 months following the crime ($N = 26$). At 9 months postassault, none of the 15 crime victims interviewed met criteria for PTSD. Thus, like the rape victims, most of the crime victims initially responded with PTSD symptoms that decreased substantially by 3 months postassault. While the pattern of gradual decrease in PTSD incidence by 3 months postassault was the same for rape and crime victims, it is important to note that rape victims are more likely to develop PTSD initially and to maintain it over time.

Evidence from other populations converge with the rape and crime victims' reactions cited above, to suggest that, once a chronic PTSD has developed, it is likely to remain relatively stable over time if treatment is not introduced (McFarlane, 1988*a*, *b*). After fire, 315 firefighters were assessed for PTSD using the General Health Questionnaire (GHQ) (Goldberg, 1972) at 4, 8, 11, and 29 months postdisaster. Of firefighters who were symptomatic at 4 months after the fire, 69% remained so at later assessments, suggesting that PTSD at 4 months posttrauma is a relatively good predictor for the chronicity of the disorder (McFarlane, 1988*b*). Support for this conclusion also comes from another study with firefighters (McFarlane, 1988*a*). Eighty-one per cent of firefighters diagnosed with PTSD at 8 months following the fire ($N = 50$) still had PTSD at 42 months. Thus, it appears that by 3–4 months posttrauma, and definitely by 6–8 months posttrauma, the course of PTSD becomes chronic and can no longer be expected to subside naturally, as in a normal reaction to trauma.

### *Prevalence of PTSD*

Several studies have assessed the incidence of PTSD using a retrospective methodology. Rape victims ($N = 33$) were interviewed 12–36 months postassault to assess the presence and duration of PTSD symptoms (Resick *et al.*, unpublished data). The results were remarkably similar to those reported by Rothbaum *et al.* (1992). Of the rape victims studied, 76% reported experiencing PTSD symptoms that lasted less than 1 month, 60.6% reported PTSD lasting at least 1 month, and 39.4% met criteria for PTSD at the time of inquiry, 12–36 months postassault.

An investigation of PTSD using a modified version of the Diagnostic

Interview Schedule (DIS) (Robins *et al.*, 1981) was conducted with rape and crime victims from a community sample of 391 adult females (Kilpatrick *et al.*, 1987). Of those who had experienced a completed rape, 57.1% suffered from PTSD at some point following the asault, and 16.5% met PTSD criteria at the time of the inquiry (average of approximately 15 years postassault). Of aggravated assault victims, 36.8% had PTSD at some point after the assault, and 10.5% were diagnosed as having PTSD at the time of the interview (average of 10.5 years postassault). Thus, again, a large number of victims initially responded to rape with PTSD symptoms, but a smaller number developed a chronic disorder. In addition, rape appeared to be more likely to induce PTSD than did other serious crimes not involving sexual assault.

In yet another retrospective study, lifetime and current prevalence of PTSD was investigated in a community sample of 214 adult family survivors of homicide victims (here called 'homicide survivors') (Kilpatrick *et al.*, 1988). Subjects were assessed for PTSD via a 30-min telephone interview. Twenty-nine per cent of survivors of criminal homicide experienced PTSD at some point, with 7.0% experiencing PTSD at the time of inquiry (which was not specified). Of the survivors of alcohol-related vehicular homicide (i.e. family members of victims), 34.1% experienced PTSD at some point, with 2.2% experiencing PTSD at the time of inquiry. Thus, approximately one-third of homicide survivors evidenced an occurrence of PTSD at some point following the death, but a very small percentage developed a chronic disorder.

The prevalence of PTSD in Vietnam veterans was assessed thoroughly, although retrospectively, in the National Vietnam Veteran Readjustment Study. Using multiple measures of PTSD, it was found that 15.2% of the men and 8.5% of the women who served in Vietnam, nearly 500 000 people, were suffering from PTSD at the time of inquiry, more than 15 years postservice (Schlenger *et al.*, 1992). This average prevalence rate was found to differ among subgroups, with Hispanic men experiencing the highest rate of PTSD (27.9%), followed by African American men (20.6%), with Caucasian or other men experiencing the lowest rate of PTSD (13.7%).

As would be expected, the lifetime prevalence of PTSD in the men and women who served in Vietnam was much higher than rates in the general population. Among male veterans, 30.9% reported experiencing PTSD at some point following their service. The lifetime prevalence for female veterans was 26%. This study found that 'of the 1.7 million veterans who ever experienced significant symptoms of PTSD after the Vietnam war, approximately 830 000 (49%) still experience clinically significant distress and disability from symptoms of PTSD' (p. 365, Weiss *et al.*, 1992).

A different picture emerged from data collected on civilians who experienced heavy shelling during wartime. Saigh (1988) assessed 12 undergraduate and graduate students at the American University of Beirut in 1983 and 1984 before and after a major offensive involving heavy shelling of the areas near the university. Structured interviews aimed at diagnosing PTSD retrospectively (approximately one year following the shelling) revealed that nine of the 11 (81.8%) students interviewed experienced PTSD symptoms immediately following the shelling. However, the symptoms of eight of these nine spontaneously remitted within 1 month after the shelling; the remaining student developed chronic PTSD. These results are consistent with reports from World War II, demonstrating that civilians undergoing an air raid exhibited short-lived fear reactions, but very few developed intense persistent fear reactions (Rachman, 1989). Findings corroborating this observation were also reported from Northern Ireland (Cairns & Wilson, 1984).

There are data to suggest that the course of PTSD in children may be similar to that in adults. Children aged 5 to 13 were evaluated for PTSD approximately 1 month ($N = 159$) and 14 months ($N = 100$) following a fatal sniper attack on their school playground (Pynoos *et al.*, 1987; Nader *et al.*, 1990). Using the children's version of the PTSD Reaction Index completed by an interviewer, they found that the occurrence of PTSD was significantly correlated with degree of exposure. At the 1-month assessment, 77% of the children who were on the playground during the attack were classified as severely or moderately suffering from PTSD and 67% of children who were in the school building had PTSD. At the 14-month assessment, 74% of the children who were on the playground still manifested PTSD, as compared to fewer than 19% of those who were in the school. The latter did not significantly differ from the unexposed group (children not at school during the attack). Thus, nearly all of the children studied, who were on the playground during the attack and fulfilled PTSD criteria at the 1-month assessment, were suffering from chronic PTSD at 14 months, whereas children who were less exposed to the attack (i.e. were inside the school) recovered sometime between 1 and 14 months postattack. Thus, the criterion of the revised edition of the DSM-III for 1-month duration of symptoms was an excellent predictor of chronic PTSD in the highly exposed children, but a poor predictor for the less-exposed group. Perhaps an intermediate assessment would have increased the accuracy of prediction for the entire population.

The similarities between the results of different investigations with similar populations supports the reliability of the findings. The rape and crime studies evidenced a high incidence of PTSD initially, which decreased gradually and stabilized around 3 months postassault. A certain proportion of these cases remain chronic sufferers. The civilians also responded with a high rate of PTSD initially but almost all recovered quickly. Children's reactions appeared to vary with their proximity to the original trauma. Most of the children in close proximity to the sniper responded with PTSD that remained chronic. However, most of the children who were not in close proximity to the sniper initially responded with PTSD, which tended to dissipate over time.

***Subtypes***

The DSM-III (American Psychiatric Association, 1980) distinguished two subtypes of PTSD: acute ('symptoms begin within six months of the trauma and have not lasted six months', *ibid.*, p. 237) and chronic or delayed ('symptoms either develop more than six months after the trauma or last six months or more', *ibid.*, p. 237). In the only controlled comparison available, 31 Vietnam veterans with delayed-onset PTSD were compared with 32 with acute-onset PTSD (Watson *et al.*, 1988). Veterans were assessed for PTSD using a structured interview based on DSM-III criteria. No significant differences between the two groups emerged. In addition, no evidence was found to support the hypotheses that delayed onset was related to the severity of the trauma, the severity of the symptoms, repression, or previous stress history. In the above-cited studies of school children following a fatal sniper attack (Pynoos *et al.*, 1987; Nader *et al.*, 1990), no cases of delayed PTSD reactions were noted. Thus, PTSD was present at the 14-month assessment only in those children who were diagnosed with PTSD at the 1-month assessment. It seems that the DSM-III distinction of acute, chronic, and delayed PTSD has not gained support from empirical studies.

Solomon & Mikulincer (1988) described a combat stress reaction (CSR) that often occurs during war (i.e. on the battlefield) and includes 'restlessness, psychomotor retardation, psychological withdrawal, sympathetic activity, startle reactions, confusion, nausea, vomiting, and paranoid reactions' (Solomon & Mikulincer, 1988, p. 264; from Grinker & Spiegel, 1945). Solomon & Mikulincer (1988, p. 264) noted that, 'despite the extreme variability of this phenomenon, a common denominator can be identified: the soldier ceases to function militarily and/or begins to function in a bizarre manner that usually endangers himself and/or his comrade'. In an assessment of the long-term problems of Israeli veterans from the 1982 Lebanon War, 59% of cases with CSR suffered from PTSD at 1 year postwar as compared to 16% of a veteran control group who had not manifested CSR. At 2 years postwar, 56% of cases with CSR and 14% of controls without CSR, met diagnosis criteria for PTSD. Thus, CSR appeared to be a good predictor of later development of PTSD.

### *Trauma variables*

Trauma variables, as opposed to individual variables, impact the reactions as well. For example, injury during an assault and the type of assault (rape vs non-sexual assault) were found to predict the development of PTSD (Kilpatrick *et al.*, 1989). Assault-related guilt as well as the perception of life-threat, which is going to be emphasized in the DSM-IV, were found to predict reactions to criminal assault, including PTSD severity (McCahill *et al.*, 1979; Ellis *et al.*, 1981; Sales *et al.*, 1984; Kilpatrick *et al.*, 1989; Riggs *et al.*, unpublished data).

## Neurochemical responses

One of the primary reasons to study neuropeptide-containing neurones in anxiety disorders such as PTSD is that these substances modulate the activity of hormones and neurotransmitters that have already been implicated in the pathophysiology of these disorders. The study of neuropeptides, therefore, may provide a more precise understanding of the dysregulation of neuroendocrine and neurotransmitter systems that may be closer to the primary 'source' of the biological defect.

For example, neuroendocrine abnormalities in depression and anxiety disorders have been repeatedly demonstrated in the hypothalamic–pituitary–adrenal (HPA) axis and the hypothalamic–pituitary–thyroid axis (Butler & Nemeroff, 1990; Yehuda & Nemeroff, 1993). Because the primary phsyiological control of adenohypophyseal hormone secretion is mediated by releasing and release-inhibiting neuropeptides in the hypothalamus (Owens & Nemeroff, 1993) it is of interest to study the neuropeptide systems that may ultimately be responsible for the neuroendocrine alterations in psychiatric illness.

Similarly, the study of neuropeptides in affective and anxiety disorders is important, because of findings of altered monoamine neurotransmission in these disorders. The observation that neuropeptides are widely distributed throughout the central nervous system (CNS), with each peptide showing a unique heterogeneous distribution pattern, has revealed that, in addition to their actions as releasing factors, neuropeptides act as neuroregulators within the CNS. Many of the classical monoamine neurotransmitter systems implicated in psychiatric illness such as norepinephrine, dopamine, and serotonin either innervate, or are innervated by neuropeptide-containing neurones. The recent demonstration of colocalization of neuropeptides and neurotransmitters (Hokfelt *et al.*, 1984; Nemeroff & Bissette, 1986) has provided additional evidence for the interaction of neuropeptides and neurotransmitters.

A third impetus for studying neuropeptides in these major psychiatric disorders is that neuropeptides are densely concentrated (with and without colocalized neurotransmitters) in brain regions thought to be involved in their pathogenesis, and, when exogenously administered, produce effects that may be related to psychiatric symptoms. For example, intraventricular injection of certain neuropeptides in laboratory animals has been found to produce profound behavioral effects, which resemble signs and symptoms of certain psychiatric disorders. Thus, some neuropeptides may be depressogenic or anxiogenic substances in and of themselves. This hypothesis is also being tested by measuring basal concentrations of peptides in plasma, cerebrospinal fluid (CSF) and tissues of depressed and anxious patients, and also by study of the effects of various neuropeptides on depressive and anxiety symptoms. These and other strategies for studying the role of neuropeptides in psychiatric disorders associated with trauma are briefly described below, as is the current state of the field.

Corticotropin-releasing factor (CRF) is a 41-amino acid residue neuropeptide that is localized in high concentrations in the parvocellular region of the paraventricular nucleus (PVN) of the hypothalamus (Olschowka *et al.*, 1982). Originally discovered by Saffran and Schally (1955) in hypothalamic extracts, CRF was sequenced 25 years later by Vale *et al.* (1981). CRF is the major physiological regulator of adrenocorticotropic hormone (ACTH), β-endorphin and other proopiomelanocortin (POMC)-derived peptides from the adenohypophysis (Rivier *et al.*, 1982), and also acts as a neurotransmitter in several extrahypothalamic brain areas (Smith *et al.*, 1986). Immunohistochemical and radioimmunoassay studies have shown that CRF is heterogeneously distributed in both hypothalamic and extrahypothalamic brain regions including the forebrain (frontal cortex, amygdala, stria terminalis) (Sawchenko & Swanson, 1985) and brainstem (e.g. locus coeruleus, parabrachial nucleus) (Chappell *et al.*, 1986).

The heterogeneous extrahypothalamic distribution of CRF receptors has been demonstrated both by autoradiographic and radioligand-binding techniques (DeSouza, 1987). It is partly because of its extrahypothalamic distribution in limbic areas that regulate emotionality, that CRF has been hypothesized to play a role in the pathogenesis of anxiety and affective disorders (Pihoker & Nemeroff, 1993).

Convergent lines of evidence support a role for CRF in the pathophysiology of affective and anxiety disorders. Intracerebroventricular (i.c.v.) administration of CRF induces behaviors in animals that resemble symptoms of depression and anxiety. For example, i.c.v. injections of CRF in rats cause a decreased food intake (Britton *et al.*, 1982), decreased sexual behaviour (Sirinathsinghju *et al.*, 1983), increases in locomotor activity (Britton *et al.*, 1986), and disruptions in normal sleep. These behavioral alterations have been suggested to be similar to many of the revised DSM-III signs and symptoms for major depression, and anxiety disorders (Pihoker & Nemeroff, 1993; Nemeroff, 1991).

Anxiety-related behaviors in response to i.c.v. CRF include an increased startle response (Swerdlow *et al.*, 1986), increased psychomotor agitation in familiar environments (Britton *et al.*, 1986), decreased exploratory behavior (Berridge & Dunn, 1987), and increased freezing (Berridge & Dunn, 1987) in novel environments in rats. Sympathoadrenal activation similar to that observed in posttraumatic stress disorder (Kosten *et al.*, 1987; Yehuda *et al.*, 1990*b*) is also enhanced following injection of CRF. Specifically, CRF injection increases both brain norepinephrine turnover (Berridge & Dunn, 1987) and peripheral epinephrine and norepinephrine secretion, and results in increases in heart rate and blood pressure (Brown 1986; Fisher *et al.*, 1983). It is of interest that many of the anxiogenic effects of CRF can be reversed by clinically effective anxiolytics, such as chlordiazepoxide (Britton *et al.*, 1985). Furthermore, the $\beta$-adrenergic antagonist propranolol can reverse CRF-stimulated increases in anxiety in response to conditioned emotional stress (Cole & Koob, 1988).

Another line of evidence supporting a role for CRF in the pathogenesis of anxiety disorders is that CRF produces effects in brain areas believed to be directly involved in the pathophysiology of these diseases. For example, CRF has been shown to increase the neuronal firing rate of noradrenergic neurones (Valentino & Foote, 1987), as well as norepinephrine turnover (Butler *et al.*, 1990*a*) after direct microinjection in the locus coeruleus. Noradrenergic neurones in this region mediate behavioral activation to stress, and have been implicated in the pathophysiology of both affective and anxiety disorders (Redmond & Huang, 1979). The finding that CRF increases noradrenergic neuronal firing in this region suggests that CRF may mediate not only the neuroendocrine activation, but also the behavioral arousal in response to stress. Furthermore, alterations in local coeruleus activity in affective and anxiety disorders may in part be secondary to increased CRF secretion. Indeed, there is evidence from preclinical studies that CRF neuronal systems are altered following both acute and chronic stress; in fact, CRF concentrations are markedly increased in the locus coeruleus after stress (Chappell *et al.*, 1986). Because noradrenergic projections from the locus coeruleus innervate many brain areas in the forebrain, it is plausible that increased noradrenergic activation in response to CRF hypersecretion could be involved in the pathophysiology of affective and anxiety symptoms in humans.

The preclinical data clearly support the hypothesis that increased CRF synaptic availability may occur in affective and/or anxiety disorders. This hypothesis is also rendered plausible by the evidence of increased hyperactivity of the HPA axis in depressive disorders, and increased activation of the locus coeruleus in anxiety disorders (i.e. specifically, panic disorder and PTSD), both phenomena likely mediated by CRF.

That hyperactivity of the HPA axis occurs in approximately 40–60% of patients with major depressive disorders has been one of the most often replicated findings in biological psychiatry. This hyperactivity is manifested by increased basal plasma cortisol concentrations (Sachar *et al.*, 1973), increased urinary free cortisol excretion (Carroll *et al.*, 1976), and a decreased number of lymphocyte glucocorticoid receptors (Whalley *et al.*, 1986). Depressed patients show a high rate of cortisol non-suppression in response to dexamethasone (Evans & Nemeroff, 1983), and a blunted ACTH response to exogenously administered CRF (Gold & Chrousos, 1985; Kilts *et al.* 1987).

CRF concentrations in the CSF have now been measured in several separate studies. While measurements of peptide concentrations alone are insufficient to determine whether changes in synthesis, storage, or release are present, they do likely represent alterations in the activity of peptide-containing neurones and/or altered clearance. Nemeroff *et al.* (1984) were the first to report CSF CRF-like immunoreactivity in depressed patients compared to healthy subjects, schizophrenics and demented patients. Subsequently, in five additional studies, the finding of increased CRF concentrations in the CSF of depressed patients has been confirmed (for a review see Owens & Nemeroff, 1993). Furthermore, Nemeroff *et al.* (1991) determined that the elevation in CSF of CRF concentrations in depression was most likely state-dependent. Whereas depressed patients showed an elevated CSF level of CRF prior to electroconvulsive therapy (ECT), CSF concentrations of CRF were decreased 24 h following their final ECT treatment.

Although the findings of increased CSF concentrations of CRF in depression are of interest and consistent with a role for CRF hypersecretion in affective disorders, it is important to recognize the fact that CSF measures represent a relatively crude sampling of overall brain CRF function. Thus, these CSF measures, in and of themselves, are not informative in localizing the specific CRF neural circuits that may be responsible for the increased CSF levels of CRF in depression. For example, the proportion in CSF of CRF that derives from extrahypothalamic CRF-containing neurones is unclear.

Further verification of increased CRF secretion in depression has come from post-mortem studies of CRF receptor density in suicide victims. Nemeroff *et al.* (1988) demonstrated a 23% decrease in CRF receptor number in the frontal cortex of 26 suicide completers compared with 28 control subjects.

Given the plethora of preclinical information suggesting that CRF in the locus coeruleus can mediate anxiety-related symptoms (see above), it is plausible to hypothesize that CSF concentrations of CRF in patients with generalized anxiety and/or PTSD would be increased, especially when patients are symptomatic. We have not observed increases in CSF concentrations of CRF in patients with panic disorder (Jokonninen *et al.*, 1993). However, data from test studies of CRF stimulation in PTSD have tended to support the idea of increased CRF secretion in anxiety disorders. These are described below.

The CRF-stimulation test has been utilized in the study of depression, primarily as a tool to scrutinize the mechanism responsible for the hypercortisolemia commonly observed in this disorder. When administered intravenously, CRF (1 μg/kg) produces a robust ACTH and cortisol response in normal humans (Schuemeyer *et al.*, 1984). In drug-free patients with major depressive disorder, the ACTH response to CRF is attenuated (Gold *et al.*, 1984; Holsboer *et al.*, 1984). While the exact mechanism leading to the blunted pituitary response in depression is not known, one explanation for this phenomenon is that the attenuated ACTH secretion is a result of a decreased pituitary responsiveness to CRF caused by long-term hypersecretion of CRF from the median eminence, and resultant downregulation of anterior pituitary CRF receptors. A second explanation that has been invoked to explain the blunted ACTH response to CRF, is that of an increased negative feedback inhibition of the pituitary corticotroph secondary to hypercortisolemia. Although the blunted ACTH response to CRF plausibly could be secondary to hypercortisolemia, recent findings cast doubt on this theory. Von Bardeleben & Holsboer (1989) and our group (Krishnan & Nemeroff, personal communication) found that depressed patients, unlike normal controls, continued to exhibit an ACTH and cortisol response to CRF if pretreated with high doses of dexamethasone. If the blunted pituitary–adrenal response to CRF occurred because of hypercortisolemia and increased negative feedback, pretreatment with dexamethasone would have abolished the ACTH and cortisol responses to CRF. Thus, the blunted ACTH response to CRF in depression likely reflects pituitary densensitization secondary to hypothalamic CRF hypersecretion.

In patients with panic disorder (Roy-Byrne *et al.*, 1986) and PTSD (Smith *et al.*, 1989), the ACTH response to CRF is also blunted. However, the mechanisms underlying this effect may well be distinct from the mechanism described above for major depressive disorder, primarily because these patients do not exhibit chronic HPA axis hyperactivity. In panic disorder, cortisol secretion has been reported to be either normal (Liebowitz *et al.*, 1985) or increased (Goldstein *et al.*, 1987). However, the cortisol response to dexamethasone has consistently been reported to be normal (Goldstein *et al.*, 1987). In PTSD, recent evidence suggests that, in contrast to depression, there is decreased activity of the HPA axis (Yehuda *et al.*, 1991*b*) as evidenced by low baseline urinary cortisol excretion (Mason *et al.*, 1986; Yehuda *et al.*, 1990*a*), an increased number of lymphocyte glucocorticoid receptors (Yehuda *et al.*, 1991*b*), and an exaggerated inhibitory cortisol response (i.e. supersuppression) to dexamethasone (Yehuda *et al.*, 1991*a*). In panic disorder and PTSD, the attenuated ACTH response to CRF in the absence of hypercortisolemia may be due to hyperresponsiveness of the pituitary gland to normal circulating concentrations of cortisol resulting directly from an increased number of glucocorticoid receptors on the adenohypophysis. Further studies examining glucocorticoid receptors in anxiety and affective disorders are clearly warranted to determine the extent to which major depression and each of the anxiety disorders are similar in regards to HPA axis abnormalities.

Cholecystokinin (CCK), a gut–brain peptide containing 33 amino acid residues, also exists in tetrapeptide and octapeptide forms. Long known to be a gastrointestinal peptide, CCK was discovered to exist in the CNS only recently (Vanderhaegen *et al.*, 1981). CCK has now been localized in several brain regions, including the cerebral cortex, amygdala, and hippocampus (Reeve *et al.*, 1984), and, importantly, is colocalized with other neurotransmitters, particularly dopamine in the midbrain.

Although earlier studies focused on a role for CCK in satiety, nociception, and schizophrenia, recent evidence suggests that this peptide may be involved in anxiety disorders. Preclinical studies have shown that microiontophoretic application of both CCK-8 and CCK-r results in electrophysiological excitation in several brain regions and these effects are reversed by benzodiazepines (Bradwejn & de Montigny, 1984). CCK administration in the amygdala was found to produce anxiety in behavioral paradigms (Hendrie & Dourish, 1990).

CCK-produced symptoms of anxiety (de Montigny, 1989) and actual panic attacks (Bradwejn *et al.*, 1990, 1991) both in normal controls and in patients with panic disorder. Patients with panic disorder are unusually susceptible to the anxiogenic effects of this peptide. It remains to be determined whether endogenous CCK neuronal activity is abnormally altered in panic disorder, and the extent to which the finding of an enhanced sensitivity to the anxiogenic effects of CCK is specific to this psychiatric disorder.

The differences between major depressive disorders and PTSD have been documented in studies of the HPA axis (see above). An interesting question that arises concerns the similarities between PTSD and other anxiety disorders such as panic disorder. There is evidence to suggest similarities between panic disorder and PTSD in noradrenergic dysregulation. Thus, Southwick *et al.* (1991) reported an increased incidence of panic attacks in patients with panic disorder and those with PTSD following intravenous (i.v.) infusion of the $\alpha_2$-antagonist yohimbine. A subset of patients with PTSD also reported experiencing flashbacks during the yohimbine infusion.

Clearly, further studies of neuropeptide and monoaminergic dysregulation in patients with PTSD is warranted.

## Psychophysiological reactions

As for many anxiety disorders, increased arousal is one of the prominent characteristics of PTSD. The revised edition of DSM-III (American Psychiatric Association, 1980) lists symptoms of increased arousal in PTSD, including sleep disturbance, irritability and anger, difficulty concentrating, hypervigilance, exaggerated startle response, and physiological reactivity to reminders of the traumatic event.

Psychophysiological studies of most of these symptoms of increased arousal in PTSD sufferers are scarce, despite the fact that a minimum of two arousal symptoms are required for a PTSD diagnosis. Laboratory documentation is lacking for sleep disturbance (Ross *et al.*, 1989), irritability, distractability, and hypervigilance, even though they are common symptoms of PTSD. Although the exaggerated startle response has been studied, the results provide equivocal evidence for increased reactivity. Physiological reactions to reminders of the trauma have been the only symptom repeatedly tested and demonstrated in the laboratory.

### *Startle reactions*

Psychophysiological studies of startle responses in PTSD present a mixed picture. Combat veterans with PTSD were found to have larger eyeblink startle responses to unsignalled stimuli than did controls (Butler *et al.*, 1990*b*). Traumatized children actually demonstrated smaller eyeblinks than non-traumatized controls, with an unsignalled acoustic stimulus (Ornitz & Pynoos, 1989). The traumatized children showed less startle inhibition with brief prestimulus signals and more startle facilitation with long prestimulus signals. However, another study of combat veterans found no difference in habituation of the startle response between PTSD and control subjects (Ross *et al.*, 1989). Such equivocal results measuring startle reactions are likely attributable to differences in the paradigms used to study the phenomenon. Although it is impossible to describe the typical effect on the startle reaction of trauma, based on the current state of knowledge, it is definitely worthy of future study.

### *Cardiac, electrodermal and muscular reactions to reminders*

Physiological hyperresponsiveness of combat veterans with PTSD to stimuli associated with their trauma has been well documented (Blanchard *et al.*, 1982, 1986; Malloy *et al.*, 1983; Pallmeyer *et al.*, 1986; Pitman *et al.*, 1987, 1990). Combat veterans with PTSD were compared to different groups including veterans without PTSD, non-veterans, and psychiatric patients without PTSD, and were exposed to audiotaped combat sounds or videotaped combat scenes. In general, veterans with PTSD were more reactive on cardiac, electrodermal, cardiovascular, and/or muscular measures than controls in response to trauma-specific stimuli but not to general fear stimuli.

In a typical paradigm, Blanchard *et al.* (1982) compared Vietnam veterans with PTSD to matched non-veteran controls on heart rate (HR), blood pressure (BP), forehead muscle activity (EMG), skin resistance level (SRL), and peripheral temperature. Measures were taken during baseline periods, mental arithmetic tests (non-combat stressor), rest (return to baseline), music, and increasing intensities of combat sounds. PTSD individuals were more reactive than normal controls to auditory presentations of combat sounds as measured by HR, systolic BP, and forehead EMG. Blanchard *et al.* (1986) replicated these findings with regards to HR using a similar paradigm comparing Vietnam combat veterans with PTSD to veterans without any disorder. Differences in HR, systolic and diastolic BP, SRL, and frontal EMG between Vietnam combat veterans with and without PTSD during presentation of combat sounds were also found by Gerardi *et al.* (1989). Similarly, Malloy *et al.* (1983) compared Vietnam veterans with and without PTSD to psychiatric inpatients without PTSD and found the subjects with PTSD more reactive on HR and skin-resistance responses to videotapes of combat scenes and sounds than the comparison groups.

In a different paradigm, Vietnam veterans with and without PTSD were compared on skin conductance response (SCR) in response to stress words related to Vietnam (e.g. 'kill', 'Nam', 'jungle'), words phonetically related to the stress words (e.g. 'kin' 'none', 'junkyard'), and neutral words (e.g. 'mix', 'brief', 'shop') (McNally *et al.*, 1987). The veterans with PTSD exhibited enhanced SCRs in response to the stress words as compared to the other target words and compared to the group without PTSD. However, in a similar paradigm, Trandel & McNally (1987) failed to replicate the above study, finding no differences between Vietnam combat veterans with PTSD and non-combat veterans without PTSD on SCR in response to any category of stimulus word.

The specificity of this hyperresponsiveness to traumatic material has been further demonstrated by Pitman *et al.* (1987). Vietnam combat veterans with PTSD were more reactive than normal combat veteran controls on skin conductance and forehead EMG to imagery of their individualized combat experiences, but not to other non-PTSD-related stressful imagery. Moreover, anxiety-disordered combat veterans without PTSD were *not* hyperresponsive to their combat imagery (Pitman *et al.*, 1990). It is interesting to note that the veterans with PTSD were significantly more responsive (on SCR, EMG, trend for HR) than their anxiety-disordered counterparts, but only to their individualized combat scripts and not to standardized combat scripts or general fear scripts.

All of the above studies collected autonomic data after the trauma, so it is possible that people who developed PTSD had higher tonic arousal prior to the trauma and that such arousal may have predisposed them to developing the disorder. In order to explore this hypothesis, Pitman *et al.* (unpublished data) examined military records of inductees' pulse rates and blood pressure prior to combat activity and related it to their later PTSD status. They found that combat veterans with PTSD were no more aroused on these measures prior to their traumatic combat events than were veterans, without PTSD, indicating that the increased autonomic arousal is a response to the trauma rather than an individual trait or cause for PTSD.

### *Chronic increased arousal*

Several experiments have focused on tonic autonomic activity in PTSD combat veterans, with equivocal results. Veterans with PTSD have been found to have elevated tonic HR and BP (Blanchard *et al.*, 1986; Pitman *et al.*, 1987), whereas in other studies base levels were not significantly elevated in PTSD (Malloy *et al.*, 1983; Pitman *et al.*, 1990). Several studies have failed to find baseline differences between PTSD Vietnam combat veterans and normal combat veteran controls (Malloy *et al.*, 1983; Pitman *et al.*, 1987), anxiety-disordered combat veterans without PTSD (Pitman *et al.*, 1990), and psychiatric inpatients without PTSD (Malloy *et al.*, 1983). In yet two other studies the means appeared higher for PTSD, but statistical tests were not reported (Blanchard *et al.*, 1982; Pallmeyer *et al.*, 1986). In female rape victims with PTSD, compared to victims without PTSD and non-victimized controls, the resting-level HR tended to be highest for the PTSD group, and the number of spontaneous fluctuations lowest, but these apparent differences were not statistically significant (Kozak *et al.*, unpublished data). Davidson & Baum (1986) found that individuals living within 8 kilometers of the Three Mile Island nuclear power station had elevated HR and BP as compared to controls living 80 miles away. The inconsistencies among the results suggest that elevations in basal physiological activity may not occur in all sufferers from PTSD.

One hypothesis that has been put forward to account for these inconsistent findings concerns the presumed phasic shifting between periods of increased arousal and periods of numbing (van der Kolk, 1984). It is possible that individuals tested during a numb phase would not appear more aroused than controls, but those same individuals tested during an aroused phase would demonstrate increased arousal when compared to controls. This phasic shifting has not been taken into account in physiological studies of PTSD to this point, resulting in likely methodological errors contributing to differences in findings.

### *Impaired physiological habituation*

It appears that tendencies for elevated autonomic hyperreactivity in response to fear-relevant stimuli characterize victims with chronic PTSD, but not traumatized individuals without PTSD. One possible mechanism to account for this difference is an impaired capacity for physiological habituation. Foa *et al.* (1989) hypothesized that failure to habituate to routine encounters with situations that evoke traumatic memories could account in part for the persistence of PTSD. To explore this hypothesis, habituation of autonomic reactions to auditory tones in rape survivors with and without PTSD and a non-victimized control group were compared. On two measures of electrodermal activity (i.e. number of trials to habituation and percentage of non-habituators in each group), the PTSD group showed less habituation than the other two groups. The PTSD group had significantly more trials to extinction than the other groups, and the percentage of non-habituators was significantly higher for the PTSD group than for the other two groups. Overall HR acceleration to the tones was higher for the two assault groups than for the non-victim control group. Although the PTSD and non-PTSD individuals appeared to show more trials to habituation than the non-victims, these differences were not statistically significant. This resistance to habituation may account for the increased physiological arousal found in other studies of PTSD, particularly with male combat veterans.

## Affective reactions

### *Rape trauma syndrome*

Burgess & Holmstrom (1974) described a two-phase reaction to rape, consisting of an acute phase and a reorganization phase, which they termed 'rape trauma syndrome' The acute phase, characterized by disorganization lasting from several hours to several weeks, included both 'impact reactions' (e.g. shock, disbelief) and 'somatic reactions' (e.g. physical trauma). The reorganization phase was depicted as a long-term process of active lifestyle changes (e.g. changing residences) and long-term chronic disturbances such as nightmares and fears.

### *Anxiety and depression*

The most incessant reactions documented following rape appear to be intense fears of rape-related situations and general diffuse anxiety, having been noted up to 16 years postassault (Ellis *et al.*, 1981; Kilpatrick *et al.*, 1981; Calhoun *et al.*, 1982). In one study, only 23% of victims were asymptomatic at 1 year after rape on fear measures (Veronen & Kilpatrick, 1982). Similarly, in another study, although victims' fearfulness declined somewhat over time, they remained more fearful than non-victim controls one year postassault (Calhoun *et al.*, 1982). While depression is also a common reaction to rape, it appears to be less persistent (Frank *et al.*, 1979; Kilpatrick *et al.*, 1979; Atkeson *et al.*, 1982; Frank & Stewart, 1984). Nevertheless, a sizeable percentage of the post-Vietnam PTSD patients exhibit comorbid major depression.

### *Anger*

Anger has been repeatedly observed in rape and crime victims and war veterans with PTSD (Kilpatrick *et al.*, 1981; Lee & Rosenthal, 1983; Yassen & Glass, 1984; Hyer *et al.*, 1986; Woolfolk & Grady, 1988). In a prospective study, 116 rape and crime victims were compared to a matched non-victimized control group ($N = 50$) on measures of anger and anger expression (Riggs *et al.*, unpublished data). Results indicated that in general, victims were angrier than non-victims. Certain assault variables, such as the use of a weapon and the victim's response to the attack, predicted the anger response. In addition, it was found that elevated anger predicted the development of PTSD. The authors speculate that intense anger may interfere with the modification of the traumatic memory by inhibiting fear responses that would lead to habituation and by allowing the victim to avoid feelings of anxiety. That is, the victims who are more prone to experience anger than anxiety would not have the opportunity to confront fearful situations and have that fear decrease (habituate), which thereby leaves the anxiety-provoking cues and responses unchanged.

***Dissociation***

Dissociation is described as a 'disturbance or alteration in the normally integrative functions of identity, memory, or consciousness' (American Psychiatric Association, 1980, p. 269). Mild forms of dissociation are common, such as driving along a familiar route and realizing that you have not been paying attention to where you were driving (being on 'automatic pilot'). The most extreme form of dissociation recognized in the revised edition of DSM-III is multiple personality disorder (MPD) described as 'the existence within the person of two or more distinct personality or personality states (American Psychiatric Association, 1980, p. 269). A continuum of pathology lies between these two extremes.

It is commonly held that dissociation in the more extreme forms is the result of trauma (Putnam, 1985). As a coping mechanism, dissociation serves psychologically to remove the individual from an extremely aversive event when physical escape appears impossible. Wartime dissociative phenomena, especially psychogenic amnesia and psychogenic fugue reactions, have been estimated to be present in from 5% to 14% of all psychiatric combat patients (Sargent & Slater, 1941; Grinker & Spiegel, 1943; Henderson & Moore, 1944; Torrie, 1944; Fisher, 1945), in some cases, finding a direct relationship between the degree of combat-induced stress and the degree of dissociation. In a study of 100 MPD cases, 97% were found to have experienced significant childhood trauma (Putnam *et al.*, 1986). The most commonly reported trauma was incest (68%), followed by physical abuse, physical and sexual abuse combined, extreme neglect, witness to violent death, other abuses, and extreme poverty. Individuals with PTSD scored almost as high as individuals with MPD on a measure of dissociation (Bernstein & Putnam, 1986). In that sample, the PTSD sufferers scored higher than patients with alcohol dependence, anxiety disorders, and schizophrenia, and normal subjects including adolescents. In a prospective study, adult female rape and non-sexual assault victims with and without PTSD were compared for dissociation (Dancu *et al.*, 1990). Victims with PTSD scored significantly higher than victims without PTSD on measures of dissociation, intrusion, avoidance and assault-related distress. Higher levels of dissociation were related to greater levels of post-assault distress.

At this time, the causal role of dissociation in PTSD is unclear. It is possible that a tendency to dissociate predisposes traumatized individuals to develop PTSD by inhibiting the emotional processing of the traumatic material. On the other hand, individuals with PTSD may tend to dissociate as a coping response to intrusive images and fears. It has been proposed that PTSD is, in fact, a disorder that falls somewhere between anxiety disorders and dissociative disorders (Foa *et al.*, 1992).

## Conclusion

Perhaps what is most remarkable is how little we know about the long-term consequences, either psychological or neurobiological, of trauma, either acute or chronic. The most important information we currently lack is that from long-term longitudinal studies of both psychological and biological alterations in patients who have been exposed to trauma. In addition, we know very little about the effects of different types of trauma; for example, virtually nothing is known about the trauma associated with miscarriage in pregnant women. It is evident that the area of comorbidity of posttraumatic stress disorder and other psychiatric and medical entities is an important avenue for study. This includes drug and alcohol abuse, preexisting affective disorder, vulnerability to affective disorder (i.e. patients with a marked family history) and comorbidity of post-traumatic stress disorder with medical illnesses such as cardiovascular disease, cancer, diabetes, etc. We know little about the genetics of susceptibility to trauma, though it seems rather evident that genetics plays an important role. Similarly, the role of prior experience, both positive and negative, needs to be systematically explored. Although considerable attention has been paid to categorical measures, relatively few studies have focused on validated dimensional measures of either the nature of the trauma or the nature of the dysfunction after the trauma; indeed, it is evident that new rating scales will have to be developed. Such activities are being pursued, for example, by the National Center for PTSD in the USA, funded by the Veterans' Administration Medical Centers.

Last, and perhaps most important, is the issue of treatment. We know very little about psychopharmacological management of these patients, and clinical experience thus far indicates that patients who have sustained severe trauma do not do terribly well with standard antidepressant or anxiolytic treatment. Although certain psychological therapies seem promising, the combination of pharmacotherapy and psychotherapy in this population of patients has not been systematically studied to a similar extent as that to which such combination therapies have been scrutinized in patients with unipolar depression. The advent of new tools to study biological alterations, such as functional and structural brain imaging, coupled with advances in both nosology and the measurement of treatment response, suggests that rapid advances are possible in this field.

## References

American Psychiatric Association (1980). *Diagnostic and Statistical Manual of Mental Disorders*, 3rd edn, revised. Washington, DC: American Psychiatric Association.

Atkeson, B., Calhoun, K., Resick, P. & Ellis, E. (1982). Victims of rape: repeated assessment of depressive symptoms. *J. Consult. Clin. Psychol.*, **50**, 96–102.

Baum, A., Gatchel, R. J. & Schaeffer, M. A. (1983). Emotional, behavioral, and physiological effects of chronic stress at Three Mile Island. *J. Consult. Clin. Psychol.*, **41**, 565–72.

Bernstein, E. M. & Putnam, F. W. (1986). Development, reliability and validity of a dissociation scale. *J. Nerv. Ment. Dis.*, **174**, 727–34.

Berridge, C. W. & Dunn, A. J. (1987). A corticotropin-releasing factor antagonist reverses the stress-induced changes of exploratory behavior in mice, *Horm. Behav.*, **21**, 393–401.

Blanchard, E. B., Kolb, L. C., Gerardi, R. J., Ryan, D. & Pallmeyer, T. P. (1986). Cardiac response to relevant stimuli as an adjunctive tool for diagnosing post-traumatic stress disorder in Vietnam veterans. *Behav. Ther.*, **17**, 592–606.

Blanchard, E. B., Kolb, L. C., Pallmeyer, T. P. & Gerardi, R. J. (1982). A psychophysiological study of post-traumatic stress disorder in Vietnam veterans. *Psychiatr. Q.*, **54**, 220–9.

Bradwejn, J. & De Montigny, C. (1984). Benzodiazepines antagonize cholecystokinin-induced activation of rat hippocampal neurons. *Nature*, **312**, 363–4.

Bradwejn, J., Koszychi, D. & Meterissian, G. (1990). Cholecystokinin tetrapeptide induces panic attacks in patients with panic disorder, *Can. J. Psychiatry*, **38**, 83–5.

Bradwejn, J., Koszychi, D. & Shriqui, C. (1991). Enhanced sensitivity of cholecystokinin tetrapeptide in panic disorder: clinical and behavioral findings, *Arch. Gen. Psychiatry*, **48**, 603–10.

Bravo, M., Rubio-Stipec, M., Canino, G. J., Woodbury, M. A. & Ribera, J. C. (1990). The psychological sequelae of disaster stress prospectively and retrospectively evaluated. *Am. J. Community Psychol.*, **18**, 661–80.

Britton, D. R., Koob, G. F., Rivier, J. & Vale, W. (1982). Intraventricular corticotropin-releasing factor enhances behavioral effects of novelty, *Life Sci.*, **363**–7.

Britton, K. T., Lee, G., Vale, W. *et al.* (1986). Corticotropin-releasing factor (CRF) receptor antagonist blocks activating and anxiogenic actions of CRF in the rat. *Brain Res.*, **369**, 303–6.

Britton, K. T., Morgan, J., Rivier, J. *et al.* (1985). Chlordiazepoxide attenuates response suppression induced by corticotropin-releasing factor in the conflict test. *Psychopharmacology*, **86**, 170–4.

Bromet, E. J., Hough, L. & Connell, M. (1984). Mental health of children near

the Three Mile Island reactor. *J. Prev. Psychiatry*, **2**, 275–301.
Brown, M. R. (1986). Corticotropin-releasing factor: central nervous system sites of action. *Brain Res.*, **399**, 10–14.
Burgess, A. W. & Holmstrom, L. L. (1974). The rape trauma syndrome. *Am. J. Psychiatry*, **131**, 981–6.
Burstein, A., Ciccone, P. E., Greenstein, R. A., Daniels, N., Olsen, K., Mazarek, A., Decatur, R. & Johnson, N. (1988). Chronic Vietnam PTSD and acute civilian PTSD: a comparison of treatment experiences. *Gen. Hosp. Psychiatry*, **10**, 245–9.
Butler, P. D. & Nemeroff, C. B. (1990). Corticotropin-releasing-factor as a possible cause of comorbidity in anxiety and depressive disorders. In *Comorbidity of Mood and Anxiety Disorders*, ed. J. D. Maser & C. R. Cloniger, pp. 413–38. Washington, DC: American Psychiatric Press.
Butler, P. D., Weiss, J. M., Stout, J. C. & Nemeroff, C. B. (1990*a*). Corticotropin-releasing-factor produces fear-enhancing and behavioral activation effects following infusion into the locus coeruleus. *J. Neurosci.*, **10**, 176–83.
Butler, R. W., Braff, D. L., Rausch, J. L., Jenkins, M. A., Sproch, J. & Geyer, M. A. (1990*b*). Physiological evidence of exaggerated startle response in a subgroup of Vietnam veterans with combat related PTSD. *Am. J. Psychiatry*, **147**, 1308–12.
Cairns, E. & Wilson, R. (1984). The impact of political violence on mild psychiatric morbidity in Northern Ireland. *Br. J. Psychiatry*, **145**, 631–5.
Calhoun, K. S., Atkeson, B. M. & Resick, P. A. (1982). A longitudinal examination of fear reactions in victims. *J. Counsel. Psychology*, **29**, 655–61.
Carroll, B. J., Curtis, G. C., Davies, B. M. *et al.* (1976). Urinary free cortisol excretion in depression. *Psychol. Med.*, **6**, 43–50.
Chappell, P. B., Smith, M. A., Kilts, C. D. *et al.* (1986). Alterations in corticotropin-releasing factor-like immunoreactivity in discrete rat brain regions after acute and chronic stress. *J. Neurosci.*, **6**, 2908–14.
Cole, B. J. & Koob, G. F. (1988). Propranolol antagonizes the enhanced conditioned fear produced by corticotropin-releasing factor. *J. Pharmacol. Exp. Ther.*, **247**, 902–10.
Dancu, C., Rothbaum, B. O., Riggs, D. & Foa, E. (1990). The relationship between dissociation and PTSD. Poster presented at the *23rd Annual Convention of the Association for the Advancement of Behavior Therapy*, November, San Francisco, CA.
Davidson, L. M. & Baum, A. (1986). Chronic stress and post-traumatic stress disorders. *J. Consult. Clin. Psychol.*, **54**, 303–8.
de Montigny, C. (1989). Cholecystokinin-4 tetrapeptide induces panic-like attacks in healthy volunteers: preliminary findings. *Arch. Gen. Psychiatry*, **46**, 511–17.
DeSouza, E. B. (1987). Corticotropin-releasing factor receptors in the rat central nervous system: characterization and regional distribution. *J. Neurosci.*, **7**, 88–100.
Ellis, E. M., Atkeson, B. M. & Calhoun, K. S. (1981). An assessment of long-term reaction to rape. *J. Abnormal Psychol*, **90**, 263–66.
Evans, D. L. & Nemeroff, C. B. (1983). Use of the dexamethasone suppression test using DSM-III criteria on an inpatient psychiatric unit. *Biol. Psychiatry*, **18**, 505–11.
Fisher, C. (1945). Amnestic states in war neuroses: the psychogenesis of fugues. *Psychoanal. Q.*, **14**, 437–68.

Fisher, L. A., Jesson, G. & Brown, M. R. (1983). Corticotropin-releasing-factor: mechanisms to elevate mean arterial pressure and heart rate, *Regul. Pept.*, **5**, 153–61.

Foa, E. B., Steketee, G. & Rothbaum, B. O. (1989). Behavioral–cognitive conceptualization of post-traumatic stress disorder. *Behav. Ther.*, **20**, 155–76.

Foa, E. B., Zinbarg, R. & Rothbaum, B. O. (1992). Uncontrollability and unpredictability in PTSD: an animal model. *Psychol. Bull.*, **112**, 218–38.

Frank, E. & Stewart, B. D. (1984). Depressive symptoms in rape victims. *J. Affective Disord.*, **1**, 269–77.

Frank, E., Turner, S. M. & Duffy, B. (1979). Depressive symptoms in rape victims. *J. Affect. Dis.*, **1**, 269–77.

Gerardi, R. J., Blanchard, E. B. & Kolb, L. C. (1989). Ability of Vietnam veterans to dissimulate a psychophysiological assessment for PTSD. *Behav. Ther.*, **20**, 229–44.

Gold, P. W. & Chrousos, P. (1985). Clinical studies with corticotropin-releasing factor: implications for the diagnosis and pathophysiology of depression, Cushing's disease and adrenal insufficiency. *Psychoneuroendocrinology*, **10**, 401–19.

Gold, P. W., Chrousos, G., Kellner, C. *et al.* (1984). Psychiatric implications of basic and clinical studies with corticotropin-releasing factor. *Am. J. Psychiatry*, **141**, 619–27.

Goldberg, D. P. (1972). *The Detection of Psychiatric Illness by Questionnaire.* London: Oxford University Press.

Goldstein, S., Halbreich, U., Asnis, G. *et al.* (1987). The hypothalamic–pituitary–adrenal system in panic disorder. *Am. J. Psychiatry*, **144**, 1320–5.

Green, B. L., Grace, M. C., Lindy, J. D., Gleser, G. C., Leonard, A. C. & Kramer, T. L. (1990). Buffalo Creek survivors in the second decade: comparison with unexposed and nonlitigant groups. *J. Appl. Soc. Psychology*, **20**, 1033–50.

Green, B. L., Korol, M., Grace, M. C., Vary, M. G., Leonard, A. C., Gleser, G. C. & Smitson-Cohen, S. (1991). Children and disaster: age, gender, and parental effects on PTSD symptoms. *J. Am. Acad. Child Adolesc. Psychiatry*, **30**, 945–51.

Grinker, R. R. & Spiegel, J. P. (1943). *War Neuroses in North Africa.* New York: Josiah Macy, Jr., Foundation.

Grinker, R. R. & Spiegel, J. P. (1945). *Men under Stress.* Philadelphia, Blakistan.

Henderson, J. L. & Moore, M. (1944). The psychoneuroses of war. *New England J. Med.*, **230**, 273–9.

Hendrie, C. A. & Dourish, C. T. (1990). Anxiolytic profile of the cholecystokinin antagonist devazepide in mice. *Brit. J. Pharmacol.*, **99**(Suppl.), 138.

Hokfelt, T., Everitt, B. J., Theodorsson-Norheim, T. *et al.* (1984). Neurotensin and NPT-like immunoreactivities in central catecholamine neurons. In *Neuropharmacology and Central Nervous System: Theoretical Aspects*, ed. E. Usdin, A. Carlsson & A. Dahlstron, pp. 231–7. New York: Alan R. Liss.

Holsboer, F., vonBardeleben, U., Gerken, A. *et al.* (1984). Blunted corticotropin and normal cortisol responses to human corticotropin-releasing factor in depression. *New Engl. J. Med.*, **311**, 1127.

Hyer, L., O'Leary, W. C., Saucer, R. T., Blount, J., Harrison, W. R. & Boudewyns, P. A. (1986). Inpatient diagnosis of posttreatment stress disorder. *J. Consult. Clin. Psychol.*, **54**, 698–702.

Jokonninen, J., Lepola, U., Bissette, G., Nomeroff, C. B. & Rickinen, P. (1993). CSF corticotropin-releasing factor is not affected in panic disorder. *Biol. Psychiatry*, **33**, 136–8.

Kilpatrick, D. G., Amick, A. & Resnick, H. S. (1988). Preliminary research data on post-traumatic stress disorder following murders and drunk driving crashes. Presented at the *14th Annual Meeting of the National Organization for Victim Assistance*, September, Tucson, Arizona.

Kilpatrick, D. G., Resick, P. A. & Veronen, L. J. (1981). Effects of a rape experience: a longitudinal study. *J. Soc. Issues*, **37**, 105–22.

Kilpatrick, D. G., Saunders, B., Amick-McMullan, A., Best, C., Veronen, L. & Resnick, H. (1989). Victim and crime factors associated with the development of post-traumatic stress disorder. *Behav. Ther.*, **20**, 199–214.

Kilpatrick, D. G., Saunders, B. E., Veronen, L. J., Best, C. L. & Von, J. M. (1987). Criminal victimization: lifetime prevalence, reporting to police, and psychological impact. *Crime Delinquency*, **33**, 479–89.

Kilpatrick, D. G. & Veronen, L. J. (1984). *Treatment of Fear and Anxiety in Victims of Rape*, Final Report, Grant No. R01 MH29602. Rockville, MD: National Institute of Mental Health.

Kilpatrick, D. G., Veronen, L. J. & Resick, P. A. (1979). The aftermath of rape: recent empirical findings. *Am. J. Orthopsychiatry*, **49**, 658–9.

Kilts, C. D., Bissette, G., Krishnan, K. R. R. *et al.* (1987). The preclinical and clinical neurobiology of corticotropin-releasing factor (CRF). In *Hormones and Depression*, ed. U. Halbreich, pp. 297–311. New York: Raven Press.

Kosten, T. R., Mason, J. W., Giller, E. *et al.* (1987). Sustained urinary norepinephrine elevation in post-traumatic stress disorder, *Psychoneuroendocrinology*, **12**, 13–20.

Lee, J. A. B. & Rosenthal, S. J. (1983). Working with victims of violent assault. *J. Contemp. Soc. Work*, December, 593–601.

Liebowitz, M. R., Gorman, J. M., Fryer, A. J. *et al.* (1985). Lactate provocation of panic attacks. II. Biochemical and physiological findings. *Arch. Gen. Psychiatry*, **42**, 709–10.

Lindy, J. D., Green, B. L., Grace, M. & Titchener, J. (1983). Psychotherapy with survivors of the Beverly Hills Supper Club fire. *Am. J. Psychother.*, **4**, 593–610.

Malloy, P. E., Fairbank, J. A. & Keane, T. M. (1983). Validation of a multimethod assessment of post-traumatic stress disorder in Vietnam veterans. *J. Consult. Clin. Psychol.*, **51**, 488–94.

Mason, J. W., Giller, E. L., Kosten, T. R. *et al.* (1986). Urinary free cortisol levels in post traumatic stress disorder patients. *J. Nerv. Ment. Dis.*, **174**, 145–59.

McCahill, T. W., Meyer, L. C. & Fischman, A. M. (1979). *The Aftermath of Rape*. Lexington, MA: Health.

McFarlane, A. C. (1988*a*). The phenomenology of posttraumatic stress disorders following a natural disaster. *J. Nerv. Ment. Dis.*, **176**, 22–9.

McFarlane, A. C. (1988*b*). The longitudinal course of posttraumatic morbidity: the range of outcomes and their predictors. *J. Nerv. Ment. Dis.*, **176**, 30–9.

McNally, R. J., Luedke, D. L., Besyner, J. K., Peterson, R. A., Bohm, K. & Lips, O. J. (1987). Sensitivity to stress-relevant stimuli in PTSD. *J. Anxiety Disord.*, **1**, 105–116.

Muse, M. (1986). Stress-related, posttraumatic chronic pain syndrome: behavioral treatment approach. *Pain*, **25**, 389–94.

Nadelson, C. C., Notman, M. T., Zackson, H. & Gornick, J. (1982). A follow-up study of rape victims. *Am. J. Psychiatry*, **139**, 1266–70.

Nader, K., Pynoos, R., Fairbanks, L. & Frederick, C. (1990). Children's PTSD reactions one year after a sniper attack on their school. *Am. J. Psychiatry*, **147**, 1526–30.

Nemeroff, C. B. (1991). The neurobiology of neuropeptides: an introduction. In *Neuropeptides and Psychiatric Disorders*, ed. C. B. Nemeroff, pp. 3–14. Washington, DC: American Psychiatric Press.

Nemeroff, C. B. & Bissette, G. (1986). Neuropeptides in psychiatric disorders. In *American Handbook of Psychiatry*, ed. P. A. Berger & H. K. H. Brodie, pp. 64–110. New York, NY: Basic Books.

Nemeroff, C. B., Bissette, G., Akil, H. & Fink, M. (1991). Neuropeptide concentrations in the cerebrospinal fluid of depressed patients treated with electroconvulsive therapy: corticotropin-releasing factor, β-endorphin and somatostatin. *Br. J. Psychiatry*, **158**, 59–63.

Nemeroff, C. B., Owens, M. J., Widerlov, E., Bissette, G. *et al.* (1988). Reduced corticotropin-releasing factor binding sites in the frontal cortex of suicides. *Arch. Gen. Psychiatry*, **45**, 577–9.

Nemeroff, C. B., Widerlov, E., Bissette, G., *et al.* (1984). Elevated concentrations of CSF corticotropin-releasing factor-like immunoreactivity in depressed patients, *Science*, **226**, 1342–4.

Olschowka, J. A., O'Donhue, T. L. & Meuller, G. P. (1982). The distribution of CRF-like immunoreactive neurons in rat brain. *Neuroendocrinology*, **35**, 305–8.

Ornitz, E. M. & Pynoos, R. S. (1989). Startle modulation in children with post traumatic stress disorder. *Am. J. Psychiatry*, **146**, 866–70.

Owens, M. J. & Nemeroff, C. B. (1993). The role of CRF in the pathophysiology of affective disorders: laboratory and clinical studies. In *Corticotropin-releasing Factor*, CIBA Foundation Symposium 172, pp. 296–316. New York: John Wiley & Sons.

Pallmeyer, T. P., Blanchard, E. B. & Kolb, L. C. (1986). The psychophysiology of combat-induced post-traumatic stress disorder in Vietnam veterans. *Behav. Res. Ther.*, **24**, 645–52.

Pihoker, C. & Nemeroff, C. B. (1993). The role of corticotropin-releasing factor in the pathophysiology of anxiety disorders. In *Biology of Anxiety Disorders, Recent Developments*, Progress in Psychiatry, ed. H. Saric. APA Press.

Pitman, R. K., Orr, S. P., Forgue, D. F., Altman, B. & Herz, L. R. (1990). Psychophysiologic responses to combat imagery of Vietnam veterans with post-traumatic stress disorders vs. other anxiety disorders. *J. Abnorm. Psychol.*, **99**, 49–54.

Pitman, R. K., Orr, S. P., Forgue, D. F., deJong, J. B. & Claiborn, J. M. (1987). Psychophysiologic assessment of post-traumatic stress disorder imagery in Vietnam combat veterans. *Arch. Gen. Psychiatry*, **44**, 970–5.

Putnam, F. W. (1985). Dissociation as a response to extreme trauma. In *The Childhood Antecedents of Multiple Personality*, ed. R. P. Kluft. Washington, DC: American Psychiatric Press.

Putnam, F. W., Guroff, J. J., Silberman, E. K., Barban, L. & Post, R. M. (1986). The clinical phenomenology of multiple personality disorder: a review of 100 recent cases. *J. Clin. Psychiatry*, **47**, 285–93.

Putnam, J. J. (1881). Recent investigations into patients of so-called concussion of the spine. *Boston Med. Surg. J.*, **109**, 217.

Pynoos, R. S., Frederick, C., Nader, K., Arroyo, W., Steinberg, A., Eth, S.,

Nunez, F. & Fairbanks, L. (1987). Life threat and posttraumatic stress in school-age children. *Gen. Psychiatry*, **44**, 1057–63.
Rachman, S. (1989). *Fear and Courage*, 2nd edn. New York: W. H. Freeman.
Rado, S. (1942). Pathodynamics and treatment of traumatic war neurosis (traumatophobia). *Psychosom. Med.*, **42**, 363–8.
Redmond, D. E. Jr & Huang, Y. (1979). Current concepts. II. New evidence for a locus coeruleus-norepinephrine connection with anxiety. *Life Sci.*, **25**, 2149–62.
Reeve, J. R., Eysselein, V. E., Walsh, H. *et al.* (1984). Isolation and characterization of biologically active and inactive cholecystokinin octapeptide from human brain. *Peptides*, **5**, 459–66.
Resick, P. (1987). *Reactions of female and male victims of rape or robbery*, Final Report, Grant No. MH37296. Washington, DC: National Institute of Justice.
Rigler, R. (1879). Bever die Folgen der Verletzungen auf Eisenbahnen, inbesondere der Verletzungen des Ruckenmarks. In *Mit Hinblick auf das Haftpflichfgesetz dargestellf*, vol. VIII, p. 80. Berlin.
Rivier, C., Rivier, J. & Vale, W. (1982). Inhibition of adrenocorticotropic hormone secretion in the rat by immunoneutralization of corticotropin-releasing factor. *Science*, **218**, 377–8.
Robins, L. N., Helzer, J. C., Croughan, J. & Ratcliff, K. S. (1981). The NIMH Diagnostic Interview Schedule: its history, characteristics, and validity. *Arch. Gen. Psychiatry*, **38**, 381–9.
Ross, R. J., Ball, W. A., Sullivan, K. A. & Caroll, S. N. (1989). Sleep disturbances as the hallmark of post-traumatic stress disorder. *Am. J. Psychiatry*, **146**, 697–707.
Rothbaum, B. O., Foa, E. B., Murdock, T., Riggs, D. & Walsh, W. (1992). A prospective examination of post-traumatic stress disorder in rape victims. *J. Traum. Stress*, **5**, 455–75.
Roy-Byrne, P., Uhde, T. W., Post, R. M. *et al.* (1986). The corticotropin-releasing hormone stimulation test in patients with panic disorder. *Am. J. Psychiatry*, **143**, 896–9.
Sachar, E. J., Hellman, L., Roffwarg, H. *et al.* (1973). Disrupted 24-hr. patterns of cortisol secretion in psychotic depression. *Arch. Gen. Psychiatry*, **28**, 19–24.
Saffran, M. & Schally, A. V. (1955). Release of corticotropin by anterior pituitary tissue *in vitro*. *Can. J. Biochem. Physiol.*, **33**, 408–15.
Saigh, P. A. (1988). Anxiety, depression, and assertion across alternating intervals of stress. *J. Abnorm. Psychol.*, **97**, 338–41.
Sales, E., Baum, M. & Shore, B. (1984). Victim readjustment following assault. *J. Soc. Issues*, **40**, 17–36.
Sargent, W. & Slater, E. (1941). Amnestic syndromes in war. *Proc. Roy. Soc. Med.*, **34**, 757–64.
Sawchenko, P. E. & Swanson, L. W. (1985). Localization, colocalization and plasticity of corticotropin-releasing factor immunoreactivity in rat brain. *Fed. Proc.*, **44**, 221–7.
Schlenger, W. E., Kulka, R. A., Fairbank, J. A., Hough, R. L., Jordan, B. K., Marmar, C. R. & Weiss, D. S. (1992). The prevalence of post-traumatic stress disorder in the Vietnam generation: a multimethod, multisource assessment of psychiatric disorder. *J. Trauma. Stress*, **5**, 333–64.
Schuemeyer, H., Avgerinos, P. W., Gold, W. T. *et al.* (1984). Human corticotropin-releasing factor dose response and time course of ACTH and cortisol secretion in man. *J. Clin. Endocrinol. Metab.*, **59**, 1103–8.

Shore, J. H., Tatum, E. L. & Vollmer, W. M. (1986). Psychiatric reactions to disaster: the Mount St. Helens experience. *Am. J. Psychiatry*, **143**, 590–5.

Sirinathsinghju, D. J. S., Rees, L. H., Rivier, J. *et al.* (1983). Corticotropin-releasing factor is a potent inhibitor of sexual receptivity in the female rat. *Nature*, **305**, 232–5.

Smith, E. M., Robins, L. N., Pryzbeck, T. R., Goldring, E. & Solomon, S. D. (1986). Psychosocial consequences of a disaster. In *Disaster Stress Studies: New Methods and Findings*, ed. J. Shore, pp. 49–76. Washington, DC: American Psychiatric Press.

Smith, M. A., Bissette, G., Slotkin, T. A. *et al.* (1986). Release of corticotropin-releasing factor from rat brain regions *in vitro*. *Endocrinology*, **118**, 1997–2001.

Smith, M. A., Davidson, J., Ritchie, J. C. *et al.* (1989). The corticotropin-releasing hormone test in post traumatic stress disorder. *Biol. Psychiatry*, **26**, 349–55.

Solomon, Z. & Mikulincer, M. (1988). Psychological sequelae of war: a two-year follow-up study of Israeli combat stress reaction (CSR) casualties. *J. Nerv. Ment. Dis.*, **176**, 264–9.

Southwick, S. M., Krystal, J. H. & Charney, D. S. (1991). Yohimbine in PTSD. *APA New Res. Abstr.*, p. 143.

Swerdlow, N. R., Geyer, M. A., Vale, W. W. & Knob, G. F. (1986). Corticotropin-releasing factor potentiates acoustic startle in rats: blockade by chlordiazepoxide. *Psychopharmacology*, **88**, 147–52.

Torrie, A. (1944). Psychosomatic casualties in the Middle East. *Lancet*, **29**, 139–43.

Trandel, D. V. & McNally, R. J. (1987). Perception of threat cues in PTSD: semantic processing without awareness. *Behav. Res. Ther.*, **25**, 469–76.

Vale, W., Speiss, J., Rivier, C. *et al.* (1981). Characterization of a 41-residue ovine hypothalamic peptide that stimulates secretion of corticotropin and β-endorphin. *Science*, **213**, 1394–7.

Valentino, R. J. & Foote, S. L. (1987). Corticotropin-releasing factor disrupts sensory response of brain noradrenergic neurones. *Neuroendocrinology*, **45**, 28–36.

Vanderhaegen, J. J., Lofstra, P. & Vierendeels, G. (1981). Cholecystokinin in the central nervous system and neurohypophysis. *Peptides*, **2**, 81–8.

van der Kolk, B. A. (ed.) (1984). *Post-traumatic Stress Disorder: Psychological and Biological Sequelae*. Washington, DC: American Psychiatric Press.

Veronen, L. J. & Kilpatrick, D. G. (1982). Stress inoculation training for victims of rape: efficacy and differential findings. Presented in a symposium entitled 'Sexual Violence and Harassment' at the *16th Annual Convention of the Association for Advancement of Behavior Therapy*, November, Los Angeles, CA.

von Bardeleben, J. & Holsboer, F. (1989). Cortisol response to a combined dexamethasone–human corticotropin-releasing hormone challenge in patients with depression. *J. Neuroendocrinol.*, **1**, 485–8.

Watson, C. G., Kucala, T., Manifold, V., Vassar, P. & Juba, M. (1988). Differences between posttraumatic stress disorder patients with delayed and undelayed onsets. *J. Nerv. Ment. Dis.*, **176**, 568–72.

Weiss, D. S., Marmar, C. R., Schlenger, W. E., Fairbank, J. A., Jordan, B. K., Hough, R. L. & Kulka, R. A. (1992). The prevalence of lifetime and partial post-traumatic stress disorder in Vietnam theater veterans. *J. Traum. Stress*, **5**, 365–76.

Whalley, L. J., Borthwick, N., Copolov, D. *et al.* (1986). Glucocorticoid receptors and depression, *Br. Med. J.*, **292**, 859–61.

Wilkinson, C. B. (1983). Aftermath of a disaster: the collapse of the Hyatt Regency Hotel skywalks. *Am. J. Psychiatry*, **140**, 1134–9.

Woolfolk, R. L. & Grady, D. A. (1988). Combat-related posttraumatic stress disorder: patterns of symptomatology in help-seeking Vietnam veterans. *J. Nerv. Mental. Dis.*, **176**, 107–11.

Yassen, J. & Glass, L. (1984). Sexual assault survivors groups: a feminist practice perspective. *Soc. Work*, **May–June**, 252–7.

Yehuda, R., Giller, E. L., Boisoneau, D. *et al.* (1991*a*). The low dose DST in PTSD. *New Res. Abstr. APA*, 144.

Yehuda, R., Lowy, M. T., Southwick, S. J. *et al.* (1991*b*). Lymphocyte glucocorticoid receptor number in post-traumatic stress disorder. *Am. J. Psychiatry*, **149**, 499–504.

Yehuda, R. & Nemeroff, C. B. (1993). Neuropeptide alterations in affective and anxiety disorders. In *Handbook of Depression and Anxiety*, ed. J. A. denBoer & A. Sitsen. New York: Marcel Dekker.

Yehuda, R., Southwick, S. M., Nussbaum, G. *et al.* (1990*a*). Low urinary cortisol excretion in patients with PTSD. *J. Nerv. Ment. Dis.*, **178**, 366–409.

Yehuda, R., Southwick, S. M., Perry, B. D. *et al.* (1990*b*). Hypothalamic–pituitary–adrenal and noradrenergic interactions in PTSD. In *Biological Assessment and Treatment of PTSD*, Progress in Psychiatry, ed. E. Giller. Washington, DC: APA Press.

# 7

# Central nervous system control of sickness behavior

STEPHEN KENT, ROSE-MARIE BLUTHE, GLYN GOODALL, KEITH W. KELLEY and ROBERT DANTZER

I feel sick. What is usually meant by this deceptively simple statement? The non-specific symptoms of infectious diseases include profound behavioral and psychological changes. Sick individuals are febrile, hypersomnic, depressed and lethargic. In addition, they experience malaise, generalized aches and pains, an inability to concentrate, loss of appetite, and a lack of interest in usual activities, including social contacts and sex. This constellation of non-specific symptoms is collectively referred to as 'sickness behavior' (Hart, 1988; Kent *et al.*, 1992*a*). Regardless of, or perhaps more precisely, because of their commonality, they are frequently ignored by physicians because they contribute little in facilitating a diagnosis. In fact, they are more often considered as an uncomfortable, but generally banal, part of the pathogen-induced debilitative process. Their commonality and their evolutionary conservation, however, suggest other reasons for their presence.

Fever, for example, is not merely a symptom but is an adaptive response that enables a host to defend itself against, and survive, infection by a pathogen. It is an evolutionary response that has now been demonstrated in fish, reptiles, and even invertebrates, such as mollusks and insects (for a review, see Kluger, 1991). The medical dogma of the twentieth century has suggested that fever should be prevented; however, strong evidence now suggests otherwise. Preventing the manifestation of fever in poikilothermic animals by placing them in a cool environment, or in homeostatic animals by the administration of prostaglandin (PG) synthesis inhibitors, is detrimental to their survival (for a review, see Kluger, 1991). Although, for the most part, experimental evidence is lacking, arguments can also be made for the contribution of sickness behavior to the survival of infected organisms (Hart, 1988). Recent evidence is that these non-specific symptoms are induced and controlled by the proinflammatory cytokines released by an activated immune system, and that they play a role in the recuperative process. This review focuses on the role of the central nervous system in regulating sickness behavior.

## Communication between the immune and central nervous systems

The cells of the immune system release a plethora of soluble factors in response to infection, tissue injury, neoplastic growth, or immunological disorders. The principal proinflammatory compounds are the cytokines, interleukin (IL)-1, IL-6, tumor necrosis factor alpha (TNF-$\alpha$), and the interferons (IFN). In addition, these cells also release several anti-inflammatory compounds, for example, IL-1 receptor antagonist (IL-1ra), IL-4, IL-10, and transforming growth factor $\beta$. Immunologists have focused on determining their role in coordinating the local response of phagocytic cells, lymphocytes, and other accessory cells of the immune system, especially during the acute phase reaction. This response, known as the acute phase response (Kushner, 1991), is characterized by leukocytosis, increased sedimentation rate of red blood cells, activation of complement and clotting cascades, synthesis and release by hepatocytes of acute phase proteins (e.g. fibrinogen, C-reactive protein, ceruloplasmin, $\alpha_1$-antitrypsin), negative nitrogen balance, and decreased serum levels of iron and zinc. In addition to their autocrine and paracrine effects, cytokines act in a hormonal fashion on distant target cells. During the last decade, physiologists have begun to examine the role and mechanisms of action by which cytokines activate the pituitary–adrenal axis, and induce fever and sickness behavior.

## Assessing sickness behavior

The main problem in trying to implicate cytokines in the induction of sickness behavior is the lack of any standard objective and quantitative measures. This is explained by the fact that psychologists are not accustomed to studying, and pathologists are rarely interested in, the behavior of infected animals.

Sickness or malaise has been studied indirectly using the conditioned taste aversion (CTA) paradigm. This paradigm is based on the association that an individual develops between the taste of a novel food or fluid recently eaten or drunk and a subsequent bout of gastrointestinal illness (Garcia *et al.*, 1974). In a typical experiment, animals are trained to drink their daily allocation of water during a 30 min presentation of a water bottle. On the day of conditioning, they are presented with a saccharin solution instead of water and are subsequently injected with a toxic dose of lithium chloride or another poison. After recovery, they are presented with the saccharin solution that was originally paired with the episode of sickness, either alone or concurrently with water. Conditioned animals refrain from drinking the saccharin solution and the amount ingested is negatively related to the intensity of the previously experienced sickness, i.e. the more severe the illness, the stronger the aversion to the taste.

Another way of assessing sickness is to look for alterations of ongoing spontaneous or learned behavior. As an example, the sickness developed by morphine-dependent rats upon challenge with naloxone can be measured in a very precise way as disruption of operant responding in animals trained to press a lever for food in a Skinner box (Babbini *et al.*, 1972; Gellert & Sparber, 1977). This measure is much more sensitive and specific than the physical symptoms that are often used to assess withdrawal (e.g. body-weight loss and wet-dog shakes).

The choice of behavioral end-points to be used as indicators of cytokine-induced sickness can be guided by what is already known about the nature of fever symptoms. The reduction in body care activities that leads to the scruffy-looking hair coat that is characteristic of sick animals (Hart, 1988) is not easy to quantify, and has therefore not yet been used. In contrast, changes in general activity, feeding behavior and social interactions are easier to assess, using automated recording or direct observation.

All of the above measures are based on a reduction or elimination of a behavior; however, it is not yet known whether sickness behavior can be assessed more directly by use of positive indicators instead of negative ones. Pain-motivated behavior, for example, can be best elucidated by the occurrence of recuperative behaviors such as licking and protection of the body areas that are affected. Quantifying the curled posture animals adopt to minimize heat loss could be a way to solve this problem. Another example of a positive behavior was first demonstrated 30 years ago by Neal Miller and colleagues. They had remarked on the fact that endotoxin suppressed all ongoing activity, including bar pressing. They were, however, able to demonstrate that this was not always the case. Rats placed in a rotating drum were trained to press a bar to briefly stop its rotation; after administration with endotoxin, they actually increased their rate of bar pressing in order to stop the rotation (Holmes & Miller, 1963; Miller, 1964).

## Cytokines induce sickness behavior

### *Clinical studies*

The first indication in favour of the role of cytokines in sickness behavior came from clinical trials with purified or recombinant cytokines. Due to their wide range of immune effects and widespread availability due to recombinant technology, these molecules were thought to have a high potential as therapeutics by enhancing immune defenses in cancer, viral illness, and immunodeficient states. Their large-scale use, however, turned out to be impractical, due to their severe physiological and neurological side-effects. Early clinical trials focused on the use of IFN in the treatment of malignant disease. These clinical studies resulted in anecdotal evidence of central nervous system (CNS) toxicity manifested by sleepiness and confusion. For this reason, Rohatiner *et al.* (1983) undertook a controlled study of the CNS side-effects of IFN. They observed that of 11 leukaemia patients continuously infused with IFN-$\alpha$ (100 million units per day) for seven days, 'all patients became pyrexial and complained of anorexia, fatigue and general malaise, describing symptoms similar to those of influenza'. Furthermore, although they appeared intellectually intact, they were 'withdrawn, slow to answer questions and totally disinterested in their surroundings'. Another study observed similar changes developing after one or two weeks of therapy with recombinant human IFN-$\alpha$ (5 million units per day) (Renault *et al.*, 1987). Moreover, they documented 'overt emotional and psychiatric problems' ranging from depression to irritability and delirium. The psychiatric side-effects, however, generally did not appear until the second or third month of treatment.

These neurotoxic effects are not limited to IFN-$\alpha$. Similar effects were observed during the treatment of metastatic cancer patients with recombinant IL-2 and IL-2-activated killer cells. Most patients experienced 'decreased energy, fatigue, anorexia, and malaise', which they compared to 'an influenza-like syndrome'. In addition, they 'frequently became apathetic with drowsiness, loss of interest, and frequent daytime sleeping and sleep disturbances'. More alarming was the fact that some patients developed clinically significant neuropsychiatric symptoms, including delirium, hallucinations, paranoid delusions, impaired memory, and irritability (Denicoff *et al.*, 1987). The onset of these symptoms appeared almost exclusively at the end of each treatment phase (i.e. day 5). More recently, IL-1$\beta$ (1–100 ng/kg, intravenously (i.v.)) has been administered to cancer patients as a bone-marrow stimulant. Although all patients became febrile with chills and rigor, and the majority experienced nausea and vomiting, headaches, and mild-to-moderate musculoskeletal pain, no psychic disturbances were observed (Smith *et al.*, 1990; Tewari *et al.*, 1990; Crown *et al.*, 1991). In each of the above-described cases, all toxic effects were dose-related and were eliminated shortly after therapy was discontinued.

***Animal studies***

Experimental studies in animals have confirmed that systemic or intracerebral injections of recombinant cytokines have profound behavioral effects in addition to their pyrogenic and metabolic activity. In nearly all of these studies, spontaneous locomotor activity and food intake have been used as indices of neurotoxicity. It is only in the past five to six years that more systematic studies have addressed the mechanisms and significance of the effects of cytokines on behavior. Most of these studies have concentrated on IL-1, since this molecule is available in bulk quantities due to recombinant technology, and there are immunopharmacological and molecular tools to interfere specifically with its biological activity.

Several studies have concentrated on the ability of cytokines to induce CTA. For example, recombinant rat IL-1$\beta$ (rrIL-1$\beta$) administered intraperitoneally (i.p.) induced a dose-dependent (1–10 µg/rat) decreased preference for saccharin in a two-bottle test in rats, accompanied by dose-dependent impairment of weight gain (Tazi *et al.*, 1988). This effect was comparable in strength and duration to that resulting from the peripheral administration of lipopolysaccharide (LPS) (Figure 7.1). Administration of 50 ng rrIL-1$\beta$ into the lateral ventricle resulted in similar effects (Tazi *et al.*, 1990).

Learned aversions to a specific diet associated with the development of tumors have been observed in cancer patients and in rats (Bernstein & Sigmundi, 1980). It was postulated that these effects were due to TNF, since tumors are associated with elevated levels of TNF-$\alpha$. Subsequently, it was shown that TNF administration (50 µg/kg twice a day for 3 days) led to the development of a strong aversion to a novel diet in rats (Bernstein *et al.*, 1991).

In contrast to IL-1$\beta$ and TNF-$\alpha$, murine IFN-$\alpha$ administered at doses that induce anorexia (800–1600 U/g) failed to induce CTA in mice in a two-bottle test after either one or three pairings with chocolate milk. Furthermore, the combination of IFN-$\alpha$ with LiCl (an illness-inducing agent) failed to modify the LiCl-induced CTA (Segall & Crnic, 1990*a*).

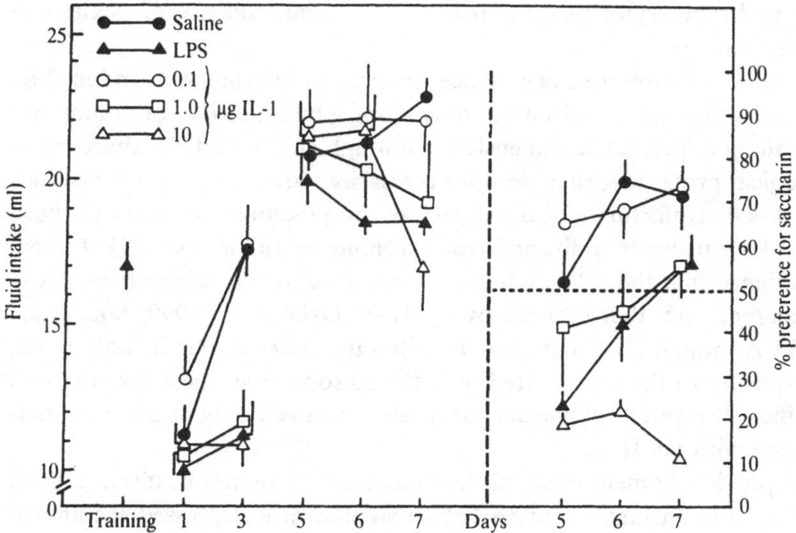


Figure 7.1. Aversive effects of IL-1 and LPS in rats. LPS (20 mg/kg) or rhIL-1$\beta$ (0.1–10 μg/rat) were injected i.p. after a 30-min session of saccharin presentation on days 1 and 3. The left graph represents the overall mean intake of water during the last two days of training and, for each experimental group, the mean intake of saccharin during the course of conditioning (days 1 and 3) and the mean fluid (saccharin + water) intake during preference tests (days 5–7). The right graph represents for each experimental group the mean percentage preference for saccharin during preference tests on days 5–7. Each experimental group contained 6–7 rats. Vertical bars represent ±SEM. (From Tazi *et al.*, 1988.)

These results demonstrate that at least in the case of IFN-α, different mechanisms are responsible for a decrease in food intake and the development of CTA.

It should be noted that the relative importance of malaise and changes in internal state as the determining factors in the development of CTA is not clear (Goudie, 1979; Dantzer *et al.*, 1988). The fundamental assumption is that CTA is induced by the 'toxicity' or 'sickness' induced by the treatment; however, little evidence exists to support it. Early studies supported this assumption by demonstrating the induction of CTA by toxic compounds acting peripherally and centrally (e.g. lead and mercury). It was subsequently demonstrated that CTA can be induced by compounds that are not generally considered to be toxic and by drugs of abuse, such as amphetamine and morphine, at doses that are self-administered (Goudie, 1979). Consequently, the CTA paradigm can be used to investigate the nature of changes in internal states caused by

IL-1 and other cytokines, but it is not sufficient evidence of sickness in treated animals.

In terms of subjective experience, changes in internal state induced by aversive drugs are perceived not only along a quantitative continuum but also along a qualitative dimension. Although IL-1 and TNF share many biological properties, they do not necessarily induce the same experience of sickness. Unfortunately, direct tests of this possibility have not yet been carried out using drug discrimination techniques. In the case of IL-1, there is evidence that the CTA induced by intracerebroventricular (i.c.v.) IL-1 is different from that induced by i.p. IL-1 (Dyck *et al.*, 1990; Janz *et al.*, 1991). Although IL-1 activates the pituitary–adrenal axis in both cases, re-exposure to the taste paired with the episode of sickness resulted in a significant elevation of plasma corticosterone levels only in those animals injected with i.p. IL-1.

As previously mentioned, proinflammatory cytokines decrease general activity. For instance, murine IFN-$\alpha$ significantly depressed locomotor activity, head pokes into a food tray, and food intake of mice, for up to 24 h after i.p. injection of a single dose of 1600 U/g (Segall & Crnic, 1990*b*). Murine IFN-$\alpha$, under the same test conditions, produced more extensive, although later-occurring, effects (Crnic & Segall, 1992*a*). Administration of recombinant human (rh) IL-1$\alpha$ or rhIL-1$\beta$ either centrally in picogram or peripherally in nanogram quantities to mice reduced, in a dose-dependent manner, the duration of contacts with novel objects mounted slightly below floor level in a hole-board apparatus divided into nine interconnecting compartments, without altering grooming, scratching, or measures of locomotor activity, such as movements between the compartments or rears (Spadaro & Dunn, 1990; Dunn *et al.*, 1991).

Social exploration of conspecific juveniles by adult animals is very sensitive to sickness. It is decreased in a time- and dose-dependent manner after either peripheral or central injection of rhIL-1$\beta$ to rats (Dantzer *et al.*, 1991) and mice (Bluthé *et al.*, 1991*c*; Crestani *et al.*, 1991). Similar results were obtained after treatment with LPS, IL-1$\alpha$, and TNF-$\alpha$ (Bluthé *et al.*, 1991*a*, *c*, 1992*a*) (Figure 7.2). As previously mentioned, disruption of lever pressing for food is a sensitive index of sickness. Peripheral and central injections of rhIL-1$\beta$ produce dramatic time- and dose-dependent decreases in the number of operant responses of rats trained to press a lever for food according to a fixed ratio 10 schedule of food reinforcement (i.e. one food pellet for every ten presses) (Bluthé *et al.*, 1989; Crestani *et al.*, 1991). Peripheral administration of LPS induces a comparable

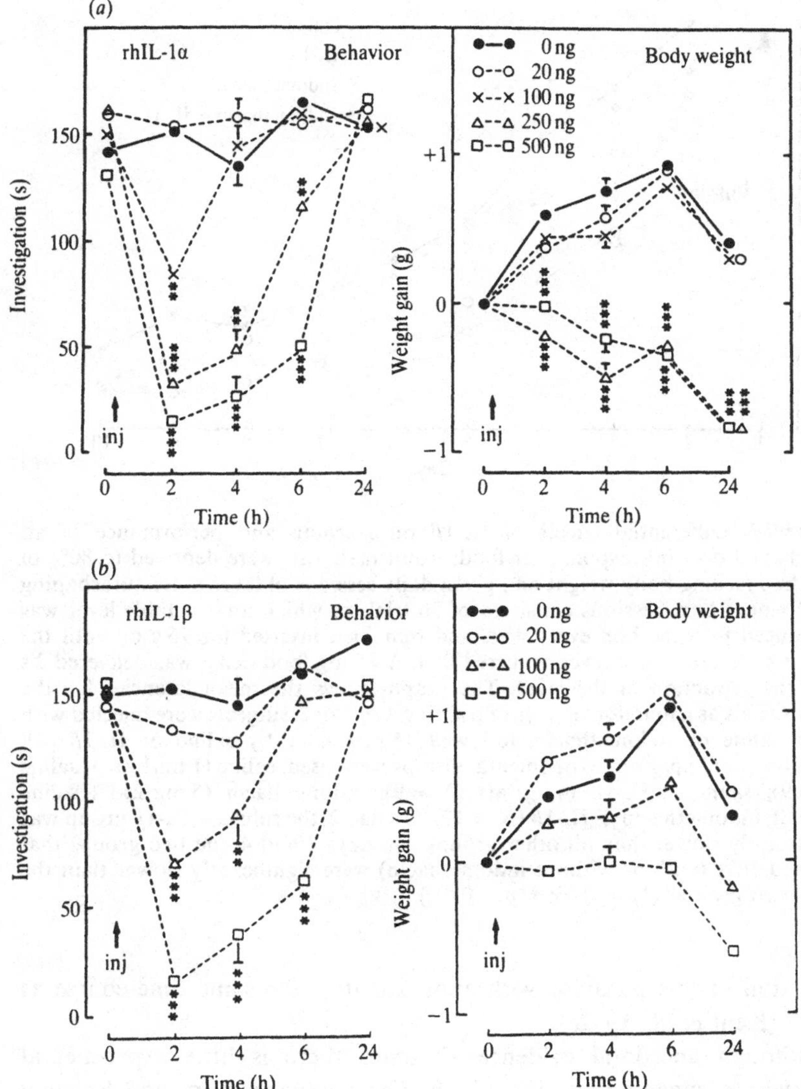


Figure 7.2. Effects of rhIL-1$\alpha$ (*a*) and rhIL-1$\beta$ (*b*) on social exploration and body weight in mice. Individually housed males DBA/2 were presented with a juvenile conspecific at time 0 (baseline) and the duration of olfactory investigation of this social stimulus was assessed during a 4-min test. They were then injected i.p. with saline or various doses of the cytokine under investigation and presented again with another juvenile at different time intervals. Body weight was measured at the end of each test session. For clarity of representation, SEM is presented only for the third point of each curve; $N = 8$ for IL-1$\alpha$, $N = 7$ for IL-1$\beta$; $**p < 0.01$, $***p < 0.001$ compared with baseline value. (From Bluthé *et al.*, 1991*c*.)

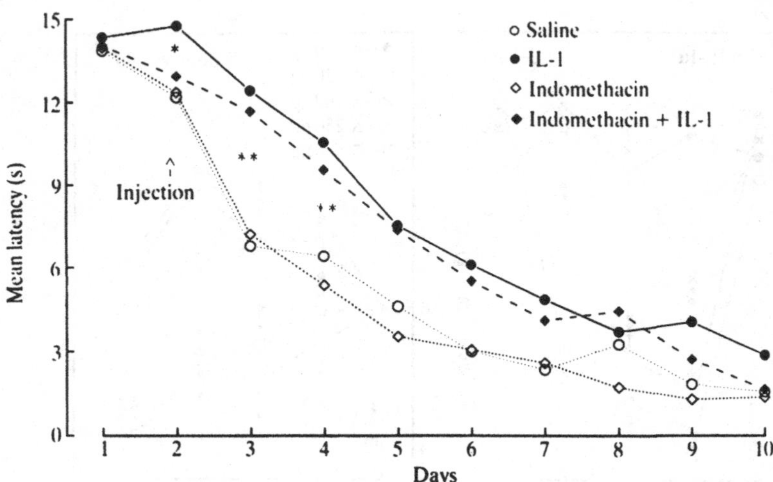


Figure 7.3. Differential effects of IL-1$\beta$ on learning and performance of an autoshaped operant response for food. Adult male rats were deprived to 80% of their free-feeding body weight and given daily sessions of lever press autoshaping in a Skinner box. Sessions consisted of 36 trials in which a retractable lever was introduced into the box every 45 s, and remained inserted for 15 s or until the lever was pressed, whichever occurred first. A 45-mg food pellet was delivered 2 s after the retraction of the lever. The graph shows the mean latencies for the 36 15-s trials as a function of days of training. On day 2, subjects were injected with either saline or indomethacin, followed 15 min later by saline or IL-1$\beta$. All injections were i.p. Four experimental groups were used: saline (1 ml/kg) + saline ($N = 9$); saline + IL-1$\beta$ (4 μg/rat) ($N = 9$); indomethacin (5 mg/kg) + saline ($N = 8$); indomethacin + IL-1$\beta$ ($N = 12$). On day 2, the saline + IL-1$\beta$ group was significantly slower than all other groups. On days 3 and 4, the two groups that received IL-1 (with or without indomethacin) were significantly slower than the other two groups. (*$p < 0.05$; **$p < 0.01$.)

reduction of this behavior with approximately the same time-course as IL-1$\beta$ (Kent *et al.*, 1992*c*).

Although anecdotal evidence abounds, there is little experimental evidence to suggest that sickness interferes with memory and learning ability. Our group has preliminary evidence that IL-1$\beta$ and LPS dramatically affect the learning of an autoshaped operant response for food, whereas it has little or no effect on performance once the response has been learned. Interestingly, these effects on learning are PG-independent. Pretreatment with indomethacin blocks the performance effects induced by IL-1, but not the learning deficit (Goodall *et al.*, in preparation) (Figure 7.3).

***Experimental studies in humans***

Based on their earlier work demonstrating that infection with upper respiratory viruses decreased the efficiency with which psychomotor tasks are performed (Smith *et al.*, 1987*a*, *b*, 1988*a*), Smith *et al.* (1988*b*) observed the effects of three doses of IFN-α (0.1–1.5 million units) on performance. Subjects injected with the largest dose of IFN produced symptoms and performance changes that closely resembled those found in volunteers with influenza. They displayed hyperthermia and experienced feelings of sickness. In addition, they were significantly slower at responding in a reaction-time task when they were uncertain when a target stimulus would appear, but were not impaired on pursuit tracking or syntactic reasoning tasks.

In view of these results, more studies are clearly warranted to examine the behavioral effects of subclinical doses of IFN and other cytokines.

***Illness in humans***

The central cytokinergic system has recently been implicated in the etiology of three disorders: chronic fatigue syndrome, dementia of the acquired immunodeficiency syndrome (AIDS), and the wasting syndrome of AIDS. The evidence is primarily theoretical for the first, but clinical for the last two. The chronic fatigue syndrome has been described following various infections (Bannister, 1988). This syndrome is characterized by persistent or recurrent symptoms of profound fatigue, sleep disturbances, difficulty in concentration, mood changes, and a variety of musculoskeletal aches (Sharpe *et al.*, 1991), and also manifests many of the features found in atypical depression. All these symptoms can be associated with cytokine activity and the acute-phase response. Consequently, both the IFNs (MacDonald *et al.*, 1987) and IL-1 (Ur *et al.*, 1992) have been hypothesized to be responsible for the chronic fatigue symptoms. In both cases, it has been postulated that the release of cytokines, either systemically, or centrally from glial cells or neurones, induces excessive sleepiness in the form of fatigue, and that in certain individuals, particularly where activation of the central cytokinergic system is prolonged, this manifests as chronic fatigue syndrome. Neither of these theories precludes the involvement of other cytokines (e.g. IL-6 or TNF-α). Unfortunately, at the present time, little clinical evidence exists to support either of these hypotheses.

As many as 80% of all AIDS patients have neurological abnormalities on post-mortem examination, and as many as 60% suffer from symptoms of CNS dysfunction, such as memory loss, difficulty in concentrating, slowness in thinking, and motor and behavioral difficulties (Price *et al.*, 1988). Recent evidence suggests that these effects may be due to the activation of the central cytokinergic system and the liberation of cytokines, both systemically and centrally. Human immunodeficiency virus (HIV) is neurotropic and enters neural tissue soon after infection. Strains of this virus have been demonstrated to be highly tropic for brain macrophages and microglial cells (Koenig *et al.*, 1986; Koyanagi *et al.*, 1987). Both HIV and gp120, the envelope protein of HIV that binds to the CD4 cell-surface antigen, induce IL-1 and TNF production *in vitro* in peripheral blood monocytes (Merrill *et al.*, 1989) and primary rat-brain cultures (Merrill *et al.*, 1992). Infusion of i.c.v. gp120 resulted in an elevation of brain levels of IL-1 and induced IL-1-like effects, such as an elevation in plasma corticosterone and decreasing cellular immune responses in rats, whereas i.v. administration resulted only in a decrease in cellular immune responses (Sundar *et al.*, 1991). Furthermore, elevated levels of IL-1$\beta$ and IL-6 have been detected in the cerebrospinal fluid of approximately 50% of AIDS patients (Gallo *et al.*, 1989).

Progressive weight loss and debilitation are common consequences of HIV infection. This wasting syndrome is a major cause of morbidity in the disease. The mechanisms underlying this syndrome can be divided into three categories: those that impair nutrient intake, those that interfere with nutrient absorption, and those that produce metabolic derangements (Grunfeld & Kotler, 1992). The ensemble of these symptoms is similar to that observed in other chronic infections and malignancies. As previously described, systemic or central administration of cytokines reduces food intake. In addition, it decreases gastric motility and acid secretion, leading to retention of food in the stomach and small intestine, and alters metabolism (for a review, see Grunfeld & Kotler, 1992). All of these symptoms can be induced by the central release of cytokines. However, early clinical studies with AIDS patients attempted to correlate these alterations with levels of circulating cytokines, with minimal success. This lack of success may be due to the simple fact that they were looking in the wrong place.

## Pharmacodynamic aspects of the sickness-inducing properties of cytokines

### *Pharmacokinetics*

Intravenous injection of rats with $^{125}$I-rhIL-1$\beta$ (4 μg/kg) resulted in a rapid distribution of IL-1, with a half-life of 2.9 min (Reimers *et al.*, 1991).

IL-1 was eliminated in accordance with first-order kinetics (half-life of elimination, 41.1 min) by degradation primarily in the kidney and liver, and excretion via the kidneys. Circulating, intact IL-1 was present up to 5 h following i.p. injection and was distributed in several organs. Distribution of IL-1 was similar in all organs after subcutaneous (s.c.), i.p., or i.v. administration except the pancreas, where greater levels accumulated after i.p. administration compared to s.c. or i.v. injections. In mice, the reported half-life of the distribution phase of rhIL-1$\beta$ injected i.v. was 5–10 min (Newton *et al.*, 1988). TNF-$\alpha$ had a similar half-life of distribution, but a much longer half-life of elimination (1.7–11 h) (Ferraiolo *et al.*, 1988).

### *Route of injection*

In general, peripheral and central injections of cytokines produced the same range of behavioral effects. In the case of social exploration, nanogram amounts of IL-1$\beta$ were required when this cytokine was injected i.c.v., instead of microgram amounts when administered i.p. (Dantzer *et al.*, 1991; Kent *et al.*, 1992*b*). Since the time course of the effects of IL-1 on social exploration was shorter in the first case than in the second, it is tempting to conclude that IL-1 acts centrally to alter social exploration. In contrast, ten times more IL-1 needed to be injected i.c.v. to induce significant decreases in food-motivated behavior (Kent *et al.*, 1992*b*). In addition, the latency of effect was delayed after i.c.v. treatment; the largest effects were observed 2–4 h post-injection instead of 1 h (Figure 7.4). This suggests that IL-1 does not act centrally to affect this behavior (see p. 156).

Because of the importance of the liver in the degradation of IL-1, it is likely that different routes of administration at the periphery lead to quantitatively different effects. Following the observation that s.c. IL-1$\beta$ was more effective than i.p. IL-1$\beta$ on food intake, rectal temperature, and blood-glucose level of rats (Reimers *et al.*, 1991), the effects of s.c. and i.p. rhIL-1$\beta$ on social exploration of mice were compared. Mice injected with 500 ng IL-1 were more sensitive when the cytokine was injected s.c. than when it was injected i.p. (Bluthé *et al.*, unpublished data) (Figure 7.5).

### *Chronic versus acute injections*

Chronic administration of rhIL-1$\beta$ (2 μg/day) via an osmotic mini-pump implanted s.c. resulted in the development of tolerance to the anorexic and weight-depressing effects of IL-1 within a few days (Mrosovsky *et al.*,

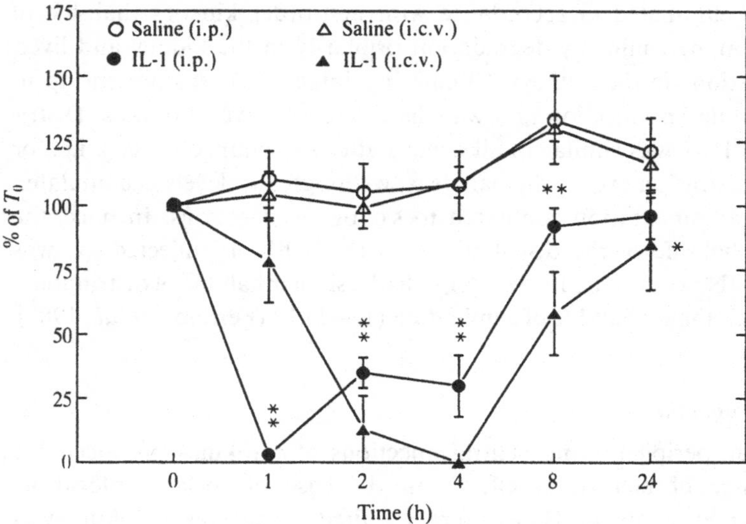


Figure 7.4. Effects of i.p. and i.c.v. IL-1$\beta$ on food-motivated behavior. Adult male rats were deprived to 85% of their free-feeding body weight before being trained to press a bar for a 45-mg food pellet in a Skinner box on a fixed ratio 10 schedule (i.e. one food pellet for every 10 presses). Each rat served as its own control. Each test session lasted 5 min. Animals were injected with rhIL-1$\beta$ i.p. (4 μg/rat; $N = 5$) or i.c.v. (40 ng/rat; $N = 5$) and physiological saline (1 ml, i.p.; 1 μl, i.c.v.). Separate groups of rats were used for i.p. and i.c.v. injections. All injections were given immediately after the first test session (time 0). Data are expressed as percentage of preinjection response rate. Vertical bars represent ±SEM. (*$p < 0.05$; **$p < 0.01$ compared to respective control values.)

1989). There is evidence that tolerance does not develop at the same rate for different behavioral end-points. Tolerance developed earlier to the depressing effects of IL-1$\beta$ on social exploration than to its effects on body weight (Bluthé *et al.*, 1991*b*). Continuous administration of murine IL-1$\alpha$ (3 μg/day) to rats kept in their home cage reduced eating activity and locomotor activity, and increased drinking (Otterness *et al.*, 1988). Locomotor activity remained decreased over the 5 days of treatment. Drinking activity was significantly elevated during the light period and this effect remained constant during the observation period. In contrast, eating behavior returned to control levels on days 4 and 5 during the later, but not earlier, half of the dark period.

Because of its rapidity of appearance (1–3 days), tolerance to the effects of IL-1 did not appear to be mediated by the mounting of an immune response to the injected cytokine. Possible mechanisms include the induction

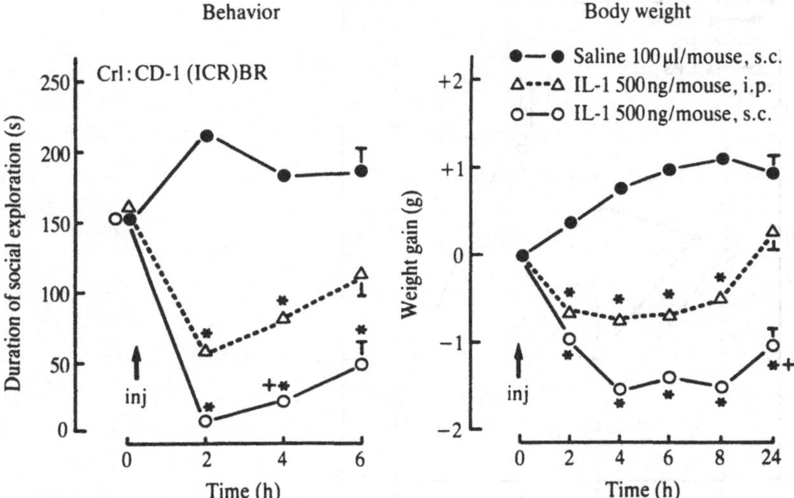


Figure 7.5. Effects of s.c. and i.p. injection of rhIL-1$\beta$ on social exploration in mice. Individually housed male Crl:CD-1 (ICR) BR mice, 7 weeks of age, were presented with a juvenile conspecific at time 0 (baseline) and the duration of social exploration was assessed during a 5-min test. Mice were then injected with physiological saline (100 µl s.c.; $N = 5$), rhIL-1$\beta$ (500 ng/100 µl s.c.; $N = 5$) or rhIL-1$\beta$ (500 ng/100 µl i.p.; $N = 5$) and tested 2, 4, and 6 h later with another juvenile. Body weight was measured at the end of each test session and 8 and 24 h later. $*p < 0.05$ compared to saline; +, $p < 0.05$ compared to IL-1 injected i.p.

of IL-1-degrading enzymes, downregulation of IL-1 receptors, induction of IL-1 soluble receptors, synthesis of IL-1ra, or altered CNS mechanisms.

In contrast to what was seen during continuous administration, repeated injections of IL-1 did not appear to lead to important changes in the magnitude of the observed behavioural response (Figure 7.6). The same does not apply to LPS, since repeated administration of endotoxin led to the rapid development of tolerance.

## Mechanisms of the behavioral effects of cytokines

### *Role of endogenous cytokines*

The demonstration that LPS induced behavioral effects similar to those of IL-1 in endotoxin-sensitive, but not endotoxin-resistant, mice, together with the observation that IL-1 was active in both lines of mice (Crestani, 1990), suggests that the secretion of proinflammatory cytokines is responsible

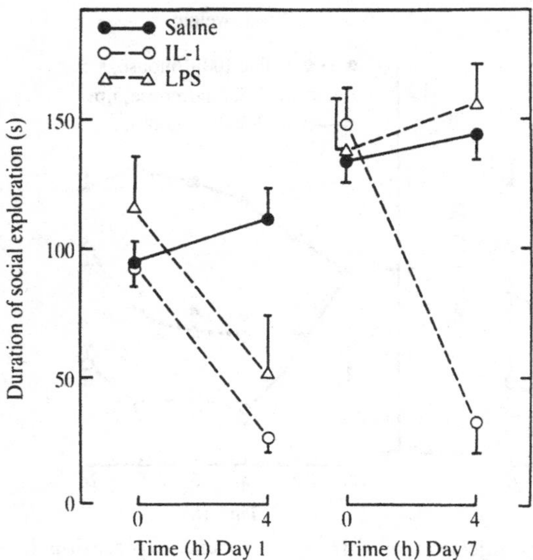


Figure 7.6. Tolerance develops to the depressing effects of injections of LPS but not IL-1 in social exploration in rats. Rats were injected with physiological saline ($N = 8$), LPS (20 mg/kg; $N = 4$), or rhIL-1$\beta$ (5 µg/rat; $N = 8$) four times at 48 h intervals. On the first day (day 1) and the last day (day 7) of injections, their interest toward a juvenile conspecific was measured. Each treatment was administered immediately after the first test session (time 0) and the rats were retested 4 h later. Note that LPS and IL-1 had similar depressing effects on social exploration on the first day of treatment but that LPS was no longer effective on day 7, in contrast to IL-1.

for the development and maintenance of sickness behavior in response to LPS. The exact cellular targets that are responsible for these effects, however, have not yet been identified. In the case of the pituitary–adrenal axis, depletion of macrophages by peripheral injection of liposomes encapsulated with dichloromethylene diphosphonate completely abrogated the hormonal response to a subpyrogenic dose of LPS (De Rijk *et al.*, 1991). The same strategy has not yet been used for assessing the role of macrophages in the behavioral effects of LPS.

Another strategy for identifying the mediators that are responsible for the effects of LPS is to use cytokine antagonists acting at the receptor level. Administration of rhIL-1ra at doses that blocked the behavioral effects of IL-1$\beta$ attenuated the depressing effect of LPS on social exploration and on body weight when injected i.p., but not i.c.v. (Bluthé *et al.*, 1992*b*) (Figure 7.7). In contrast, the same treatment had no effect on the LPS-induced disruption of food-motivated behavior, regardless of

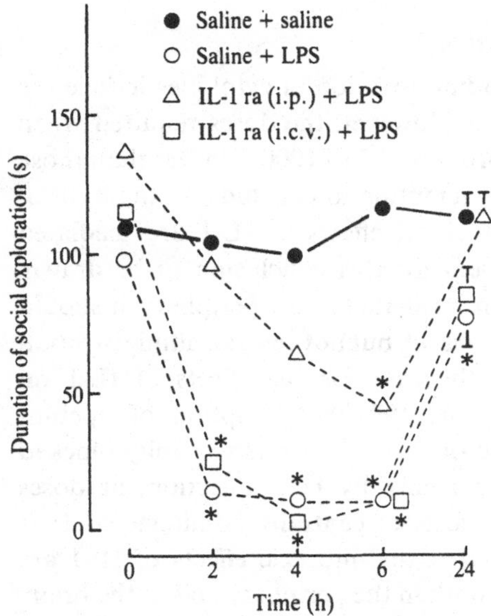


Figure 7.7. Effects of IL-1ra on the effects of LPS on social exploration in rats. Rats were injected with either saline or IL-1ra followed by saline or LPS. Four experimental groups were used: saline (i.p.) + saline (i.p.) ($N = 5$); saline (i.p.) + LPS (250 μg/kg i.p.) ($N = 6$); IL-1ra (3 mg/rat i.p.) + LPS (250 μg/kg i.p.) ($N = 5$); IL-1ra (60 μg/rat i.c.v.) + LPS (250 μg/kg i.p.) ($N = 7$). Injections were administered immediately after the first session, in which their interest toward a juvenile conspecific was measured, and animals were tested again after 2, 4, 6, and 24 h. SEM is represented only for the last time point. $^*p < 0.05$ compared with baseline values. (From Bluthé *et al.*, 1992*c*)

the route of injection, suggesting that IL-1 is not the principal mediator of these effects (Kent *et al.*, 1992*c*).

Cytokines have the ability to induce the synthesis and release of other cytokines and themselves in a cascade-like manner (Dinarello, 1991). This cascade serves to amplify the local effects of cytokines into a global effect, due to the multiplicity of targets and the overlapping biological effects of the cytokines. To test which cytokine is predominant in a given effect, the same pharmacological strategy based on the administration of cytokine antagonists, antibodies, or soluble receptors can be used. For example, pretreatment with IL-1ra blocked the depressive effects of TNF-α on social exploration, but only partially attenuated the accompanying weight loss. These results suggest that TNF-induced sickness behavior is mediated primarily by endogenously released IL-1, whereas the metabolic changes are independent of IL-1 (Bluthé *et al.*, 1991*a*).

***Peripheral versus central sites of action***

In general, peripheral and central administration of cytokines induce the same range of behavioral symptoms. However, the doses required when they were injected centrally were normally 100 to 1000-fold less than those required peripherally. Although it is tempting to conclude on the basis of this dose differential that the behavioral effects of IL-1 are mediated centrally, these data are not sufficient for this conclusion to be drawn.

If the behavioral effects of IL-1 are mediated at the periphery, it should be possible to abrogate them by peripheral, but not central, administration of IL-1ra. This was found to be the case for the effects of IL-1 on food-motivated behavior (Kent *et al.*, 1992*b*). Disruption of operant responding induced by i.p. injection of rhIL-1$\beta$ in rats was fully blocked by i.p.-injected IL-1ra, but only partially by i.c.v. injection, at doses that fully blocked the behavioral effects of centrally administered IL-1 (Figure 7.8). These results suggest that the anorexic effects of IL-1 are mediated by IL-1 receptors located both in the periphery and in the brain. In contrast, centrally injected IL-1ra was able to fully block the effects of peripherally injected rhIL-1$\beta$ on social behavior (Figure 7.8) (Kent *et al.*, 1992*b*). Consequently, it can be proposed that either peripherally injected IL-1 is able to enter the brain, or endogenous IL-1 is produced and released in the brain in response to peripheral IL-1.

This begs the question of how peripherally released cytokines access the brain. IL-1 and the other proinflammatory cytokines are large, hydrophilic peptides (17 kDa) that are unlikely to cross the blood–brain barrier in significant amounts without the aid of a transport system. Such a system has been proposed, based on the fact that radiolabeled IL-1$\alpha$ injected i.v. in mice was determined to cross the blood–brain barrier with an entry rate 44-fold greater than that predicted by leakage alone (Banks *et al.*, 1989). IL-1 entered virtually every brain region examined, including areas such as the cerebellum and cortex. The highest rate of entry, but not the largest amount, was found in the hypothalamus.

Despite these results, it is more commonly agreed that IL-1 and other cytokines act at the level of the circumventricular organs, where the blood–brain barrier is absent or leaky. Circumventricular organs are specialized neural structures that lie outside the blood–brain barrier and have sensory and neurosecretory functions (Weindl, 1972). One of these structures is the organum vasculosum of the lamina terminalis (OVLT). It is located within the rostral wall of the third ventricle, adjacent to the preoptic area and septum. The consensus is that IL-1 does not enter the

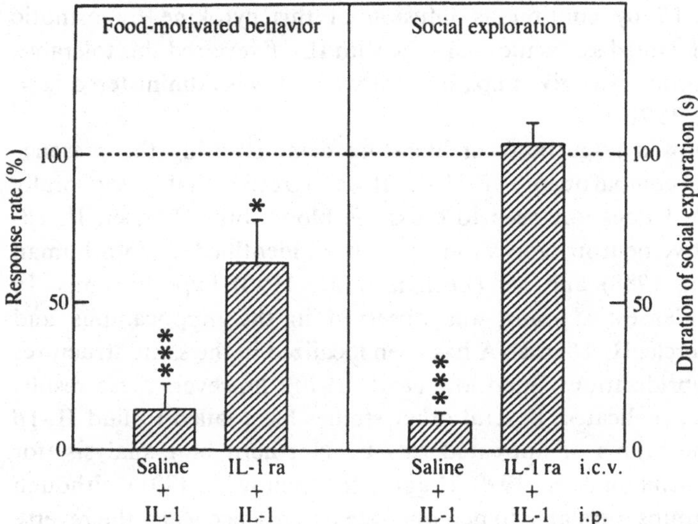


Figure 7.8. Differential blockade of central IL-1 receptors on food-motivated behavior and on social exploration. IL-1ra or saline was injected i.c.v. into rats trained to press a lever for food on a fixed ratio 10 schedule (24 μg/rat IL-1ra) or to rats presented with a juvenile conspecific (4 μg/rat IL-1ra). This injection was followed by i.p. rhIL-1$\beta$ (4 $\mu$g/rat) or saline. Injections were given immediately after the first test session and animals were tested again after 1 h (food-motivated behavior) or 2 h (social exploration). The figure represents percentage variation with regard to baseline values (*$p < 0.01$, ***$p < 0.001$). Note that pretreatment with IL-1ra blocked the effects of IL-1 on social exploration but only partially attenuated the effects of this cytokine on food-motivated behavior. (Modified from Kent *et al.*, 1992*b*.)

brain, but binds to cells on the vascular side of the OVLT, thereby inducing the synthesis and release of $PGE_2$, which then freely diffuses to nearby neural structures, and acts on them either directly or by promoting the local synthesis and release of IL-1 and other cytokines (Katsuura *et al.*, 1990). A third possibility is that peripheral IL-1 activates substance P-containing primary sensory afferents which transmit this information to the central IL-1 compartment (Kent *et al.*, 1992*a*).

Evidence exists for the differential regulation of peripheral and central cytokine levels and IL-1 receptors. In bacterial meningitis, high concentrations of IL-1, IL-6, and TNF-$\alpha$ in the cerebrospinal fluid did not correlate with high systemic levels of these same cytokines (Waage *et al.*, 1989). Central administration of IL-1$\beta$ resulted in a much more marked elevation of circulating levels of IL-6 than either i.v. or i.p. injections (De Simoni *et al.*, 1990). In addition, in rats made tolerant to the behavioral effects of IL-1$\beta$ by continuous infusion of this cytokine by osmotic mini-pump inplanted s.c., acute challenge with IL-1$\beta$ reversed this tolerance when the injection was given i.p., but not when it was administered i.c.v. (Bluthé *et al.*, 1991*b*).

There is now a large body of literature demonstrating the presence of a central compartment of IL-1. It is agreeed that peripherally circulating IL-1 does not need to cross the blood–brain barrier. IL-1$\beta$-immunoreactive neurons and axons have been identified in both human (Breder *et al.*, 1988) and rat (Lechan *et al.*, 1990) hypothalamus. In the rat, the densest staining was observed in the hippocampus and olfactory tubercle. IL-1$\beta$ mRNA has been localized in the same structures by *in situ* hybridization (Bandtlow *et al.*, 1990); however, these results have yet to be replicated. Several other studies have failed to find IL-1$\beta$ mRNA in the brains of untreated rats by Northern blot analysis (for example, see Minami *et al.*, 1990; Higgins & Olschowka, 1991), although these same groups were able to demonstrate its presence using the reverse transcription–polymerase chain reaction (Higgins & Olschowka, 1991; Minami *et al.*, 1991). Therefore, it appears that IL-1$\beta$ mRNA is present in the brains of untreated rats, but in limited quantities.

Several groups have investigated the ability of peripherally administered endotoxin to induce IL-1 in the CNS. Van Dam *et al.* (1992) observed immunoreactive IL-1$\beta$ in large numbers of macrophages in the meninges and choroid plexus and ramified microglia within the parenchyma of the brain after peripheral injection of endotoxin in rats. Similarly, increases in bioactive IL-1 were detected in mouse and rabbit brain tissue after the same treatment (Fontana *et al.*, 1984; Clark *et al.*, 1991). In contrast, i.v. injections of endotoxin or crude monocyte supernate containing IL-1 had no influence on cerebrospinal fluid levels of IL-1 in cats, whereas i.c.v. administration of endotoxin increased them (Coceani *et al.* 1988).

IL-1 receptors have been identified in the mouse brain by classical binding techniques (Takao *et al.*, 1990) and by quantitative autoradiography (Haour *et al.*, 1990). The highest densities of receptors were found in the hippocampus, choroid plexus and pituitary. In the hippocampus, they were likely to be on intrinsic neurones, since their density decreased following quinolinic acid lesions, which destroy neurones but leave glia intact (Takao *et al.*, 1990). In accordance with their similar biological activities, the two molecular forms of IL-1, IL-1$\alpha$ and IL-1$\beta$, bound with the same affinity to brain IL-1 receptors. The binding characteristics of brain IL-1 receptors appear to be similar to those of T cells and fibroblasts, but the molecular identity of these receptors has not yet been confirmed. On immune targets, two types of IL-1 receptors have been characterized, an 80 kDa form present on T lymphocytes and fibroblasts (type I) and a 68 kDa form present on B lymphocytes and macrophages (type II) (Dinarello, 1991). Messenger RNA for the type I IL-1 receptor has been localized in the hippocampus by *in situ* hybridization (Cunningham *et al.*, 1992). The same technique has been used to demonstrate that the pituitary contains both type I and type II receptors (Parnet *et al.*, 1993).

An important element for the discussion concerning the role of central IL-1 is the observation that hippocampal, but not pituitary, receptors are downregulated following peripheral administration of LPS (Haour *et al.*, 1990). This supports the previously mentioned possibility that IL-1 is released in the brain under conditions leading to peripheral production of this cytokine.

Although it is clear that the behavioral effects of IL-1 and other proinflammatory cytokines can be mediated peripherally or centrally, depending on the behavioral end-point, there is clearly a need for a better delineation of the cellular targets. In the case of central targets, a micropharmacological approach consisting of local injections of agonists and/or antagonists would be the best way to address this issue. For example, microinjections of 5 ng rhIL-1$\beta$ directly into the ventromedial nucleus of the hypothalamus decreased response to food to the same degree as injections of 40 ng of this cytokine into the lateral ventricle (Kent *et al.*, unpublished data).

### *Role of corticotropin-releasing factor*

Because of the potent activating effects of IL-1 on hypothalamic corticotropin-releasing factor (CRF) and the role played by this neuropeptide in IL-1-induced thermogenesis (Rothwell, 1989), the possible involvement of CRF in the behavioral effects of IL-1 has been assessed using CRF antiserum or $\alpha$-helical $CRF_{9-41}$ (ahCRF), an antagonist of CRF receptors.

Immunoneutralization of endogenous CRF in the brain attenuated the anorexic effects of IL-1$\beta$ (Uehara *et al.*, 1989*b*). In the same manner, i.c.v. administration of CRF antiserum blocked the reduction of immobility induced by i.c.v. rhIL-1$\beta$ in rats forced to swim in a confined space, and IL-1-induced sinking (Del Cerro & Borrell, 1990). The reduction of exploratory behavior of mice placed in a multicompartment chamber induced by peripherally administered rhIL-1$\alpha$ and rhIL-1$\beta$ was reversed by prior i.c.v. administration of ahCRF (Dunn *et al.*, 1991).

Although these findings suggest that brain CRF modulates the behavioral effects of IL-1, contradictory evidence exists. In particular, the decrease in food-motivated behavior induced in rats by i.p. injection of rhIL-1$\beta$ was not altered by i.c.v. administration of either ahCRF or CRF (Bluthé *et al.*, 1989), although CRF administered by itself did induce a slight reduction in operant responding. When IL-1 was injected centrally, ahCRF did not alter the peak effect, but facilitated the return toward baseline (Bluthé *et al.*, 1992*b*). In addition, Opp *et al.* (1989) observed that i.c.v. injections of CRF attenuated the somnogenic effects of i.c.v. IL-1$\beta$ in rabbits.

The exact factors that are responsible for these differences are still unknown, although differences in species and dose may play a role. However, it is clear that the involvement of CRF in the behavioral effects of IL-1 is not a general phenomenon.

### *Role of prostaglandins*

IL-1 and other cytokines are potent inducers of PG production in the gastrointestinal tract (Robert *et al.*, 1991), astrocyte cultures (Katsuura *et al.*, 1989), and the hypothalamus (Sirko *et al.*, 1989; Komaki *et al.*, 1992). Administration of cyclooxygenase inhibitors, such as indomethacin, at doses that abolish the synthesis of PGs, attenuated the pyrogenic and anorexic effects of IL-1 (Hellerstein *et al.*, 1989; Uehara *et al.*, 1989*a*). Furthermore, a diet rich in fish-oil, which decreases endogenous $PGE_2$ production, also abolished the anorexic effects of rhIL-1$\beta$ (Hellerstein *et al.*, 1989). In addition, pretreatment with indomethacin or piroxicam, another cyclooxygenase inhibitor, blocked the depressing effects of peripherally injected rhIL-1$\beta$ on food-motivated behavior in rats and on social exploration in mice (Crestani *et al.*, 1991).

Evidence suggests that the decrease in food intake induced by administration of IL-1 did not involve the central release of PGs. Central administration of ibuprofen blocked the fever, but not the anorexia, induced by centrally injected IL-1$\beta$, whereas this compound was effective when administered peripherally (Shimizu *et al.*, 1991). Acetaminophen, which preferentially inhibits brain cyclooxygenase relative to that in peripheral tissues, did not block the decrease in food intake observed after i.p. IL-1$\beta$ (Hellerstein *et al.*, 1989).

Therefore, although peripheral, but not central, PGs are responsible for some of the behavioral effects of IL-1, PGs do not appear to be responsible for all the behavioral effects of IL-1 or other cytokines. For example, in rats continuously infused with murine IL-1$\alpha$, piroxicam completely inhibited the stimulation of drinking behavior, but had no effect on the reduction in eating activity and locomotor activity induced by the cytokine (Otterness, 1991). Similarly, pretreatment with indomethacin had no effect on IL-1-induced CTA (Tazi *et al.*, 1990) or the depression of general activity and food intake induced in mice by peripheral injection of IFN-α (Crnic & Segall, 1992*b*).

### *Role of nitric oxide*

The sustained vasodilatation and hypotension induced by IL-1 and other proinflammatory cytokines are mediated by the local synthesis and release of nitric oxide (NO), via induction of an NO synthase in both endothelial and vascular smooth muscle cells (Moncada *et al.*, 1991). In addition to its potent vasodilatory effects, NO behaves as an effector molecule in immunological reactions and as a neurotransmitter in the central and peripheral nervous systems.

Administration of agents that block the synthesis of NO from L-arginine has been shown to attenuate the dramatic fall in blood pressure that occurs during septic shock in response to exogenously administered LPS or TNF (Kilbourn *et al.*, 1990; Thiemermann & Vane, 1990). To test whether NO production is also involved in the behavioral effects of IL-1, mice were pretreated with various doses of *N*-nitro-L-arginine methyl ester, a selective inhibitor of the brain and endothelial NO synthase (Bluthé *et al.*, 1992*c*). Administration of high doses of the antagonist (30 mg/kg) potentiated the depressing effects of rhIL-1β on social exploration, whereas lower doses (5 mg/kg) had no effect. This potentiation was attenuated by pretreatment with L-arginine, but not by D-arginine (Figure 7.9). Administration of the antagonist had no effect on the IL-1-induced weight loss. Inhibition of NO synthase also potentiated the effects of IL-1β on food-motivated behavior (Kent *et al.*, unpublished data). Although these results suggest that NO production has a protective role in the behavioral effects of IL-1, they need to be complemented by further studies elucidating the effect of IL-1 on brain NO synthase and the further contribution of the different isoforms of this enzyme to the observed effects.

## Cryogens oppose behavioral effects of cytokines

Brain arginine vasopressin (AVP) (Kasting, 1989) and α-melanocyte-stimulating hormone (α-MSH) (Lipton, 1989) have been characterized as

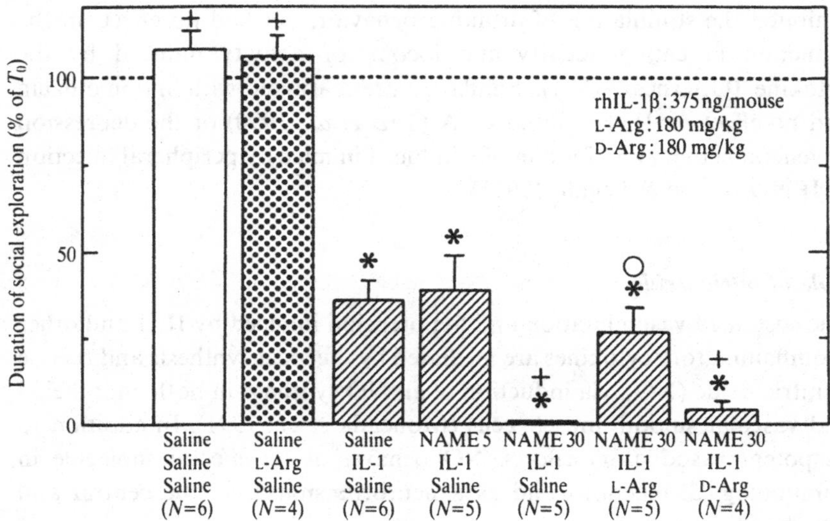


Figure 7.9. Potentiation of IL-1 induced changes in social exploration by pretreatment with L-NAME, an inhibitor of nitric oxide synthase, and the effect of L-arginine or D-arginine. The interest of each mouse expressed towards a juvenile conspecific was measured. Each column represents the mean variation measured 4 h after injection of rhIL-1$\beta$. The number of mice in each group is given in parentheses. *$p < 0.05$ compared to saline; +, $p < 0.05$ compared to IL-1; ○, $p < 0.05$ compared to the IL-1 + L-NAME group). Previous experiments had established that the doses of L-NAME (5 or 30 mg/kg) had no effect on social exploration. (From Bluthé *et al.*, 1992c.)

physiological inhibitors of fever, and are accordingly named endogenous antipyretics or cryogens. These peptides are released in the brain in response to endogenous pyrogens and function to suppress fever. They therefore appear to be part of a negative feedback loop regulating the thermogenic properties of cytokines.

The possibility that AVP counteracts the behavioral effects of IL-1 was tested by studying the interaction between AVP and IL-1 in rats during social exploration (Dantzer *et al.*, 1991). Central injection of AVP attenuated the suppression of behavior induced by i.c.v. rhIL-1$\beta$. Conversely, central injection of an antagonist of the vasopressor receptors of AVP, dPTyr(Me)AVP, potentiated the behavioral effects of IL-1. These last results are important because they suggest that endogenous AVP plays a physiological modulatory role in the behavioral effects of IL-1. The vasopressinergic neurones that are responsible for these effects are certainly those that are located in the bed nucleus of the stria terminalis

(BNST) and that project to the septum. These neurones possess the peculiarity of being highly sensitive to circulating androgens. Castration led to a dramatic reduction in the content of AVP mRNA in the BNST neuronal cell bodies (Miller *et al.*, 1989) and a reduction in immunoreactive AVP of the terminal areas of the septum (De Vries *et al.*, 1984). These changes were reversed by treatment with testosterone. Castration potentiated the depressing effects of continuous infusion of rhIL-1$\beta$ on social exploration in rats, as well as the effect of an acute central injection of IL-1 (Dantzer *et al.*, 1991). Furthermore, i.c.v. administration of AVP was more effective in attenuating the behavioral effects of IL-1 in castrated than in intact male rats, and, conversely, i.c.v. administration of the antagonist of AVP receptors was unable to counteract the behavioral effects of IL-1 in castrated male rats in which the vasopressinergic innervation of the septum was reduced. Similarly, the depressing effects of an acute i.c.v. injection of IL-1 on social exploration were attenuated by chronic infusion of AVP in castrated males and augmented by chronic infusion of the AVP antagonist in intact males (Bluthé & Dantzer, 1992). Although the stimulatory action of IL-1 and other endogenous pyrogens on AVP is well established, much more remains to be learned about the way AVP interacts with the effects of the cytokines, to better understand the mechanisms that are responsible for these effects.

Although $\alpha$-MSH antagonizes some of the physiological effects of IL-1, its ability to block the behavioral effects of IL-1 has not yet been explored in depth. Central infusion of this peptide blocks the increase in plasma ACTH and corticosterone and the suppression of cellular immune responses induced by IL-1$\beta$ (Weiss *et al.*, 1991). In addition, the decrease in food intake observed after i.c.v. IL-1$\beta$ was attenuated by the simultaneous infusion of $\alpha$-MSH (Uehara *et al.*, 1992). It may be that $\alpha$-MSH competes for IL-1 receptors, since it selectively inhibits the specific binding of $^{125}$I-rhIL-1$\beta$ to the IL-1 type I receptors (Mugridge *et al.*, 1991). It is of interest to determine whether $\alpha$-MSH is able to block the other behavioral effects of IL-1 and other cytokines.

## Conclusion

The presence of cytokines and their receptors in neural elements and the potential role of cytokines in brain development and regulation of central functions has opened an entirely new area of research in neuroimmunomodulation. The number of articles addressing the effects of cytokines on the central nervous system is expanding tremendously, and sufficient evidence is now available to support acceptance of the notion that cytokines are intepreted by the brain as signals of sickness. Sickness can actually be considered as a motivation, i.e. a central state that organizes perception and action. A sick individual does not have the same priorities as a well person, and this reorganization of priorities appears to be mediated by the effects of cytokines on a number of peripheral and central targets. The possibility that the defense reaction to infection and inflammation is organized at different levels of regulation in the organism has turned out to be heuristically fruitful, both in terms of adaptation and homeostasis, and in terms of mechanisms. The continuing elucidation of these mechanisms should provide new insight into the way sickness is represented in the brain.

## Acknowledgements

Supported by INSERM, INRA and DRET (RD: 90-166). S.K. was partially supported by a Bourse Chateaubriand and a fellowship from Sanofi Recherche.

## References

Babbini, M., Gaiardi, M. & Bartoletti, M. (1972). Changes in operant behavior as an index of withdrawal state from morphine in rats, *Psychonomic Sci.*, **29**, 142–4.

Bandtlow, C. E., Meyer, M., Lindholm, D., Spranger, M., Heumann, R. & Thoenen, H. (1990). Regional and cellular codistribution of interleukin 1$\beta$ and nerve growth factor mRNA in the adult rat brain: possible relationship to the regulation of nerve growth factor synthesis. *J. Cell Biol.*, **111**, 1701–11.

Banks, W. A., Kastin, A. J. & Durham, D. A. (1989). Bidirectional transport of interleukin 1$\alpha$ across the blood brain barrier. *Brain Res. Bull.*, **23**, 433–7.

Bannister, B. A. (1988). Post-infectious disease syndrome. *Postgrad. Med. J.*, **64**, 559–67.

Bernstein, I. L. & Sigmundi, R. A. (1980). Tumor anorexia: a learned food aversion? *Science*, **209**, 416–18.

Bernstein, I. L., Taylor, E. M. & Bentson, K. L. (1991). TNF-induced anorexia and learned food aversions are attenuated by area postrema lesions. *Am. J. Physiol.*, **260**, R906–R910.

Bluthé, R. M., Crestani, F., Kelley, K. W. & Dantzer, R. (1992*a*). Mechanisms of the behavioral effects of interleukin 1. *Ann. NY Acad. Sci.*, **650**, 268–75.

Bluthé, R. M. & Dantzer, R. (1992). Chronic intracerebral infusions of vasopressin and vasopressin antagonist modulate behavioral effects of interleukin-1 in rat. *Brain Res. Bull.*, **29**, 897–900.

Bluthé, R. M., Dantzer, R. & Kelley, K. W. (1989). CRF is not involved in the behavioural effects of peripherally injected interleukin 1 in the rat. *Neurosci. Res. Commun.*, **5**, 149–54.

Bluthé, R. M., Dantzer, R. & Kelley, K. W. (1991*a*). Interleukin-1 mediates behavioral but not metabolic effects of tumor necrosis factor α in mice. *Eur. J. Pharmacol.*, **209**, 281–3.

Bluthé, R. M., Dantzer, R. & Kelley, K. W. (1991*b*). Dissociation entre les composantes périphérique et centrale de la tolérance aux effets comportementaux de l'interleukine-1 chez le rat. *C. R. Acad. Sci. Paris*, **312**, 689–94.

Bluthé, R. M., Dantzer, R. & Kelley, K. W. (1992*b*). Effects of interleukin-1 receptor antagonist on the behavioral effects of lipopolysaccharide in rat. *Brain Res.*, **573**, 318–20.

Bluthé, R. M., Parnet, P., Dantzer, R. & Kelley, K. W. (1991*c*). Interleukin-1 receptor antagonist blocks effects of IL-1α and IL-1β on social behaviour and body weight in mice. *Neurosci. Res. Commun.*, **15**, 151–8.

Bluthé, R. M., Sparber, S. & Dantzer, R. (1992*c*). Modulation of the behavioural effects of interleukin-1 in mice by nitric oxide. *Neuroreport*, **3**, 207–9.

Breder, C. D., Dinarello, C. A. & Saper, C. B. (1988). Interleukin-1 immunoreactive innervation of the human hypothalamus. *Science*, **240**, 321–4.

Clark, B. D., Bedrosian, I., Schindler, R., Cominelli, F., Cannon, J. G., Shaw, A. R. & Dinarello, C. A. (1991). Detection of interleukin 1α and 1β in rabbit tissues during endotoxemia using sensitive radioimmunoassays. *J. Appl. Physiol.*, **71**, 2412–18.

Coceani, F., Lees, J. & Dinarello, C. A. (1988). Occurrence of interleukin-1 in cerebrospinal fluid of the conscious cat. *Brain Res.*, **446**, 245–50.

Crestani, F. (1990). Effets comportementaux de l'endotoxine et de l'interleukine-1 chez la souris: bases cellulaires. Ph.D. thesis, University of Bordeaux II.

Crestani, F., Seguy, F. & Dantzer, R. (1991). Behavioural effects of peripherally injected interleukin-1: role of prostaglandins. *Brain Res.*, **542**, 330–5.

Crnic, L. S. & Segall, M. A. (1992*a*). Behavioral effects of mouse interferons-α and -γ and human interferon-α in mice. *Brain Res.*, **590**, 277–84.

Crnic, L. S. & Segall, M. A. (1992*b*). Prostaglandins do not mediate interferon-α effects on mouse behavior. *Physiol. Behav.*, **51**, 349–52.

Crown, J., Jakubowski, A., Kemeny, N., Gordon, M., Gasparetto, C., Wong, G., Sheridan, C., Toner, G., Meisenberg, B., Botet, J., Applewhite, J., Sinha, S., Moore, M., Kelsen, D., Buhles, W. & Gabrilove, J. (1991). A phase I trial of recombinant human interleukin-1β alone and in combination with myelosuppressive doses of 5-fluorouracil in patients with gastrointestinal cancer. *Blood*, **78**, 1420–7.

Cunningham, E. T., Wada, E., Carter, D. B., Tracey, D. E., Battey, J. F. & De Souza, E. B. (1992). *In situ* localization of type I interleukin-1 receptor messenger RNA in the central nervous system, pituitary, and adrenal gland of the mouse. *J. Neurosci.*, **12**, 1101–14.

Dantzer, R., Bluthé, R. M. & Kelley, K. W. (1991). Androgen-dependent vasopressinergic neurotransmission attenuates interleukin-1 induced sickness behavior. *Brain Res.*, **557**, 115–20.

Dantzer, R., Bluthé, R. M. & Le Moal, M. (1988). Experimental assessment of drug-induced changes in cognitive function: vasopressin as a case study. *Neuro. Toxicol.*, **9**, 471–8.

Del Cerro, S. & Borrell, J. (1990). Interleukin-1 affects the behavioral despair response in rats by an indirect mechanism which requires endogenous CRF. *Brain Res.*, **528**, 162–4.

Denicoff, K. D., Rubinow, D. R., Papa, M. Z., Simpson, C., Seipp, C. A., Lotze, M. T., Chang, A. E., Rosenstein, D. & Rosenberg, S. A. (1987). The neuropsychiatric effects of treatment with interleukin-2 and lymphokine-activated killer cells. *Ann. Intern. Med.*, **107**, 293–300.

De Rijk R. H., Van Rooijen, N., Tilders, F. J. H., Besedovsky, H. O., Del Rey, A. & Berkenbosch, F. (1991). Selective depletion of macrophages prevents pituitary–adrenal activation in response to subpyrogenic, but not pyrogenic, doses of bacterial endotoxin. *Endocrinology*, **129**, 330–8.

De Simoni, M. G., Sironi, M., De Luigi, A., Manfridi, A., Mantovani, A. & Ghezzi, P. (1990). Intracerebroventricular injection of interleukin 1 induces high circulating levels of interleukin 6. *J. Exp. Med.*, **171**, 1773–8.

De Vries, G. J., Buijs; R. M. & Sluiter, A. A. (1984). Gonadal hormone actions on the morphology of the vasopressinergic innervation of the adult rat brain. *Brain Res.*, **298**, 141–5.

Dinarello, C. A. (1991). Interleukin-1 and interleukin-1 antagonism. *Blood*, **77**, 1627–52.

Dunn, A. J., Antoon, M. & Chapman, Y. (1991). Reduction of exploratory behavior by intraperitoneal injection of interleukin-1 involves brain corticotropin-releasing factor. *Brain Res. Bull.*, **26**, 539–42.

Dyck, D. G., Janz, L., Osachuk, T. A. G., Falk, J., Labinsky, J. & Greenburg, A. H. (1990). The Pavlovian conditioning of IL-1-induced glucocorticoid secretion. *Brain Behav. Immun.*, **4**, 93–104.

Ferraiolo, B. L., Moore, J. A., Crase, D., Gribling, P., Wilking, H. & Baughman, R. A. (1988). Pharmacokinetics and tissue distribution of recombinant human tumor necrosis factor in mice. *Drug Met. Disp.*, **16**, 270–5.

Fontana, A., Weber, E. & Dayer, E. (1984). Synthesis of interleukin 1/endogenous pyrogen in the brain of endotoxin-treated mice: a step in fever induction? *J. Immunol.*, **133**, 1696–8.

Gallo, P., Frei, K., Rordorf, C., Lazdins, J., Tavolato, B. & Fontana, A. (1989). Human immunodeficiency virus type 1 (HIV-1) infection of the central nervous system: an evaluation of cytokines in cerebrospinal fluid. *J. Neuroimmunol.*, **23**, 109–16.

Garcia, J., Hankins, W. G. & Rusiniak, K. W. (1974). Behavioral regulation of the milieu interne in man and rat. Science, **185**, 824–31.

Gellert, V. F. & Sparber, S. B. (1977). A comparison of the effects of naloxone upon body weight loss and suppression of fixed-ratio operant behavior in morphine-dependent rats. *J. Pharmacol. Exper. Ther.*, **201**, 44–54.

Goudie, A. J. (1979). Aversive stimulus properties of drugs. *Neuropharmacology*, **18**, 971–9.

Grunfeld, C. & Kotler, D. P. (1992). Pathophysiology of the AIDS wasting syndrome. In *AIDS Clinical Review 1992*, ed. P. Volberding & M. A. Jacobson, pp. 191–224. New York: Marcel Dekker.

Haour, F., Ban, E., Milon, G., Baran, D. & Fillion, G. (1990). Brain interleukin 1 receptors: characterization and modulation after lipopolysaccharide injection. *Prog. NeuroEndocrin. Immunol.*, **3**, 196–204.

Hart, B. L. (1988). Biological basis of the behavior of sick animals. *Neurosci. Biobehav. Rev.*, **12**, 123–37.

Hellerstein, M. K., Meydani, S. N., Meydani, M., Wu, K. & Dinarello, C. A. (1989). Interleukin-1-induced anorexia in the rat. *J. Clin. Invest.*, **84**, 228–35.

Higgins, G. A. & Olschowka, J. A. (1991). Induction of interleukin-1$\beta$ mRNA in adult rat brain. *Mol. Brain Res.*, **9**, 143–8.

Holmes, J. E. & Miller, N. E. (1963). Effects of bacterial endotoxin on water intake, food intake, and body temperature in the albino rat. *J. Exp. Med.*, **118**, 649–58.

Janz, L. J., Brown, R., Zuo, L., Falk, J., Greenberg, A. H. & Dyck, D. G. (1991). Conditioned taste aversion but not adrenal activity develops to ICV administration of interleukin-1 in rats. *Physiol. Behav.*, **49**, 691–4.

Kasting, N. W. (1989). Criteria for establishing a physiological role for brain peptides. A case in point: the role of vasopressin in thermoregulation during fever and antipyresis. *Brain Res. Rev.*, **14**, 143–53.

Katsuura, G., Arimura, A., Koves, K. & Gottschall, P. E. (1990). Involvement of organum vasculosum of lamina terminalis and preoptic area in interleukin 1$\beta$-induced ACTH release. *Am. J. Physiol.*, **258**, E163–E171.

Katsuura, G., Gottschall, P. E., Dahl, R. R. & Arimura, A. (1989). Interleukin-1 beta increases prostaglandin $E_2$ in the rat astrocyte cultures: modulatory effect of neuropeptides. *Endocrinology*, **124**, 3125–7.

Kent, S., Bluthé, R. M., Kelley, K. W. & Dantzer, R. (1992*a*). Sickness behavior as a new target for drug development. *Trends Pharmacol. Sci.*, **13**, 24–8.

Kent, S., Bluthé, R. M., Dantzer, R., Hardwick, A. J., Kelley, K. W., Rothwell, N. J. & Vannice, J. L. (1992*b*). Different receptor mechanisms mediate the pyrogenic and behavioral effects of interleukin-1. *Proc. Natl. Acad. Sci. USA*, **89**, 9117–120.

Kent, S., Kelley, K. W. & Dantzer, R. (1992*c*). Effects of lipopolysaccharide on food-motivated behavior in the rat are not blocked by an interleukin-1 receptor antagonist. *Neurosci. Lett.*, **145**, 83–6.

Kilbourn, R. G., Gross, S. S., Jubran, A., Adams, J., Griffith, O. W., Levi, R. & Lodato, R. F. (1990). $N^G$-Methyl-L-arginine inhibits tumor necrosis factor-induced hypotension: implications for the involvement of nitric oxide. *Proc. Natl. Acad. Sci. USA*, **87**, 3629–32.

Kluger, M. J. (1991). Fever: role of pyrogens and cryogens. *Physiol. Rev.*, **71**, 93–127.

Koenig, S., Gendelman, H. E., Orenstein, T. M., dal Canto, M. C., Pezeshkpour, G. H., Yungbluth, M., Janotta, F., Aksamit, A., Martin, M. A. & Fauci, A. S. (1986). Detection of AIDS virus in macrophages in brain tissue from AIDS patients with encephalopathy. *Science*, **233**, 1089–93.

Komaki, G., Arimura, A. & Koves, K. (1992). Effect of intravenous injection of IL-1$\beta$ on $PGE_2$ levels in several brain areas as determined by microdialysis. *Am. J. Physiol.*, **262**, E246–E251.

Koyanagi, Y., Miles, S., Mitsuyasu, R. T., Merrill, J. E., Vintners, H. V. & Chen, I. S. Y. (1987). Dual infection of the central nervous system by AIDS viruses with distinct cellular tropisms. *Science*, **236**, 819–22.

Kushner, I. (1991). The acute-phase response: from Hippocrates to cytokine biology. *Eur. Cytokine Net.*, **2**, 75–80.

Lechan, R. M., Toni, R., Clark, B. D., Cannon, J. G., Shaw, A. R., Dinarello, C. A. & Reichlin, S. (1990). Immunoreactive interleukin-1$\beta$ localization in the rat forebrain. *Brain Res.*, **514**, 135–40.

Lipton, J. M. (1989). Neuropeptide alpha-melanocyte stimulating hormone in control of fever, the acute phase response and inflammation. In *Neuroimmune Networks: Physiology and Diseases*, ed. E. J. Goetzl & N. H. Spector, pp. 243–50. New York: Alan R. Liss.

MacDonald, E. M., Mann, A. H. & Thomas, H. C. (1987). Interferons as mediators of psychiatric morbidity. An investigation in a trial of recombinant alpha-interferons in hepatitis B carriers. *Lancet*, **ii**, 1175–8.

Merrill, J. E., Koyanagi, Y. & Chen, I. S. Y. (1989). Interleukin-1 and tumor necrosis factor α can be induced from mononuclear phagocytes by human immunodeficiency virus type I binding to the CD4 receptor. *J. Virol.*, **63**, 4404–8.

Merrill, J. E., Koyanagi, Y., Zack, J., Thomas, L., Martin, F. & Chen, I. S. Y. (1992). Induction of interleukin-1 and tumor necrosis factor alpha in brain cultures by human immunodeficiency virus type 1. *J. Virol.*, **66**, 2217–25.

Miller, M. A., Vician, L., Clifton, D. K. & Dorsa, D. M. (1989). Sex differences in vasopressin neurones in the bed nucleus of the stria terminalis by *in situ* hybridization. *Peptides*, **10**, 615–20.

Miller, N. E. (1964). Some psychophysiological studies of motivation and of the behavioral effects of illness. *Bull. Br. Psychol. Soc.*, **17**, 1–20.

Minami, M., Kuraishi, Y. & Satoh, M. (1991). Effects of kainic acid on messenger RNA levels of IL-1β, IL-6, TNFα and LIF in the rat brain. *Biochem. Biophys. Res. Commun.*, **176**, 593–8.

Minami, M., Kuraishi, Y., Yamaguchi, T., Nakai, S., Hirai, Y. & Satoh, M. (1990). Convulsants induce interleukin-1β messenger RNA in rat brain. *Biochem. Biophys. Res. Commun.*, **171**, 832–7.

Moncada, S., Palmer, R. M. J. & Higgs, E. A. (1991). Nitric oxide: physiology, pathophysiology, and pharmacology. *Pharmacol. Rev.*, **44**, 109–42.

Mrosovsky, N., Molony, L. A., Conn, C. A. & Kluger, M. J. (1989). Anorexic effects of interleukin 1 in the rat. *Am. J. Physiol.*, **257**, R1315–R1321.

Mugridge, K. G., Perretti, M., Ghiara, P. & Parente, L. (1991). α-Melanocyte-stimulating hormone reduces interleukin-1β effects on rat stomach preparations possibly through interference with a type I receptor. *Eur. J. Pharmacol.*, **197**, 151–5.

Newton, R. C., Uhl, J., Covington, M. & Back, O. (1988). The distribution and clearance of radiolabelled human interleukin-1β in mice. *Lymphokine Res.*, **7**, 207–15.

Opp, M., Obal, F. & Krueger, J. M. (1989). Corticotropin-releasing factor attenuates interleukin 1-induced sleep and fever in rabbits. *Am. J. Physiol.*, **257**, R528–R535.

Otterness, I. G., Golden, H. W., Seymour, P. A., Eskra, J. D. & Daumy, G. O. (1991). Role of prostaglandins in the behavioral changes induced by murine IL 1 alpha in the rat. *Cytokine*, **3**, 333–38.

Otterness, I. G., Seymour, P. A., Golden, H. W., Reynolds, J. A. & Daumy, G. O. (1988). The effects of continuous administration of murine interleukin-1α in the rat. *Physiol. Behav.*, **43**, 797–804.

Parnet, P., Brunke, D. L., Goujon, E., Demotes Mainard, J., Biragyn, A., Arkins, S., Dantzer, R. & Kelley, K. W. (1993). Molecular identification of two types of interleukin-1 receptors in the murine pituitary gland. *J. Neuroendocrinol.*, **5**, 213–19.

Price, R. N., Brew, B., Sidtis, J., Rosenblum, U., Scheck, A. C. & Cleary, P. (1988). The brain in AIDS: central nervous system HIV-1 infection and AIDS dementia complex. *Science*, **239**, 586–92.

Reimers, J., Wogensen, L. D., Welinder, B., Hejnæs, K. R., Poulsen, S. S., Nilsson, P. & Nerup, J. (1991). The pharmacokinetics, distribution and degradation of human recombinant interleukin 1β in normal rats. *Scand. J. Immunol.*, **34**, 597–617.

Renault, P. F., Hoofnagle, J. H., Park, Y., Mullen, K. D., Peters, M., Jones, B., Rustgi, V. & Jones, E. A. (1987). Psychiatric complications of long-term interferon alfa therapy. *Arch. Intern. Med.*, **147**, 1577–80.

Robert, A., Olafsson, A. S., Lancaster, C. & Zhang, W. R. (1991). Interleukin-1 is cytoprotective, antisecretory, stimulates $PGE_2$ synthesis by the stomach, and retards gastric emptying. *Life Sci.*, **48**, 123–34.

Rohatiner, A. Z. S., Prior, P. F., Burton, A. C., Smith, A. T., Balkwill, F. R. & Lister, T. A. (1983). Central nervous system toxicity of interferon. *Br. J. Cancer*, **47**, 419–22.

Rothwell, N. J. (1989). CRF is involved in the pyrogenic and thermogenic effects of interleukin $1\beta$ in the rat. *Am. J. Physiol.*, **256**, E111–E115.

Segall, M. A. & Crnic, L. S. (1990*a*). A test of conditioned taste aversion with mouse interferon-$\alpha$. *Brain Behav. Immun.*, **4**, 223–31.

Segall, M. A. & Crnic, L. S. (1990*b*). An animal model for the behavioral effects of interferon. *Behav. Neurosci.*, **104**, 612–18.

Sharpe, M. C., Archard, L. C., Banatvala, J. E., Borysiewicz, L. K., Clare, A. W., David, A., Edwards, R. H., Hawton, K. E., Lambert, H. P., Lane, R. J., McDonald, E. M., Mombray, J. F., Pearson, D. J., Peto, T., Preedy, V. R., Smith, A. P., Smith, D. G., Taylor, D. J., Tyrrell, D. A. J., Wessely, S. & White, P. D. (1991). A report – chronic fatigue syndrome: guide-lines for research. *J. R. Soc. Med.*, **84**, 118–21.

Shimizu, H., Uehara, Y., Shimomura, Y. & Kobayashi, I. (1991). Central administration of ibuprofen failed to block the anorexia induced by interleukin-1. *Eur. J. Pharmacol.*, **195**, 281–4.

Sirko, S., Bishai, I. & Coceani, F. (1989). Prostaglandin formation in the hypothalamus *in vivo:* effect of pyrogens. *Am. J. Physiol.*, **256**, R616–R624.

Smith, A. P., Tyrrell, D. A. J., Al-Nakib, W., Coyle, K. B., Donovan, C. B., Higgins, P. G. & Williams, J. S. (1987*a*). Effects of experimentally-induced virus infections and illness on psychomotor performance. *Neuropsychobiology*, **18**, 144–48.

Smith, A. P., Tyrrell, D. A. J., Al-Nakib, W., Coyle, K. B., Donovan, C. B., Higgins, P. G. & Williams, J. S. (1988*a*). The effects of experimentally-induced respiratory virus infections on performance. *Psychol. Med.*, **18**, 65–71.

Smith, A. P., Tyrell, D. A. J., Coyle, K. B. & Higgins, P. (1988*b*). Effects of interferon alpha on performance in man: a preliminary report. *Psychopharmacology*, **96**, 414–16.

Smith, A. P., Tyrrell, D. A. J., Coyle, K. B. & Willmans, J. S. (1987*b*). Selective effects of minor illness on human performance. *Br. J. Psychol.*, **78**, 183–8.

Smith, J., Urba, W., Steis, R., Janik, J., Fenton, B., Sharfman, W., Conlon, K., Sznol, M., Creekmore, S., Wells, N., Elwood, L., Keller, J., Hestdal, K., Ewal, C., Rossio, J., Kopp, W., Shimuzu, M., Oppenheim, J. & Longo, D. (1990). Interleukin-1 alpha (IL-1$\alpha$): results of a phase I toxicity and immunomodulatory trial. *Proc. Am. Soc. Clin. Oncol.*, **9**, 186–90.

Spadaro, F. & Dunn, A. J. (1990). Intracerebroventricular administration of interleukin-1 to mice alters investigation of stimuli in a novel environment. *Brain, Behav. Immun.*, **4**, 308–22.

Sundar, S. K., Cierpial, M. A., Kamaraju, L. S., Long, S., Hsieh, S., Lorenz, C., Aaron, M., Ritchie, J. C. & Weiss, J. M. (1991). Human immunodeficiency virus glycoprotein (gp120) infused into rat brain induces interleukin 1 to elevate pituitary–adrenal activity and decrease peripheral cellular immune responses. *Proc. Natl. Acad. Sci. USA*, **88**, 11246–50.

Takao, T., Tracey, D. E., Mitchell, W. M. & De Souza, E. B. (1990). Interleukin-1 receptors in mouse brain: characterization and neuronal localization. *Endocrinology*, **127**, 3070–8.

Tazi, A., Crestani, F. & Dantzer, R. (1990). Aversive effects of centrally injected interleukin-1 are independent of its pyrogenic activity. *Neurosci. Res. Commun.*, **7**, 159–65.

Tazi, A., Dantzer, R., Crestani, F. & Le Moal, M. (1988). Interleukin 1 induces conditioned taste aversion in rats: a possible explanation for its pituitary–adrenal stimulating activity. *Brain Res.*, **473**, 369–71.

Tewari, A., Buhles, W. C. & Starnes, H. F. (1990). Preliminary report: effects of interleukin-1 on platelet counts. *Lancet*, **336**, 712–14.

Thiemermann, C. & Vane, J. (1990). Inhibition of nitric oxide synthesis reduces the hypotension induced by bacterial lipopolysaccharides in the rat *in vivo*. *Eur. J. Pharmacol*, **182**, 591–5.

Uehara, A., Ishikawa, Y., Okumura, T., Okamura, K., Sekiya, C., Takasugi, Y. & Namiki, M. (1989*a*). Indomethacin blocks the anorexic action of interleukin-1. *Eur. J. Pharmacol.*, **170**, 257–60.

Uehara, A., Sekiya, C., Takasugi, Y., Namiki, M. & Arimura, A. (1989*b*). Anorexia induced by interleukin 1: involvement of corticotropin-releasing factor. *Am. J. Physiol.*, **257**, R613–R617.

Uehara, Y., Shimizu, H., Sato, N., Tanaka, Y., Shimomura, Y. & Mori, M. (1992). Carboxyl-terminal tripeptide of α-melanocyte-stimulating hormone antagonizes interleukin-1-induced anorexia. *Eur. J. Pharmacol.*, **220**, 119–22.

Ur, E., White, P. D. & Grossman, A. (1992). Hypothesis: cytokines may be activated to cause depressive illness and chronic fatigue syndrome. *Eur. Arch. Psychiatry Clin. Neurosci.*, **241**, 317–22.

van Dam, A. M., Brouns, M., Louisse, S. & Berkenbosch, F. (1992). Appearance of interleukin-1 in macrophages and in ramified microglia in the brain of endotoxin-treated rats: a pathway for the induction of non-specific symptoms of sickness? *Brain Res.*, **588**, 291–6.

Waage, A., Halstensen, A., Shalaby, R., Brandtzaeg, P., Kierulf, P. & Espevik, T. (1989). Local production of tumour necrosis factor α, interleukin 1 and interleukin 6 in meningococcal meningitis. Relation to inflammatory response. *J. Exp. Med.*, **170**, 1859–67.

Weindl, A. (1972). Neuroendocrine aspects of circumventricular organs. In *Frontiers in Neuroendocrinology*, ed. W. F. Ganong & L. Martini, pp. 3–32. Oxford: Oxford University Press.

Weiss, J. M., Sundar, S. K., Cierpial, M. A. & Ritchie, J. C. (1991). Effects of interleukin-1 infused into brain are antagonized by α-MSH in a dose-dependent manner. *Eur. J. Pharmacol*, **192**, 177–9.

# 8

# Psychological and behavioural aspects of pain

HOLGER URSIN, INGER M. ENDRESEN, ANDERS LUND and NORMA MJELLEM

## Pain

### *Introduction*

The pathophysiological and biochemical changes in the tissue produced by trauma are detected by two systems, nervous and immune. Detection by nervous system leads to behavioural responses that may alleviate the pain and favour recovery. This includes inactivity and immobilization. The withdrawal and immobilization are often efficient behavioural precautions against predators and against further traumatization.

Detection by the immune system leads to a cascade of immunological events that also favour healing. These responses are not limited to the identification and destruction of antigens and foreign material ('non-self'). The signal substances, in particular interleukin-1 (IL-1), also affect behaviour. It is very interesting that the behaviour effect is seen as the same withdrawal or inactivity resulting from the pain itself. If the trauma leads to infection and fever, the fever itself also leads to inactivity, possibly via the IL-1 mechanism. Finally, recent data point to the interaction between these systems. The signal substances are similar or the same in the periphery and in the brain. These systems are not as stimulus-bound or 'reflexive' as believed originally. Both pain transmission and immune responses are influenced by the central nervous system (CNS), and, therefore, also by psychological factors. Traumas do not seem to hit us totally at random, and the responses to trauma are also clearly influenced by psychological factors (Malt *et al.*, 1987; Malt, 1992).

The psychological and behavioural aspects of pain are important from a general scientific point of view, since they involve basic survival mechanisms. The field is also important, since it may reveal basic mechanisms that affect therapy and prognosis for pain patients. A particularly important aspect is the possible consequences for therapy and prognosis of the increasing number of chronic pain patients.

### *Pain*

The concept of pain is used to cover a rich variety of human and animal suffering. The International Association for the Study of Pain, chaired by Merskey (1979), defined pain as 'an unpleasant sensory and emotional experience associated with actual or potential tissue damage, or described in terms of such damage'. They added crucial notes to this definition pointing to the fact that it avoids tying pain to the stimulus, and that activity induced in nociceptors and nociceptive pathways by noxious stimuli is not pain, which is always a psychological state (Merksey, 1979). Pain is always a subjective experience, and should be distinguished from nociception, which refers to activity in the nociceptors or nociceptive pathways.

It is important to distinguish between acute and chronic pain states, since these two states differ in biomedical function. Although acute pain may promote survival and restitution, chronic pain is usually destructive, physically, psychologically and socially (Sternbach, 1989). In acute pain, the clinical symptoms and signs are similar to those seen in anxiety states, whereas the symptoms and signs seen in chronic pain states are similar to those seen in depressive states (Von Knorring, 1988).

Pain should be regarded as a psychobiological event. However, even so, it is clinically and conceptually necessary to distinguish between pain states with a pathophysiological basis and pain states where there is no such basis. There is a difference between a transient noxious stimulus that does not produce any tissue damage (Woolf, 1989: 'physiological pain'), and the pain arising from tissue damage in nervous injury (Woolf, 1989: 'pathological pain'). In the latter case, the pain may occur in the absence of any apparent stimulus, the threshold for pain may decrease, and the pain response may be exaggerated. However, these characteristics also occur in conditions, prolonged or even chronic, where there is no demonstrated tissue damage or inflammation. These are called idiopathic pain disorders (Williams & Spitzer, 1982) or somatoform pain disorder (DSM-II-R; American Psychiatric Association, 1987). Whatever we call it, there is a group of patients suffering from pain, where a physical disorder cannot be detected, or the physical findings are insignificant. For the somatoform pain disorder, a very significant percentage of these patients are depressed, up to 25–50% (Kaplan & Sadock, 1991). The neurobiological substrate may be the same, but the distinction plays an important role in the attribution mechanisms for the patient and the public.

Pain occurs when tissue is damaged by a noxious agent. However, in many cases there is no evident trauma or any demonstrable tissue damage. This is the case for most cases of muscle pain. Lack of physical training and monotonous, static loads seem to favour the development of muscle pain. The tension and the lack of training may be regarded as a misuse of muscles that is initiated and maintained by the brain, i.e. by the individual him- or herself. To what extent, then, is the 'injury' detected by the afferent nerve terminals self-inflicted, and what can the brain do to alleviate the condition? Are the 'natural' behavioural responses to pain, seen after tissue damage, adequate or inadequate for musculoskeletal pain? As much as 50% of the work days lost because of sickness absence in Norway is due to diagnostic groups that solely or mainly depend on subjective statements from the patient, such as pain states in muscles and connective tissue, other ill-defined conditions, and mental disorders (Tellnes, 1989*a b*). Therefore, it has become a major political issue in health care and health promotion to prevent such states, and to treat them.

One crucial question is to what extent the behaviour of the patient and the health care system is adequate for this type of pain state. The pain state is there, with psychological and biological aspects, regardless of whether it is 'pathological' or 'physiological' The issue is whether some of these states maintain themselves, in particular the chronic idiopathic pain states. It is also possible that these factors may have effects on chronic pain even when there is tissue damage (pathological pain).

Physiological trauma leads to pain, due to activity in specific nerve fibres, called nociceptors. These fibres respond to specific chemical changes in the tissue. This chapter discusses the factors regulating the biochemical state of the tissue, the nerves that record and monitor this state and the transmission of these signals to the brain. Also discussed is the efferent control of these factors by the brain, which constitutes a potent neurobiological feed-back and feed-forward system. Many of the crucial aspects of pain should be regarded as consequences of these information loops, and it is important for us to understand which parts of the loop should be attacked by therapy.

### *Pain mechanisms*

Pain originates from activity in nociceptors, specialized sets of peripheral nerve endings that convey information about injury or threat of injury.

They differ from other receptor types in that they have a high threshold to the adequate stimulus, be it heat, or a mechanical or cooling stimulus. They are found both in the skin and in the muscles, and are divided into A-fibre and C-fibre nociceptors. The nociceptors then transmit impulses to the spinal cord, where a network of neurones ascend to the brain stem and thalamus. Further connections exist between the thalamus and the cortex, ultimately leading to perception. Distinct pathways within the central nervous system can modulate nociceptive transmission at the level of the spinal cord.

One of the behavioural characteristics of pain is hyperalgesia, an enhanced pain report to natural stimuli. Pain spreads to adjacent areas, and the injured part and those surrounding it become hypersensitive. To activate nociceptors requires intense stimuli. But, once they have been activated, the threshold decreases, both in the injured part (primary hyperalgesia), and in the surrounding tissue (secondary hyperalgesia). This clinical hyperalgesia corresponds to an increase in the responsiveness of nociceptors (peripheral sensitization). In the CNS, sensitization of synaptic transmission may occur at many levels. This, and other CNS factors, may contribute to hyperalgesia. Through efferent control of muscles, sympathetic innervation of the tissue, and CNS control of the pain transmission, CNS sensitization has an effect on a positive feed-back and feed-forward loop which is essential for the understanding of behaviour related to pain.

### *Peripheral sensitization*

Peripheral sensitization translates into an increase in the sensitivity of primary afferent nociceptors in the vicinity of the injury. It involves a reduction in the threshold and/or an increase in the depolarization of the primary afferent nociceptors. Substances such as histamine, serotonin, hydrogen ions, potassium ions, neurokinins, calcitonin-gene related peptide (CGRP), and bradykinin that are released from injured afferents, damaged tissue and inflammatory cells, probably contribute to the sensitization (Raja *et al.*, 1988; Woolf, 1989). Although the exact mechanisms are not known, the various chemicals released probably exert their effect through multiple interacting intracellular second-messenger systems, leading to an alteration in the sensitivity of receptors, and to a lowering of the threshold (Levine *et al.*, 1986*b*; Rang & Ritchie, 1988; Woolf, 1989). It is assumed that these changes may be permanent, or semi-permanent, if nociceptor stimulation is upheld over a longer time (Wall & Fitzgerald, 1982; Woolf,

1989). For instance, a long-lasting sensitizing role has been suggested for substance P in the periphery, producing sensitization of nociceptors to their own action and to the action of different mediators (Nakamura-Craig & Smith, 1989).

It should be kept in mind that the peripheral increase in substance P seems due to release from the afferent terminals, and seems to require activity in these same nociceptive fibres. Tissue sensitized with repeated injections of substance P shows intense and long-lasting hyperalgesia after small doses of dopamine, or prostacyclin (Nakamura-Craig & Smith, 1989). However, there is also interaction with the sympathetic innervation of the damaged tissue. Altered excitability in the dorsal horns will influence the activity of preganglionic sympathetic neurones. Sympathetic reflexes will be increased in amplitude and duration much as is the flexor reflex (Woolf, 1989). This affects the peripheral pain mechanisms, as is evident in the clinical findings in fibromyalgic patients (Vaerøy *et al.*, 1989).

There has been much interest in the importance of sympathetic nerves for rheumatoid arthritis. The patients show many signs of disturbed sympathetic innervation (Leden *et al.*, 1983), and surgical and chemical blocking of sympathetic activity, in particular $\beta_2$ antagonists, are effective in reducing joint injury and reducing pain (Levine *et al.*, 1986*a*). A strong involvement of the sympathetic system is also demonstrated for fibromyalgic patients (Vaerøy *et al.*, 1989), and has been postulated to be a central factor for the sensitization to pain in these patients (Vaerøy, 1990). Blockade of the sympathetic activity produces pain reduction in these patients (Bengtsson & Bengtsson, 1988).

### *Central sensitization*

Until recently it was believed that the hyperalgesia that followed injury to peripheral tissue was secondary to changes at the site of injury. However, there is evidence that the increase in pain involves altered processing and hyperexcitability in the CNS. Animal models of hyperalgesia produced by inflammation or nerve injury have been developed, and some dorsal horn neurones exhibit an increase in excitability to stimulation after an initial noxious stimulation. It has also been shown that some neurones will have an enhancement of their receptive field. The induction and maintenenance of the central sensitization produced by high-threshold primary afferent inputs involve activation of neurones at *N*-methyl-D-aspartate (NMDA) receptor sites by excitatory amino acids such as glutamate and aspartate (Woolf & Thompson, 1991). The hyperexcitability, the expansion of receptive fields and the hyperalgesia following tissue or nerve injury can be blocked or reduced by the use of NMDA antagonists. Neuropeptides, such as substance P, and also CGRP are believed to act as neuromodulators, enhancing the effect of excitatory amino acids.

Changes in central nervous system excitability have also been evoked in muscle hyperalgesia. A recent experiment, inducing a noxious stimulus of muscles with intramuscular injections of bradykinin, induced an increase in excitability of dorsal horn neurones, measured by a lowering of threshold and enlargement of receptive field of the neurones. These results were similar to those obtained when perfusing the spinal cord with a solution of substance P, and the changes observed outlasted the bradykinin-induced excitation of peripheral muscle receptors (Hoheisel & Mense, 1992). What is of great interest is that the neurophysiological sensitization persisted long after the initiating stimulus had terminated, thus demonstrating that this may represent long-lasting changes. It has been proposed that the sensitizing effects of C-fibre mediators at the level of the spinal cord may last for days (Wall, 1985).

The neuromodulatory role of substance P is not believed to be limited to the periphery. Wall (1985) has postulated trophic mechanisms in the CNS, in particular for the release of substance P in the spinal cord. Glutamate and substance P coexist in some primary afferent neurones, and a functional interaction in the spinal cord between substance P and the excitatory amino acids has been shown. A concurrent activation of spinal NMDA and substance P receptors induced an enhancement of spinal transmission of nociception, that appeared to be dependent on the intensity or the quality of the peripheral stimulus (Mjellem-Joly *et al.*, 1992, 1993). This central hypersensitivity of the dorsal horn neurones could lead to an enhanced and prolonged response to subsequent noxious stimulation, and it would seem possible that such mechanisms play a role in the development of hyperalgesia and chronic pain.

### *Modulation of nociceptive transmission*

It is obvious that the subjectively experienced intensity of pain depends not only on the stimulus intensity but to a very large extent on psychological factors. Specific pathways in the CNS control pain transmission and these pathways can be activated by psychological factors. There exists an endogenous pain-modulating system that was first indicated by the discovery of analgesia induced by electrical stimulation of sites in the brainstem (Hosobuchi *et al.*, 1977). There is now general acceptance that descending pathways inhibit nociceptive transmission on the level of the spinal cord (Basbaum & Fields, 1984). The modulatory network includes the midbrain periaqueductal grey matter and adjacent reticular formation, which projects to the spinal cord via the rostroventral medulla. This pathway inhibits spinal neurones that respond to noxious stimuli. There is also a pain-modulation pathway from the dorsolateral pons to the cord. The pathway from the rostral medulla to the cord is partly serotonergic, whereas that from the dorsolateral pons is at least partly noradrenergic (Dahlström & Fuxe, 1964). In addition to these biogenic amine-containing neurones, endogenous opioid peptides are present in all regions so far implicated in pain modulation (Gramsch *et al.*, 1979). It does seem probable that these pain-modulating systems contribute to the well-known variability of perceived pain in people with apparently similar imjuries.

### *Physiological and pathological pain*

Woolf (1987, 1989) discriminated between pathological pain, inflammatory or neuropathic, and physiological pain, where there was no demonstrable pathophysiology. Pathological pain may occur in the absence of any apparent stimulus, the response is exaggerated in amplitude or duration or both, the pain threshold is decreased, the sensation spread to non-injured tissue, and there may be interactions with the sympathetic and somatosensory systems. These criteria do not seem to make any clear distinction between what many of us experience in daily life. A sore muscle from overtraining or lower back pain may very well qualify as 'pathological' without the patient entering a long-lasting or chronic state. The issue remains, therefore, in our opinion: When does physiological muscle pain become pathological? How long is 'too long' and how strong is 'too strong'? How important are the psychological factors for preservation or termination of this state?

## Pain behaviour

### *Introduction*

Pain leads to protective behaviour, healing behaviour and expressive behaviour. All these behaviours have their survival effects and instrumental effects. They are an important part of our phylogenetic heritage. We assume, therefore, that they have an adaptive value. Whereas acute pain is associated with many of the classical signs of anxiety (increased cardiac rate, increased blood pressure, pupillary dilatation, palmar sweating, hyperventilation, hypermotility and escape behaviour), the chronic pain state is associated with depression (sleep disturbances, irritability, appetite disturbances, constipation, psychomotor retardation, social withdrawal and abnormal illness behaviour). A continuous discussion has existed regarding the relation between chronic pain and depression, ranging from chronic pain as masked depression (Lopez Ibor, 1972), via chronic pain as a variant of depressive disorders (Blumer & Heilbronn, 1982), to discoveries of some similar neurochemical findings in both chronic pain and depression (Ward *et al.*, 1982; Von Knorring, 1988). In some cultures, expression of emotional distress is traditionally discouraged and suppressed, and such distress is communicated in a somatic rather than a psychological mode (Kirmayer, 1984). This occurs not infrequently in China and other Eastern countries. Some authors have speculated that this somatization tendency is associated with poor education and lower income rather than differences in cultural background (White, 1982; Westermeyer *et al.*, 1989).

The expressive part of pain behaviour is an obvious cry for help and the instrumental effect is to obtain such help. In humans we discriminate between illness, disease and sickness. Disease is the state in which there is an objective pathophysiological change, illness is the subjective state of not being well and sickness is the role we play to obtain support and assistance. Chronic pain, therefore, is associated both with illness and with sickness. Responses from the environment, including society and welfare systems, may have an undesired effect by reinforcing sickness roles in cases where a more brutal environment might have ended the state more quickly. Some of the pain behaviour may be instrumental in obtaining help, but not in acquiring new behaviour that may be more curative in the long run. The help, the comfort of being taken care of, and the relief from duties, all have a beneficial effect on acute pain states. They also reinforce this behaviour. The question is whether the acceptance of the sickness role and the instrumental reinforcement of it leads to a prolongation of behaviours incompatible with recovery. Proper muscle use and proper muscle training are not encouraged or reinforced.

Following physical trauma, the patient should go through a phase of immobility. The issue is how long this immobility phase should last. Subjective feelings of pain may not be a good indicator for when this stage should be finalized. In modern surgery, pain is definitely not a signal that is respected when patients are mobilized. In treatment of chronic pain however, this subjective feeling of pain is given much more importance. It is often left totally to the patient, and it may be that some of us allocate too much meaning and importance to the pain itself. The subjective feelings and the subjective allocation mechanisms are often the only indication for the treatment, including the immobilization.

### *Species-specific defence behaviours*

The behaviour of the immobile animal with trauma is a display of one or several species-specific antipredatory defence behaviours. Defensive-behaviours may be defined as all the responses seen when an individual is faced with threat. This may be seen as a part of the antipredatory repertoire of the animal (Fanselow & Kim, 1992). The various patterns of behaviour observed are flight, freezing, defensive threat, attack and active as well as passive avoidance behaviour. Similar behaviours are seen in social defeat. This has been described in rats (Blanchard *et al.*, 1990), and in cats (Leyhausen, 1960; Ursin, 1981, 1985).

The various behaviours differ between species. An ethological catalogue is missing for most species. There is also no agreement on the names or the taxonomy of these behaviours within species or between species (Ursin, 1981).

The antipredatory defensive reactions may be characterized by different types of physiological response depending on whether they are active or passive. During freezing, increased blood pressure and heart rate have been described by some observers, who use this as a criterion for differentiating between freezing and other types of inactivity. However, freezing may very well be followed by a very marked drop in heart rate, seen for instance in ptarmigans (Gabrielsen *et al.*, 1985).

The animals might freeze to the extent that respiration rate and heart rate, and probably also metabolism, decrease. This decreases the risk of detection. However, the animals must also be able to leave the area whenever freezing is no longer an adequate strategy. The physiological response has many similarities with the diving reflex, and one reason why the muscles do not become paralysed may be that similar vascular responses occur as during diving: the blood is flushed through the various tissues at intervals (Blix & Folkow, 1983). The increase in heart rate and blood pressure may be regarded as a preparation for intense fighting. The blood pressure decrease may help as an antipredatory response.

It is tempting to speculate on the relationships between freezing, blood-pressure decrease, vascular shock and pain. The vagal reflex may be regarded as an extreme non-adaptive end of a programme that has a reasonable phylogenetic role, but becomes inadequate in situations where recuperative behaviour depends on the conscious state. However, shock will lead to an analgetic state, and, depending on the animal lying down and receiving enough oxygen to the brain, it may represent an adaptive response.

Behavioural inhibition has been regarded as an indicator of anxiety (Gray, 1982). This state may also be involved in pain because 'freezing' may involve analgesia. The problem is that freezing is only one aspect of behavioural inhibition, and anxiety is also only one of several behaviour states that are accompanied by behavioural inhibition. The discrimination between behavioural inhibition with high heart rate and low heart rate does not seem reliable, since both high and low heart rates may accompany anxiety states.

The behaviour inhibition system was originally treated by Kaada (1951) and McCleary (1961), and may have roles other than being a part of freezing (Ursin, 1976). Strong stress, leading to defensive behaviour, may lead to stress-induced analgesia through two seemingly independent mechanisms, one opioid and one non-opioid (Brush & Shain, 1989). The combination of analgesia and freezing may be regarded as an adaptive response to a dominating and aggressive conspecific.

The decreased activity seen after shocks or social defeat may be seen as an indicator of anxiety, or risk assessment behaviour (Blanchard *et al.*, 1990; Fanselow & Kim, 1992). It is particularly easy to observe in situations where animals have to make a choice. Blanchard *et al.* (1990) accepted this as an animal model of anxiety. This is confirmed by the blockade of this behaviour by benzodiazepine anxiolytic drugs and 5 $HT_{1A}$ receptor agonists (Rodgers & Randall, 1987; Rodgers & Shepherd, 1989).

According to Fanselow & Kim (1992), fear activates the anti-predatory system, depending on the perceived level of risk. Moderate levels of risk lead to freezing, and depend on the ventral periaqueductal grey (PAG). High levels of risk, on the other hand, lead to volatile defensive behaviours characterized particularly by activity bursts, and depend on the dorsolateral PAG. There is a nice double association between the substrates for these two behaviours. Depaulis *et al.* (1989) hold that defensive behaviour and freezing depend on the intermediate PAG.

***Coping with pain***

Confrontation with threats or any situation in which the challenge is tending to overcome the resources of the subject, gives rise to stress responses. The stress may be regarded as an alarm response that prepares the organism to face the challenge. The outcome of such situations depends on the extent to which the individual is able to reach a positive response outcome expectancy (Ursin & Olff, 1993). In other words, is the individual able to cope with the situation, how efficient is this coping, and what strategies are being used?

In a review of recent Dutch material using the most commonly used questionnaires in Holland, Olff *et al.* (1993) discriminated between four main strategies in the coping and psychological defence scales. These factors were an instrumental mastery-oriented coping, a cognitive defence factor, a factor comprising defensive hostility, and, finally, a fourth factor dealing with emotion-focused coping. These factors related differentially to psychoendocrine and psychoimmunological data, and seemed to differ in the extent to which they led to efficient coping and subjective reports of health (Olff *et al.*, 1993). In this discussion of pain behaviour we analyse coping and defence strategies and their effects on handling pain and pain experience.

Expectancy of pain influences the pain responses. Arntz *et al.* (1991) investigated the effects of incorrect intensity expectations on immediate and later responses to a painful stimulus. Underpredicted painful experiences were related to subsequent higher pain responses on the physiological level, but not on the subjective level, and to increased anticipatory responses (increased pain expectations, uncertainty, subjective fear, skin conductance responses). Skin conductance level also indicated increased fear after underpredicted experiences. Overpredicted painful experiences were related to a faster decrease in subjective fear compared to the control group.

Beliefs about pain and the meaning of pain are also an important dimension, e.g. for the prognosis in patients with chronic low back pain (Strong *et al.*, 1992). These dimensions are also important for compliance with pain treatment, and successful coping. Williams & Keefe (1991) showed that patients with the belief that pain was enduring and mysterious were less likely to use cognitive coping strategies, e.g. reinterpretation of pain sensation, were more likely to catastrophize and less likely to rate their coping strategies as effective in controlling and decreasing pain than patients believing their pain to be understandable and of short duration.

This confirms what has been found in general for survival and successful coping with serious stress. The meaning of the event is important for survival (Antonovsky, 1987). Barkwell (1991) found that, for cancer patients, the ability to cope with the pain experience was little influenced by access to a palliative care unit, or by the extent of medical care. The strongest impact on pain, depression and the coping score was made by the meaning ascribed to pain by the patients. Successful pain attenuation therefore depends in part on the understanding, by individual patients, of the cognitive processing of pain.

In the USA it was found that 14.4% of the population aged between 25 and 74 years suffered from definite chronic pain related to the joints and musculoskeletal system. Another 7.4% had some pain of uncertain duration. Using a high cut-off score for depression, 18% of these patients were found to have a depression, contrasting with 8% in the control group without chronic pain (Magni *et al*., 1990). In 1983 Kramlinger *et al.* reported that of 100 chronic-pain patients, 25 were definitely depressed, 39 were probably depressed and 36 were not depressed. Ninety per cent of the definitely depressed patients showed resolution of their depression without use of antidepressant medication. The treatment consisted of behaviour modification, physical rehabilitation measures, medication management, education, group discussion, biofeedback-relaxation techniques, family member participation, and supportive psychological treatment. Gamsa (1990) has concluded that emotional disturbance in pain patients is more likely to be a consequence than a cause of chronic pain.

It has also been shown that successful copers with high self-efficacy have fewer pain responses, and that successful coping is associated with high levels of the internal locus of control (Harkapaa *et al*., 1991). In line with these findings, there are also differences between those who seek medical advice for back pain and those who do not seek such advice. The non-consulters rated their work to be more stressful, less frequently had a spouse suffering or having suffered from chronic pain, had fewer abnormal pain-drawings in a drawing test, woke up less frequently during the night, used fewer sleeping pills, and participated more often in sports. They also had a higher frequency of repression on the Meta Contrast Technique (MCT) (Lindal & Uden, 1989). It follows from what has been said that the personality of the patient must be an important resource, an important determinant for the ways of coping with pain and the success of such coping. It is also the degree of functioning rather than the pain report itself which decides the prognosis for rehabilitation results. The degree of functioning is determined by dimensions such as the amount of impairment, disability and handicaps reported by the patient (Talo *et al.*, 1992).

### *Pain behaviour, illness and sickness*

Pain behaviour may be defined as the interaction between the pain patient and his or her direct environment. Vlaeyen *et al.* (1990) listed several pain behaviours and used this for a 78-item global rating scale used by nurses to quantify observed pain behaviour in a clinical setting. Factor analysis demonstrated six internally reliable factors: distorted mobility, verbal complaints, non-verbal complaints, nervousness, depression and day-sleeping. Illness-behaviour has been defined by Dworkin (1991), who emphasized four critical areas of conceptual interest: (1) monitoring of somatic signals; (2) cognitive processes whereby bodily symptoms are interpreted; (3) attaching meaning to symptoms in the context of emotional state and concurrent environmental events; and (4) ethnocultural influences pervading meaning and shaping coping responses. This model is generalized from a closely related model developed to guide research for specific illness behaviour for dysfunctional chronic pain behaviour. It should be understood as the most important undesirable consequence associated with suffering a persistent pain condition. Dysfunctional chronic pain is a subset of illness behaviours (or a sickness role) inconsistent with documented medical findings, while the complaint of pain is prominent. Excesses in medical care, hospitalization for surgery, and abuse of medication are further characteristics of dysfunctional chronic pain. Our position is that the insurance system and welfare state policies may contribute further to this state.

Lacroix *et al.* (1990) found in the USA that, in compensation patients who were assessed 3 to 6 months after their first back injury, several predictors were correlated with return to work. These predictors included orthopaedic evaluation of severity and prognoses, number of non-organic physical signs, age, educational level, proficiency in English, the understanding by patients of the basis of their medical condition and score on scales 1 and 3 (hypochondria and hysteria) of the Minnesota Multiphasic Personality Inventory (MMPI).

The changes in emotional status associated with chronic pain states are most typically reported as mood and behaviour changes associated with depression, such as demoralization, helplessness and social isolation. The MMPI profile from a pain patient might have indicated 'neuroticism' if it had occurred in persons without chronic or acute pain. However, in pain patients this profile may not actually reflect 'neurotic traits', since many of the items concerning bodily symptoms are a part of the pain syndrome. Still, the description of two different groups of patients with chronic muscle pain and migraine is of particular interest (Ellertsen & Kløve, 1987; Ellertsen *et al.*, 1987, 1991). The authors of these reports have demonstrated that there are two subgroups, one with a depressive profile, another with a 'psychosomatic' profile, among chronic pain patients. These MMPI subgroups seem related to prognosis and results of therapy, and may also represent risk groups for development of chronic muscle pain from localized muscle pain.

**Conclusions**

Woolf (1989) drew three important conclusions for treatment of pain from his review of the pathophysiology of acute pain. Adequate pain management requires techniques that are aimed at the changes that may occur in the central nervous system, treatment should prevent the occurrence of changes in the nervous system, and treatment should not only concentrate on the afferent limb, but also be directed at the efferent sympathetic discharges. Treatment should not simply be techniques directed at suppressing sensation, but the natural history of the different pain states must be understood in order to treat them successfully.

For chronic pain, we would like to emphasize the same points. The central aspect involves the psychology of the patient, and his or her interpretation of the pain. The apparently logical withdrawal and immobility may be right for the most acute phase of the pain, but not for the long-lasting pain states. In particular, patients with long-lasting physiological pain, most commonly found in the skeletal muscular system, should not be warned against activity and loads. Normal pains are normal pains, and there is nothing basically wrong in an aching muscle to make the patient believe that these signals signify the future muscle contractions will always be painful, and, therefore, are to be avoided. The treatment should be early and efficient, and should not be directed at analgesia, or dreams thereof.

Pain elicits more pain, and behaviour that is adequate for tissue injury. However, if there is no tissue injury, this behaviour may be maladaptive. Chronic pain states and chronic muscle pain behaviour should be treated and regarded as being as dangerous to the individual as other behavioural disorders related to life style. Muscular inactivity is probably a more important health problem numerically and economically to the welfare state than any other behavioural disorder. The patients have a serious impairment of their life quality, but they do not die from this state. But the welfare state may die due to strangulation by the cost in sickness compensation.

Pain states should be taken seriously. Pain transmission should be inhibited. There are several options open for this type of treatment. The algogen levels in the peripheral tissue might be reduced, as we believe is happening during physical exercise, with increased muscle strength, improved muscle metabolism, and improved muscle vascularization and oxygenization. The possibilities of pharmacological manipulations of the biochemical environment in the muscle should be exploited further. The possibilities of manipulating the sympathetic outflow are not exhausted. It is also possible to attack the problem from the pain-inhibiting systems. The descending pain-inhibiting system may to a large extent be influenced by central factors. These include, of course, all the clinically well known psychological effects on pain transmission and pain perception.

It is generally agreed that pain influences the psychological state, and that the psychological state and trait of the individual influences his or her responses to pain. We have tried to point out some behavioural mechanisms and the possibility of a conflict between what was phylogenetically adaptive and what is adaptive in our modern society. In addition to these mechanisms, psychological factors play a role for pain transmission at all levels, and also for the biochemical changes that occur in the periphery, regardless of whether the pain is pathological or physiological. Feelings of helplessness and hopelessness, and the accompanying depression experienced by the patients, are known to be accompanied by increased levels of activation, and possibly decreased activity in the descending, inhibitory systems. Sleep disturbances, which may be secondary to the depression, or the other way around, may also influence descending serotonin systems to the spinal cord. This might explain the close relationship between changes in the MMPI and the risks of developing a chronic pain stage.

## References

American Psychiatric Association (1987). *Diagnostic and Statistical Manual of Mental Disorders*, rev. 3rd edn. Washington, DC: American Psychiatric Association.

Antonovsky, A. (1987). *Unravelling the Mystery of Health. How People Manage Stress and Stay Well.* San Francisco: Bass Publishers.

Arntz, A., van den Hout, M. A., van den Berg, G. & Meijboom, A. (1991). *Behav. Res. Ther.*, **29**, 547–60.

Barkwell, D. P. (1991). Ascribed meaning: a critical factor in coping and pain attenuation in patients with cancer-related pain. *J. Palliative Care*, **7**, 5–14.

Basbaum, A. I. & Fields, H. L. (1984). Endogenous pain control systems: brainstem spinal pathways and endorphin circuitry. *Annu. Rev. Neurosci.*, **7**, 309–38.

Bengtsson, A. & Bengtsson, M. (1988). Regional sympathetic blockade in primary fibromyalgia. *Pain*, **33**, 161–7.

Blanchard, R. J., Blanchard, D. C., Rodgers, J. & Weiss, S. M. (1990). The characterization and modelling of antipredator defensive behaviour. *Neurosci. Biobehav. Rev.*, **14**, 463–72.

Blix, A. S. & Folkow, B. (1983). Cardiovascular responses to diving in mammals and birds. In *Handbook of Physiology: The Cardiovascular System*, vol. 3 (2), pp. 917–45. Bethesda, MD: American Physiological Society.

Blumer, D. & Heilbronn, M. (1982). Chronic pain as a variant of depressive disease. *J. Nerv. Ment. Disease*, **170**, 381–406.

Brush, F. R. & Shain, C. N. (1989). Endogenous opioids and behaviour. In *Psychoendocrinology*, ed. F. R. Brush & S. Levine, pp. 379–435. San Diego: Academic Press.

Dahlstrom, A. & Fuxe, K. (1964). Evidence for the existence of monoamine containing neurons in the central nervous system. I. Demonstration of monoamines in the cell bodies of brain stem neurons. *Acta Physiol. Scand.* **62** (Suppl. 232), 1–55.

Depaulis, A., Bandler, R. & Vergnes, M. (1989). Characterization of pretentorial periaqueductal grey matter neurons mediating intraspecific defensive behaviours in the rat by microinjections of kainic acid. *Brain Res.*, **486**, 121–32.

Dworkin, S. F. (1991). Illness behaviour and dysfunction. Review of concepts and application to chronic pain. *Can. J. Physiol. Pharmacol.*, **69**, 662–71.

Ellertsen, B. & Kløve, H. (1987). MMPI profiles in chronic muscle pain. Trends in headache and migraine. *Cephalgia*, **7**, 65–71.

Ellertsen, B., Troland, K. & Kløve, H. (1987). MMPI profiles in migraine before and after biofeedback treatment. *Cephalgia*, **7**, 101–8.

Ellertsen, B., Vaerøy, H., Endresen, I. & Førre, Ø. (1991). MMPI in fibromyalgia and local nonspecific myalgia. *New Trends Exp. Clin Psychiatry*, **27**, 53–62.

Fanselow, M. S. & Kim, J. J. (1992). The benzodiazepine inverse agonist DMCM as an unconditional stimulus for fear-induced analgesia: implications for the role of GABAA receptors in fear-related behaviour. *Behav. Neurosci.*, **106**, 336–44.

Gabrielsen, G. W., Blix, A. S. & Ursin, H. (1985). Orienting and freezing response in incubating ptarmigan hens. *Physiol. Behav.*, **34**, 925–34.

Gamsa, A. (1990). Is emotional disturbance a precipitator or a consequence of chronic pain? *Pain*, **42**, 183–95.

Gramsch, C., Hollt, V., Mehraein, P., Pasi, A. & Herz, A. (1979). Regional distribution of methionine-enkephalin- and beta-endorphin-like immunoreactivity in human brain and pituitary. *Brain Res.*, **177**, 261–70.

Gray, J. A. (1982). *The Neuropsychology of Anxiety*, p. 548. Oxford: Oxford University Press.

Harkapaa, K., Jarvikovski, A., Mellin, G., Hurri, H. & Luoma, J. (1991). Health locus of control beliefs and psychological distress as predictors for treatment outcome in low-back pain patients: results of a 3-month follow-up of a controlled intervention study. *Pain*, **46**, 35–41.

Hoheisel, U. & Mense, S. (1992). Spinal mechanisms of muscular pain and hyperalgesia. International congress on new trends in referred pain and hyperalgesia, Chieti, 12 March, Italy. Unpublished paper.

Hosobuchi, Y., Adams, J. E. & Linchitz, R. (1977). Pain relief by electrical stimulation of the central grey matter in humans and its reversal by naloxone. *Science*, **197**, 183–6.

Kaada, B. R. (1951). Somato-motor, autonomic and electrocorticographic responses to electrical stimulation of 'rhinencephalic' and other structures in primates, cat and dog. *Acta Physiol. Scand.*, **24** (Suppl. 83), 1–285.

Kaplan, H. I. & Sadock, B. J. (1991). *Synopsis of Psychiatry*, pp. 421–2. Baltimore: Williams & Wilkins.

Kirmayer, L. J. (1984). Culture, affect and somatization. *Transcultural Psychiatr. Res. Rev.*, **21**, 159–88.

Kramlinger, K. G., Swanson, D. W. & Maruta, T. (1983): Are patients with chronic pain depressed? *Am. J. Psychiatry*, **140**, 747–9.

Lacroix, J. M., Powell, J., Lloyd, G. J., Doxey, N. C. S., Mitson, G. L. & Aldam, C. F. (1990). Low-back pain factors of value in predicting outcome. *Spine*, **15**, 495–9.

Leden, I., Eriksson, A., Lilja, B., Sturfelt, G. & Sundkvist, G. (1983). Autonomic nerve function in rheumatoid arthritis of varying severity. *Scand. J. Rheumatol.*, **12**, 166–70.

Levine, J. D., Fye, K., Heller, P., Basbaum, A. I. & Whiting-O'Keefe, Q. (1986*a*). Clinical response to regional intravenous guanethone in patients with rheumatoid-arthritis. *J. Rheumatol.*, **13**, 1040–3.

Levine, J. D., Taiwo, Y. O., Collins, S. D. & Tam, J. K. (1986*b*). Noradrenaline hyperalgesia is mediated through interaction with sympathetic postganglionic neurone terminals rather than activation of primary afferent nociceptors. *Nature*, **323**, 158–60.

Leyhausen, P. (1960). *Verhaltensstudien an Katzen*. Berlin: Paul Parey.

Lindal, E. & Uden, A. (1989). Why do people seek medical advice for back pain: a comparison of consulters and nonconsulters. *Clin. J. Pain*, **5**, 351–8.

Lopez Ibor, J. J. (1972). Masked depressions. *Br. J. Psychiatry*, **120**, 245–58.

Magni, C., Caldieron, C., Rigatti-Luchini, S. & Merskey, H. (1990). Chronic musculoskeletal pain and depressive symptoms in the general population. An analysis of the 1st national health and nutrition examination survey data. *Pain*, **43**, 299–307.

Malt, U. F. (1992). Coping with accidental injury. *Psychiatr. Med.*, **10**, 135–47.

Malt, U. F., Myhrer, T., Blikra, G. & Høivik, B. (1987). Psychopathology and accidental injuries. *Acta Psychiatr. Scand.*, **76**, 261–71.

McCleary, R. A. (1961). Response specificity in the behavioral effects of limbic system lesions in the cat. *J. Comp. Physiol. Psychol.*, **54**, 605–13.

Merskey, H. (1979). Pain terms: a list with definitions and notes on usage. Recommended by the IASP Subcommittee on Taxonomy. *Pain*, **6**, 249–52.

Mjellem-Joly, N., Lund, A., Berge, O. G. & Hole, K. (1992). Potentiation of a behavioral response in mice by spinal coadministration of Substance P and excitatory amino acid agonists. *Neurosci. Lett.*, **133**, 123–4

Mjellem-Joly, N., Lund, A., Berge, O. G. & Hole, K. (1993). Intrathecal co-administration of substance P and NMDA augments nociceptive responses in the formalin test. *Pain*, **51**, 195–8.

Nakamura-Craig, M. & Smith, T. W. (1989). Substance P and peripheral inflammatory hyperalgesia. *Pain*, **38**, 91–8.
Olff, M., Brosschot, J. F. & Godaert, G. L. R. (1993). Coping styles and health. *Pers. Individ. Differences*, **15**, 81–90.
Raja, S., Meyer, J. N. & Meyer, R. A. (1988). Peripheral mechanisms of somatic pain. *Anaesthesiology*, **68**, 571–90.
Rang, H. & Ritche, J. (1988). Depolarization of nonmyelinated fibres of the rat vagus produced by activation of protein kinase. *J. Neurosci.*, **8**, 2606–17.
Rodgers, R. J. & Randall, J. I. (1987). Are the analgesic effects of social defeat mediated by benzodiazepine receptors? *Physiol. Behav.*, **41**, 279–89.
Rodgers, R. J. & Shepherd, J. K. (1989). $5HT_{1A}$ agonist, 8-hydroxy-2-(DI-*n*-propylamino) tetralin (8-OH-DPAT), inhibits non-opioid analgesia in defeated mice: influence of route of administration. *Psychopharmacology*, **97**, 163–5.
Sternbach, R. A. (1989). Acute versus chronic pain. In *Textbook of Pain*, ed. P. D. Wall & R. Melzack, pp. 242–6. New York: Churchill Livingstone.
Strong, J., Ashton, R. & Chant, D. (1992). The measurement of attitudes towards and beliefs about pain. *Pain*, **48**, 227–36.
Talo, S., Ryotokoski, U., Niitsuo, L. & Knuts, L. R. (1992). Psychological impairments, disabilities, and handicaps: a pilot study of psychological assessment of functioning in chronic pain patients. *Disabil. Rehab.*, **14**, 4–9.
Tellnes, G. (1989*a*). Legens oppgaver ved sykmelding. (Doctors' duties in sickness certification.) *Tidsskrift Norsk Laegeforening*, **109**, 2439–42.
Tellnes, G. (1989*b*). Sickness certification in general practice: a review. *Fam. Pract.*, **6**, 58–65.
Ursin, H. (1976). Inhibition and the septal nuclei: breakdown of the single concept model. *Acta Neurobiol. Exp. (Warsaw)*, **36**, 91–115.
Ursin, H. (1981). Neuroanatomical basis of aggression. In *Multidisciplinary Approaches to Aggression Research*, ed. P. F. Brain & D. Benton, pp. 269–93. Amsterdam: Elsevier.
Ursin, H. (1985). The instrumental effects of emotional behaviour. In *Perspectives in Ethology*, vol. 6, ed. P. P. G. Bateson & P-H. Klopfer, pp. 45–62. New York: Plenum Press.
Ursin, H. & Olff, M. (1994). The stress response. In *Stress: An Integrated Response*, ed. C. Stanford, P. Salmon & J. Grey, pp. 3–22. Academic Press.
Vaerøy, H. (1990). *Pain, Neuropeptides, Sympathetic Responses and Personality Factors in Patients with Fibromyalgia (Fibrositis Syndrome)*. Dr Med. thesis, Department of Rheumatology, Oslo Sanitetsforenings Rheumatism Hospital, University of Oslo, Norway.
Vaerøy, H., Qiao, Z.-G., Mørkrid, L. & Forre, Ø. (1989). Altered sympathetic nervous system response in patients with fibromyalgia (fibrositis syndrome). *J. Rheumatol.*, **16**, 1460–5.
Vlaeyen, J. W., Pernot, D. F., Kole-Snijders, A. M., Schuerman, J. A., Van-Eek, H. & Groenman, N. H. (1990). Assessment of the components of observed chronic pain behavior: the Checklist for Interpersonal Pain Behavior (CHIP). *Pain*, **43**, 337–47.
Von Knorring, L. (1988). Affect and pain: neurochemical mediators and therapeutic approaches. In *Proceedings of the Vth World Congress on Pain*, ed. R. Dubner, G. F. Gebhart & M. R. Bond, pp. 276–85. Amsterdam: Elsevier Science Publishers.
Wall, P. D. (1985). Future trends in pain research. *Phil. Trans. R. Soc. London*, **308**, 393–401.

Wall, P. D. & Fitzgerald, M. (1982). If Substance P fails to fulfil the criteria as a neurotransmitter in somatosensory afferents, what may be its function? In *Substance P in the Nervous System*, Ciba Foundation Symposium, Vol. 91, ed. R. Porter & M. O'Connor. London: Pitman.

Ward, N. G., Bloom, V. L., Dworkin, S., Fawcett, J., Narasimhachari, N. & Friedel, R. O. (1982). Psychobiological markers in coexisting pain and depression: toward a unified theory. *J. Clin. Psychiatry*, **43**, 32–9.

Westermeyer, J., Bouafuely, M., Neider, J. & Callies, A. (1989). Somatization among refugees: an epidemiologic study. *Psychosomatics*, **30**, 34–42.

White, G. M. (1982). The role of cultural explanations in 'somatization' and 'psychologization'. *Soc. Sci. Med.*, **16**, 1519–30.

Williams, D. A. & Keefe, F. J. (1991). Pain beliefs and the use of cognitive–behavioral coping strategies. *Pain*, **46**, 185–90.

Williams, J. B. W. & Spitzer, R. L. (1982). Idiopathic pain disorder: a critique of pain-prone disorder and a proposal for a revision of the DSM III category pain disorder. *J. Nerv. Ment. Dis.*, **170**, 415–19.

Woolf, C. J. (1987). Physiological, inflammatory and neuropathic pain. *Adv. Tech. Stand. Neurosurg.*, **15**, 39–62.

Woolf, C. J. (1989). Recent advances in the pathophysiology of acute pain. *Br. J. Anaesth.*, **63**, 139–46.

Woolf, C. J. & Thompson, W. N. (1991). The induction and maintenance of central sensitization is dependent on *N*-methyl-D-aspartic acid receptor activation; implications for the treatment of post-injury pain hypersensitivity states. *Pain*, **44**, 293–9.

# 9

# Central control of cardiovascular responses to injury

EMRYS KIRKMAN and RODERICK A. LITTLE

## Introduction

The aim of this chapter is to review aspects of the central nervous organisation of the cardiovascular response to peripheral (non-central nervous) trauma. Two aspects of trauma are considered, namely haemorrhage or loss of circulating fluid and tissue damage or injury. In the context of this chapter, the term 'injury' is used to denote tissue damage and the associated activation of afferent nociceptive fibres, and does not itself involve loss of circulating fluid. The responses to haemorrhage and to injury are initially considered separately, before the interaction between the two responses, and the clinical implications of this interaction, are discussed. Finally, ways in which these responses may be modified by three groups of pharmacological agents are described: opioid agonists and antagonists, 5-hydroxytryptamine (5-HT) and ethanol.

Relatively little is known of the central nervous pathways specifically involved in the response to trauma. However, there is a wealth of knowledge regarding the pathways of individual cardiovascular reflexes that together may generate the response to trauma. It is therefore pertinent to describe first the cardiovascular responses to haemorrhage and injury, and their component reflexes, before discussing the relevant central nervous pathways.

## The cardiovascular response to a progressive haemorrhage

### *The pattern of response to a 'simple' haemorrhage*

A progressive 'simple' haemorrhage (loss of blood in the absence of major tissue damage, e.g. rupture of varices) produces a biphasic pattern of response (Figures 9.1, 9.2*a*). In the initial stages there is a progressive

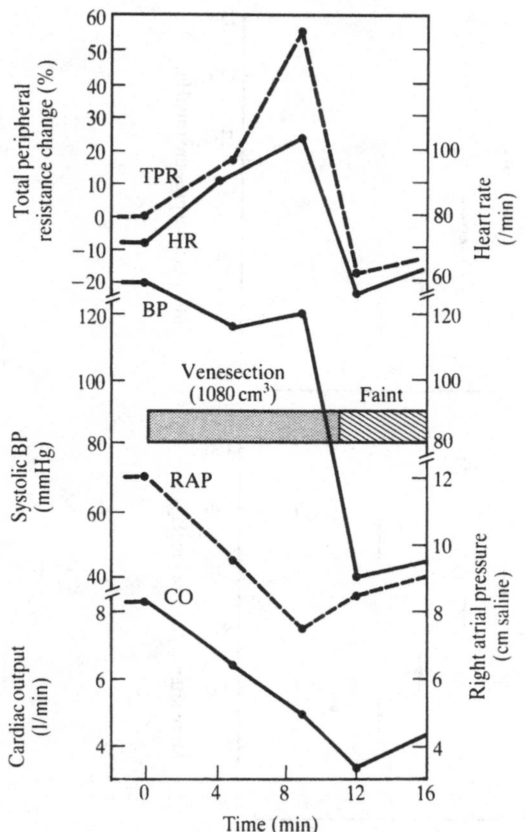


Figure 9.1. Changes in heart rate (HR), systolic arterial blood pressure (BP), cardiac output (CO), total peripheral resistance (TPR) and right atrial pressure (RAP) during a controlled haemorrhage (venesection) and subsequent faint in a human subject. (From Barcroft *et al.*, 1944.)

increase in heart rate and vascular resistance, which can maintain arterial blood pressure close to prehaemorrhage levels following blood losses of up to 10–15% of the blood volume in a young, otherwise healthy, individual (Barcroft *et al.*, 1944; Secher & Bie, 1985). However, as the severity of haemorrhage increases, and exceeds 20% of the blood volume, a very different pattern of response becomes apparent, namely a marked bradycardia and peripheral vasodilatation accompanied by a precipitous fall in blood pressure, which may lead to syncope (Barcroft *et al.*, 1944; Figures 9.1, 9.2*a*).

Since the elucidation of the mechanisms (and central nervous pathways)

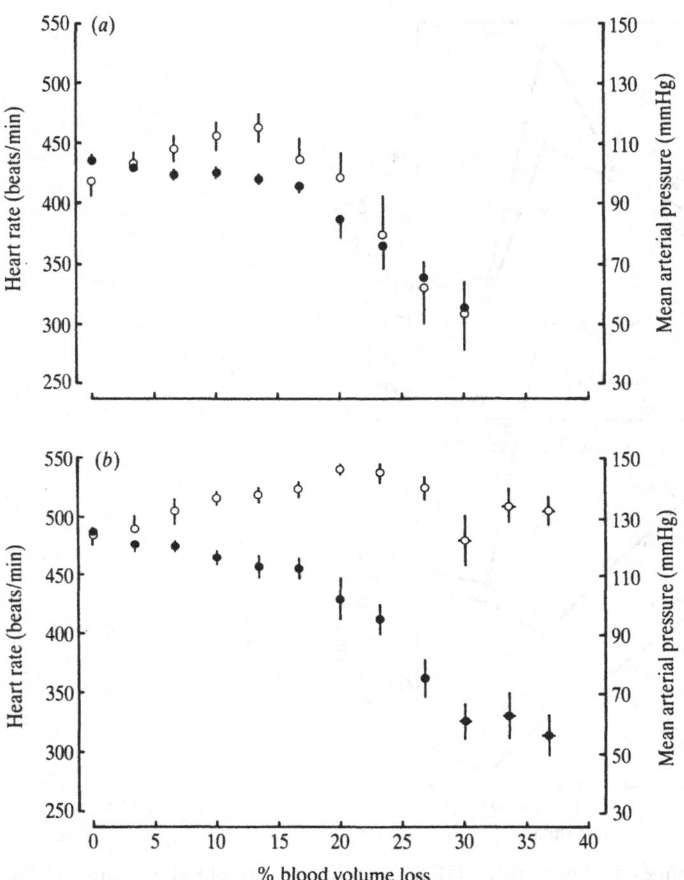


Figure 9.2. The effects of progressive 'simple' haemorrhage (*a*) and haemorrhage in the presence of bilateral hind-limb ischaemia (*b*) on heart rate (○) and mean arterial blood pressure (●) in the conscious rat. Values are shown as mean ± standard error.

of these responses to blood loss have involved investigations on animals, it should be stressed that the finer details of the response appear to vary depending on the species studied, and the choice of anaesthetic agent, if any (for example, see Schadt & Ludbrook, 1991). The pattern of response seen in the conscious rat clearly resembles that seen in the humans (Figure 9.2*a*), with the heart rate during severe haemorrhage falling below prehaemorrhage values. In contrast, severe hypovolaemia in the conscious rabbit does not generally yield a frank bradycardia, with the heart rate falling below the maximum levels seen during the early response, but remaining above the prehaemorrhage levels (for example, see Evans *et al.*, 1989*a*). Despite the modest effect on heart rate, severe hypovolaemia does result in a marked reduction in vascular resistance and hence hypotension in the conscious rabbit, as in the human (for example, Evans *et al.*, 1989*a*).

### *Reflexes involved in the response to haemorrhage*

In an explanation of the biphasic response to blood loss, three reflexes need to be considered: the arterial baroreceptor reflex, the reflex elicited by activation of cardiac C-fibre afferents, and the arterial chemoreflex.

#### *The arterial baroreceptor reflex*

The arterial baroreceptor reflex is thought to be responsible for the maintenance of arterial blood pressure following the loss of 10–15% of the blood volume. This reflex normally minimises moment-to-moment variations in blood pressure around a given 'set-point', which itself can be altered (Cowley *et al.*, 1973). The baroreceptor endings are located in the medioadventitial border of the arterial wall (Abraham, 1967; Knoche & Addicks, 1976; Krauss, 1979), in parts of the arterial system with a specialised elastic structure, mainly in the aortic arch and carotid sinus (Kirchheim, 1976). The baroreceptors themselves are slowly adapting mechanoreceptors (Bronk & Stella, 1935) that respond to the degree of stretch of the arterial wall produced by the intraluminal pressure, rather than to the intraluminal pressure itself (for example, Angell-James, 1971). Furthermore, the baroreceptors are 'rate-sensitive' and can therefore respond to the rate of change of arterial blood pressure as well as to its absolute level (Angell-James & Daly, 1970). Consequently, they can respond to a change in pulse pressure as well as changes in mean pressure.

Thus, as pulse pressure diminishes during haemorrhage, there is a decrease in baroreceptor afferent activity, even in the absence of a fall in *mean* arterial pressure. This change in baroreceptor afferent activity is signalled to the brain via the vagus nerve (from the aortic arch baroreceptors) and the sinus nerve, a branch of the glossopharyngeal nerve (from the carotid sinus baroreceptors; Heymans & Neil, 1958; Kirchheim, 1976). The efferent limb of the baroreceptor reflex is carried in the vagus and sympathetic nerves to the heart, and in the sympathetic vasoconstrictor nerves to the blood vessels (Kirchheim, 1976). When the baroreceptors are unloaded following a haemorrhage, there is a resultant reflex withdrawal of vagal-cardiac activity and an enhancement of sympathocardiac activity, leading to a tachycardia, and an increase in the activity of the sympathetic vasoconstrictor fibres leading to increased total peripheral resistance. It should be emphasised that the activation of the sympathetic supply to the various vascular beds is not uniform, with some experiencing a more intense vasoconstriction than others (Kirchheim, 1976). The activity of the baroreceptor reflex at this time is augmented by a concomitant increase in its sensitivity (Little *et al.*, 1984). The mechanism of this increase in sensitivity is unknown, although it may be due to the increases in the plasma levels of vasopressin and renin activity that occur after haemorrhage (Kirkman & Scott, 1983; Cowley *et al.*, 1984). Furthermore, the balance of pressure across the microvascular endothelium is changed in such a way that fluid moves from the extravascular to the intravascular compartment. As a consequence of these haemodynamic changes, any haemorrhage-induced falls in arterial blood pressure are minimised or prevented in the face of losses of up to 10–15% of the blood volume. Hence, the baroreceptor reflex serves to maintain blood flow to tissues critically dependent on oxygen delivery (e.g. brain) at the expense of flow to other organs (e.g. skeletal muscle) where oxygen delivery is less critical, at least in the short term.

However, as blood loss exceeds 20% of the blood volume, blood pressure falls dramatically (Figures 9.1, 9.2*a*). This is not due to a sudden failure of the baroreceptor reflex (Little *et al.*, 1984), or the imminent demise of the heart, but rather to the activation of a second reflex – possibly the reflex elicited by activation of cardiac vagal C-fibre afferents.

### *The cardiac vagal C-fibre afferents*

The cardiac vagal C-fibres form the afferent pathway from a group of receptors located mainly in the left ventricular myocardium. These receptors can be activated by mechanical and/or chemical means (e.g. prostaglandin $E_2$; Baker *et al.*, 1979), and lead to a profound reflex bradycardia, hypotension and reduction in skeletal muscle and renal vascular resistance (Öberg & Thorén, 1973; Daly *et al.*, 1988), the 'cardiac reflex'. The bradycardia is due to increased vagal efferent activity to the heart, while the reduction in vascular resistance is due to a withdrawal of sympathetic vasconstrictor tone (Öberg & Thorén, 1973; Daly *et al.*, 1988). Following a severe haemorrhage (>20% of the blood volume), it has been postulated that the mechanosensitive receptor endings of the cardiac vagal C-fibre afferents are stimulated by deformations of the ventricular wall as the heart contracts vigorously around an incompletely filled chamber (Öberg & Thorén, 1972). This is supported by the finding that sectioning the cervical vagi can reverse the bradycardia in experimental animals, and that the bradycardia and fall in blood pressure are attenuated markedly in animals that are deficient in afferent C-fibres (Little *et al.*, 1989). Furthermore, the reduction in renal sympathetic vasoconstrictor activity can be prevented by the instillation of procaine into the pericardial sac to block the afferent pathway (Burke & Dorward, 1988; Evans *et al.*, 1989*a*).

However, more recent studies have questioned the precise nature of the afferent pathway mediating the 'depressor' response associated with severe haemorrhage, since the installation of procaine into the pericardial sac may have more wide-ranging effects than simply blocking the cardiac neural pathways (Hayes *et al.*, 1992), and a similar 'depressor' response has been reported in conscious dogs that had been subjected to cardiac denervation or acute cardiac nerve blockade (Shen *et al.*, 1990, 1991). Furthermore, a case report of sympathoinhibition following the infusion of a vasodilator agent in a cardiac transplant patient with no ventricular innervation led the authors to suggest that 'stimulation of ventricular afferents is not the only mechanism that can trigger sympathoinhibition during hypovolaemic hypotension' (Scherrer *et al.*, 1990). Finally, very recent evidence suggests that aspects of the central nervous pathways mediating the 'cardiac reflex' may be different from those involved in the 'depressor' response associated with severe haemorrhage (see p. 227). However, regardless of these questions relating to the nature of the afferent pathway, it must be stressed that there is very strong evidence suggesting that the 'depressor' response associated with severe haemorrhage is reflex in nature and that the efferent limb of the reflex involves both increased vagal activity to the heart and reduced sympathetic tone to vascular beds, e.g. the kidney.

Since the efferent limb mediating the cardioinhibitory component of the depressor reflex is carried in the vagus nerve (see above), it is not surprising that the bradycardia associated with severe haemorrhage can be prevented by treatment with atropine in both humans (Lewis, 1932; Barcroft *et al.*, 1944) and experimental animals (Little *et al.*, 1989). However, the administration of atropine alone under these circumstances is not be recommended (unless there is very severe bradycardia or asystole), since it has been suggested that this 'depressor' reflex may serve to protect the heart by reducing cardiac work at a time when coronary blood flow is compromised. Indeed, there have been reports that the administration of atropine under these circumstances may be deleterious (Barriot *et al.*, 1987). The logical treatment would be to restore blood volume and hence reduce the activation of the reflex, whereupon the bradycardia should correct itself.

*The arterial chemoreceptor reflex*

The third reflex of importance in the cardiovascular response to haemorrhage is the arterial chemoreceptor reflex. The arterial chemoreceptors are found in the carotid and aortic bodies, close to the carotid sinus and aortic arch, respectively. They respond to changes in oxygen tension, a fall in oxygen tension increasing chemoreceptor afferent activity. In addition, increases in carbon dioxide tension and falls in arterial blood pH increase the sensitivity of the arterial chemoreceptors to hypoxia (Biscoe *et al.*, 1970). Stimulation of arterial chemoreceptors produces an increase in respiration (Heymans & Neil, 1958), whereas the primary cardiovascular effects are a vagally mediated bradycardia and a vasoconstriction in, for example, skeletal muscle, which is due to increased sympathetic vasoconstrictor tone (Daly, 1983). This pattern of response is subsequently modified by the increased respiratory activity, that tends to inhibit both the vagal activity to the heart and the sympathetic vasoconstrictor activity (Spyer, 1984).

Following a severe haemorrhage, the arterial chemoreceptors are activated as a result of a reduction in blood flow through the carotid and aortic bodies secondary to the fall in arterial blood pressure, and to sympathetic vasoconstriction in the bodies themselves (Daly *et al.*, 1954; Acker & O'Regan, 1981) mediated by the local release of both noradrenaline and its cotransmitter, neuropeptide Y (Potter & McCloskey, 1987). Therefore, during the hypotensive phase of a severe haemorrhage, stimulation of the arterial chemoreceptors may prevent arterial blood pressure falling even further (Kenney & Neil, 1951), and may be responsible for the increase in respiration noted following severe haemorrhage (D'Silva *et al.*, 1966). Since an increase in respiratory activity has been shown to reduce the reflex bradycardia produced by stimulation of cardiac C-fibre afferents (Daly *et al.*, 1988), it is possible that the enhanced respiratory activity seen following a severe haemorrhage may attenuate the bradycardia seen under these circumstances. This interaction between the respiratory and cardiovascular responses to chemoreceptor stimulation may also have further implications for the treatment of injured patients. For example, procedures such as intubation that inhibit respiratory activity can unmask a dangerous bradycardia (for example, see Angell-James & Daly, 1975). The role of the chemoreceptors in helping to maintain blood pressure will, of course, be increased in the injured patient with thoracic injuries, which may impair pulmonary function.

### *Central nervous pathways involved in the cardiovascular response to haemorrhage*

The central nervous pathway of the baroreceptor reflex has been studied extensively, and is the subject of numerous reviews (e.g. Spyer, 1984; Seller, 1991). Consequently, this chapter provides only a brief summary of some of the central nervous pathways involved in this reflex.

The baroreceptor afferent fibres terminate exclusively within the nucleus of the tractus solitarius (NTS) in the brainstem (Spyer, 1984). As described earlier, the efferent limb of the baroreceptor reflex is carried in both the parasympathetic nerves (vagi) to the heart and the sympathetic supply to the heart and peripheral vasculature. The cell bodies of the vagal cardiac preganglionic motor neurones are located in the nucleus ambiguus and dorsal vagal motor nucleus (McAllen & Spyer, 1976; Jordan *et al.*, 1982). The sympathetic preganglionic cell bodies are found in the intermedio-lateral columns of the thoracic and upper lumbar segments of the spinal cord (Henry & Calaresu, 1972).

#### *Control of vagal efferent activity*

The baroreceptor afferents are thought to influence vagal efferent activity via two main pathways: a short latency pathway, which is complete within the medulla, i.e. a segmental pathway travelling from the NTS to the nucleus ambiguus (Agarwal & Calaresu, 1992), and a longer latency pathway, which ascends to relay in the anterior hypothalamus before descending to the nucleus ambiguus (see Spyer, 1984) (Figure 9.3*a*). Activation of either of these pathways, following stimulation of the baroreceptors, leads to excitation of the vagal cardiac preganglionic motor neurones within the nucleus ambiguus (see Spyer, 1984), and consequently to bradycardia.

The arterial chemoreceptor afferents also terminate within the NTS (see Spyer, 1984). From the NTS there is a secondary, excitatory projection, which activates both the vagal cardiac preganglionic motor neurones and the inspiratory neurones within the nucleus ambiguus (Figure 9.3*b*). The inspiratory neurones (which project to the spinal cord and activate the

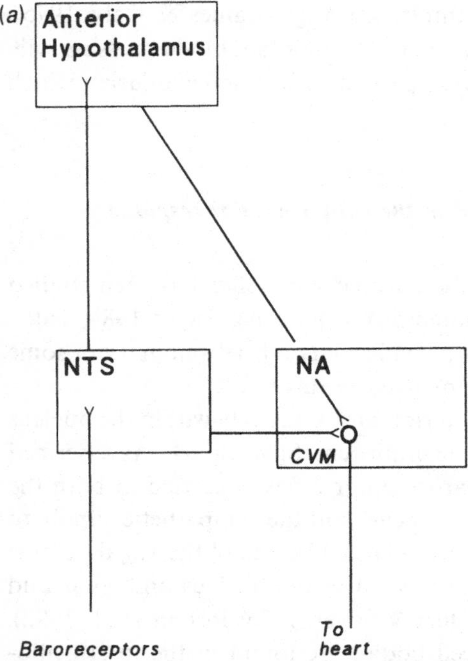


Figure 9.3. Schematic diagram indicating (*a*) two pathways whereby the baroreceptors can influence vagal efferent activity to the heart. (*continued*).

motor neurones, which cause contraction of the diaphragm; Cohen *et al.*, 1974; Ellenberger & Feldman, 1988) send a cholinergic inhibitory collateral onto the vagal cardiac preganglionic motor neurones (Garcia *et al.*, 1978). This, coupled with a second inhibitory output originating from lung stretch afferent fibres (see Daly, 1983), which are activated when the lungs inflate during inspiration, attenuates or even reverses the increase in vagal efferent activity to the heart. However, when the arterial chemoreceptor-induced respiratory stimulation is prevented, for example, during intubation, then the bradycardia becomes apparent (Angell-James & Daly, 1975).

The central nervous pathway of the reflex elicited by activation of the cardiac C-fibre afferents has been studied less extensively. Nevertheless, the afferent fibres appear to terminate within the NTS (Bennett *et al.*, 1985) where they may utilise an *n*-nitrosothiol as a neurotransmitter or neuromodulator, leading to the activation of soluble guanylate cyclase (Lewis *et al.*, 1991). A secondary pathway leads to the vagal outflow nuclei, where vagal efferent activity to the heart is stimulated via 5-$HT_{1A}$

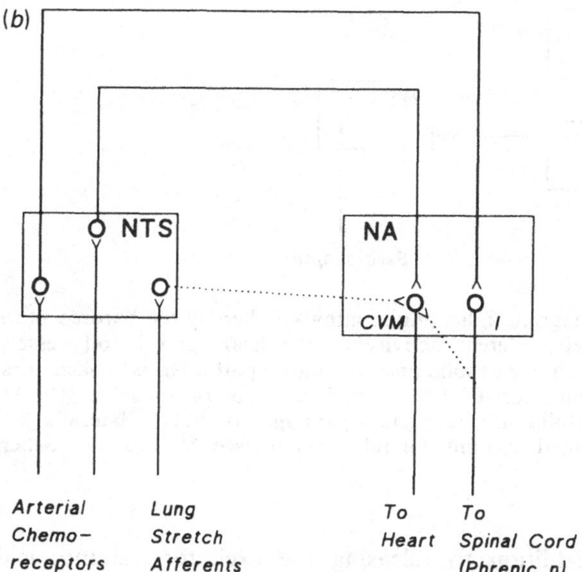


Figure 9.3 (*continued*) (*b*) Pathways whereby activation of the arterial chemoreceptors leads to excitation of vagal cardiac and inspiratory neurones, while stimulation of the lung stretch receptors leads to inhibition of the vagal cardiac neurones. Excitatory pathways are shown as solid lines, inhibitory pathways as broken lines. NTS, nucleus tractus solitarius; NA, nucleus ambiguus; CVM, vagal cardiac preganglionic motor neurone; I, inspiratory neurone. See text for details.

receptors (Bogle *et al.*, 1990). This reflex appears to be inhibited tonically via a GABA-ergic pathway (Bennett *et al.*, 1984), possibly at the level of the NTS (Bennett *et al.*, 1987).

*Control of sympathetic efferent activity: the rostral ventrolateral medulla*

The cell bodies of the sympathetic preganglionic neurones, which cause vasoconstriction, are found in the intermediolateral column of the spinal cord (Figure 9.4). They are influenced by nervous pathways descending from the brain. One such pathway, which is a major source of excitatory drive to the sympathetic preganglionic neurones, originates in the nucleus paragigantocellularis lateralis in the rostral ventrolateral medulla (RVLM) (Ross *et al.*, 1984; Brown & Guyenet, 1984). This pathway, probably by releasing the excitatory amino acid glutamate within the intermediolateral cell column (Morrison *et al.*, 1991; Kapoor *et al.*, 1992), contributes towards the maintenance of resting sympathetic tone, and hence arterial

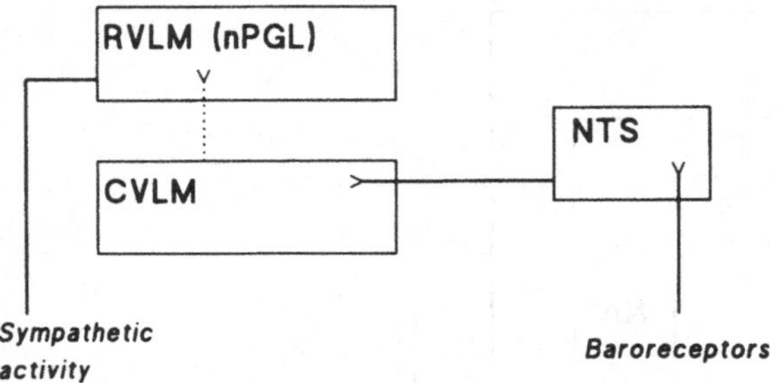


Figure 9.4. Schematic diagram indicating a pathway whereby the baroreceptors can influence sympathetic efferent activity to the heart and blood vessels. Excitatory pathways are shown as solid lines, inhibitory pathways as broken lines. NTS, nucleus tractus solitarius; CVLM, caudal ventrolateral medulla; RVLM, rostral ventrolateral medulla; nPGL, nucleus paragigantocellularis lateralis. NB This represents a simplified account; for fuller details, see, for example, Seller, 1991.

blood pressure. In addition to releasing the excitatory amino acid glutamate, it has been suggested that individual RVLM neurones may also release a number of other neurotransmitters that can influence the sympathetic vasomotor activity (Chalmers & Pilowsky, 1991). A recent study has suggested the possibility that events, e.g. haemorrhage, could cause an alteration in the synthesis, and hence possibly the relative proportion of the various cotransmitters released within the spinal cord by these RVLM neurones (McAllen *et al.*, 1992). Therefore, it may be possible that haemorrhage can modulate the effects of this neuronal pathway, merely by altering the relative proportions of transmitters and co-transmitters released by its terminations.

The sympathoexcitatory cells within the RVLM are subject to inhibition originating from baroreceptor afferent activity, which is mediated via a pathway that originates in the NTS and relays in the caudal ventrolateral medulla (CVLM) (Seller, 1991; Figure 9.4). There is evidence to suggest that this pathway involves both excitatory amino acids acting at NMDA and non-NMDA receptors in the CVLM (Jung *et al.*, 1991), and the inhibitory amino acid GABA within the RVLM (see Seller, 1991). Thus, the decrease in baroreceptor afferent activity seen during haemorrhage leads to a disinhibition of the RVLM sympathoexcitatory neurones, and a resultant increase in sympathetic efferent activity. Further studies have shown a direct enkephalinergic projection from the NTS to the RVLM (Morilak *et al.*, 1989). It has been argued that this enkephalinergic pathway may modulate the activity of the RVLM neurones, and hence alter the baroreceptor reflex and arterial blood pressure following haemorrhage or 'injury' (see below; Morilak *et al.*, 1989). This pathway could be a potential target for pharmacological interference in the traumatised patient (see below).

The central nervous pathways mediating the sympathoinhibition associated with severe hypovolaemia have been studied less extensively. The primary afferent fibres (the cardiac vagal C-fibres) terminate within the NTS. Some secondary fibres project to the CVLM, and, via an action on NMDA receptors at this site, lead to a fall in blood pressure and heart rate (Verberne *et al.*, 1989). There is also evidence for secondary projections ascending from the NTS to suprapontine levels, before descending again to the medulla (Evans *et al.*, 1991), producing a sympathoinhibitory effect involving the activation of $\delta$ opioid receptors (Evans *et al.*, 1989*a*). Again, this pathway could be a potential target for pharmacological interference in the traumatised patient (see below).

### *Role of the area postrema*

The area postrema, also found in the medulla, is anatomically connected to a number of structures implicated in the response to haemorrhage (e.g. NTS, RVLM, nucleus ambiguus) (Andrezik *et al.*, 1981; Shapiro & Miselis, 1985; Morilak *et al.*, 1989), and is thought to be involved in the response to blood loss. Following haemorrhage, neurones within the area postrema display increased activity (Kadekaro *et al.*, 1990; Badoer *et al.*, 1992). Furthermore, lesions of the area postrema impair the ability to maintain arterial blood pressure in both the dog (Katic *et al.*, 1971) and the rat (Skoog *et al.*, 1990).

It has been argued that, in the dog, the area postrema contributes to the maintenance of blood pressure following haemorrhage, by responding to increased plasma levels of angiotensin (Katic *et al.*, 1971), which, in turn, causes a pressor effect, partly due to an increase in sympathetic efferent activity (Lowe & Scroop, 1969; Scroop & Lowe, 1969). The situation in the rat, however, is less clear, since the central nervous pressor actions of blood-borne angiotensin in this species is thought not to be mediated via the area postrema (Haywood *et al.*, 1980). Therefore, it appears likely that the mechanism whereby the area postrema contributes to the maintenance of arterial blood pressure following haemorrhage extends beyond simply responding to raised plasma angiotensin levels, at least in the rat.

*The parabrachial nuclei and the caudal ventrolateral periaqueductal grey*
More rostrally in the brainstem, cells within the ventrolateral parts of the parabrachial nuclei and the Kolliker–Fuse nucleus provide a major projection to the ventrolateral medulla (Figure 9.5) (Fulwiler & Saper, 1984). These areas are of particular interest, since they receive a projection from the NTS (Loewy & Burton, 1978), and hence are likely to receive haemodynamic information. Recent studies by Ward (1989) have shown that cells in this region respond to haemorrhage. Three patterns of response could be found, which were related to the anatomical location

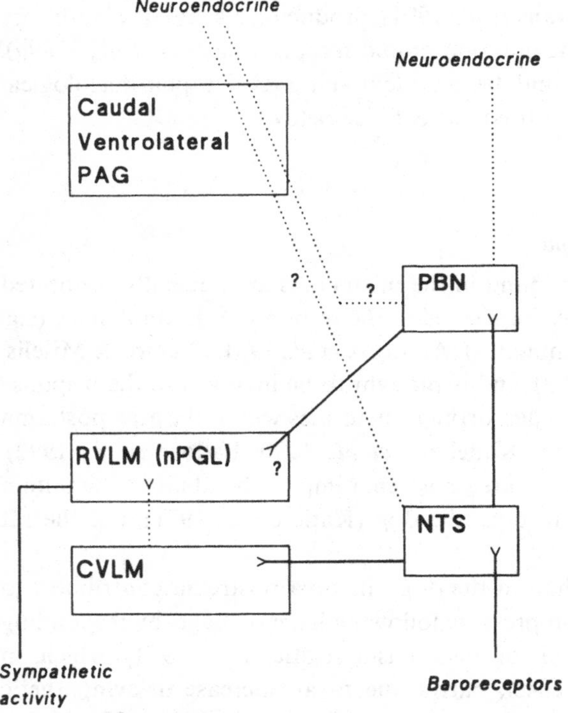


Figure 9.5. Schematic diagram indicating some of the central nervous pathways involved in an integrated cardiovascular and neuroendrocrine response to haemorrhage. Excitatory pathways are shown as solid lines, inhibitory pathways as broken lines. ?, Putative pathways which may be excitatory or inhibitory; baroreceptors are arterial baroreceptors and other cardiovascular receptors, e.g. atrial low-pressure baroreceptors; NTS, nucleus tractus solitarius; PBN, parabrachial and Kolliker–Fuse nuclei; PAG, periaqueductal grey; CVLM; caudal ventrolateral medulla; RVLM, rostral ventrolateral medulla; nPGL, nucleus paragigantocellularis lateralis. See text for details.

of the cells within the parabrachial and Kolliker–Fuse nuclei (Ward, 1989):

(a) The first group of neurones exhibited an increase in activity following haemorrhage, which was not reversed immediately during reinfusion, i.e. the neurones appeared to show a *memory* of the blood loss. Ward (1989) suggested that these cells may therefore have been responding to the neuroendrocrine as well as the haemodynamic changes induced by blood loss.
(b) A second group of neurones exhibited an increased activity during haemorrhage, which was reversed by reinfusion. These cells are thought to signal changes in blood *volume* rather than pressure.
(c) The final group of cells showed a reduction in activity during haemorrhage which was reversed on reinfusion, i.e. a mirror image of the activity in (b), above. This last group of cells may receive an input from other areas within the parabrachial nuclei, since they do not directly receive any cardiovascular afferent information.

Ward (1989) concludes by stating that although the specific functions of these parabrachial neurones are obscure at present, they may play a critical role in the control of neuroendocrine and sympathetic responses to blood loss (Figure 9.5).

Finally, the caudal ventrolateral periaqueductal grey (PAG) may also play a role in the cardiovascular response to haemorrhage, since lesions in this area markedly impair the ability to respond to a mild haemorrhage (Ward & Darlington, 1987). This region may contain cell bodies or fibres of passage transmitting information from the NTS and parabrachial nuclei to the lateral hypothalamus (Figure 9.5), and may therefore be involved in both the cardiovascular and neuroendocrine responses to haemorrhage (Ward & Darlington, 1987).

Thus, a number of central nervous pathways can be identified as being of importance in the cardiovascular response to blood loss. The functions of some of these pathways are relatively clear, while others require further investigation.

## The cardiovascular response to 'injury'

In direct contrast to haemorrhage, tissue injury/ischaemia produces an increase in arterial blood pressure accompanied by a tachycardia (Alam & Smirk, 1937, 1938; Howard *et al.*, 1955). The increase in arterial blood pressure that accompanies 'injury' is largely mediated by an increase in sympathetic outflow to the vasculature and a consequent increase in total peripheral resistance. Thus the 'injury'-induced pressor response is unaffected by complete cardiac autonomic blockade, but is abolished by the $\alpha$-adrenoceptor antagonist phentolamine (Redfern, 1981). This intense sympathetically mediated vasoconstriction induced by 'injury' could lead to a reduction in blood flow to vital organs such as the gut and kidney, and possibly lead to ischaemic damage of these organs (Overman & Wang, 1947), hence contributing to the pathophysiology of the response to 'injury' and its sequelae such as multiple organ failure.

The 'injury'-induced pressor response is accompanied by a tachycardia, rather than a bradycardia, which would be expected were the baroreceptor reflex (see above) functioning normally. This pattern of response is possible, because there is a concomitant reduction in the sensitivity and a rightward resetting (i.e. towards a higher arterial blood pressure) of the baroreflex following 'injury' (Redfern *et al.*, 1984). The reduction in baroreceptor reflex sensitivity in humans is evident within 3 h of 'injury' of moderate severity (e.g. fracture of a long bone), and persists so that only partial recovery has occurred 14 days later (Anderson *et al.*, 1990; Figure 9.6). This impairment of the baroreceptor reflex is accompanied by a persistent tachycardia which is not related to hypovolaemia, and a reduction in the variation in heart rate induced by respiration.

The afferent pathway of the response to 'injury' appears to run in somatic (including nociceptive) fibres arising in the damaged tissues. Afferent information then ascends in the spinal cord (probably via the spinothalamic tract) to the brain (Redfern *et al.*, 1984). Little is known of the precise mechanism of the reduction in the sensitivity of the baroreflex. However, recent studies have shown that activation of somatic afferent A$\delta$ fibres can lead to inhibition of baroreflex-sensitive neurones within the NTS via a GABA-ergic mechanism (McMahon *et al.*, 1992). Furthermore, it has been argued that the response to injury is reminiscent of the visceral alerting response of the defence reaction (Quest & Gebber, 1972), and that similar pathways are involved.

### *Central nervous pathways organising the cardiovascular response to 'injury'*

The most striking aspects of the response to peripheral 'injury' include the cardiovascular changes and antinociception, of which there are numerous anecdotal accounts. Unfortunately, there is very little in the literature regarding the central nervous organisation of these responses to injury. There is, however, a wealth of information concerning pathways

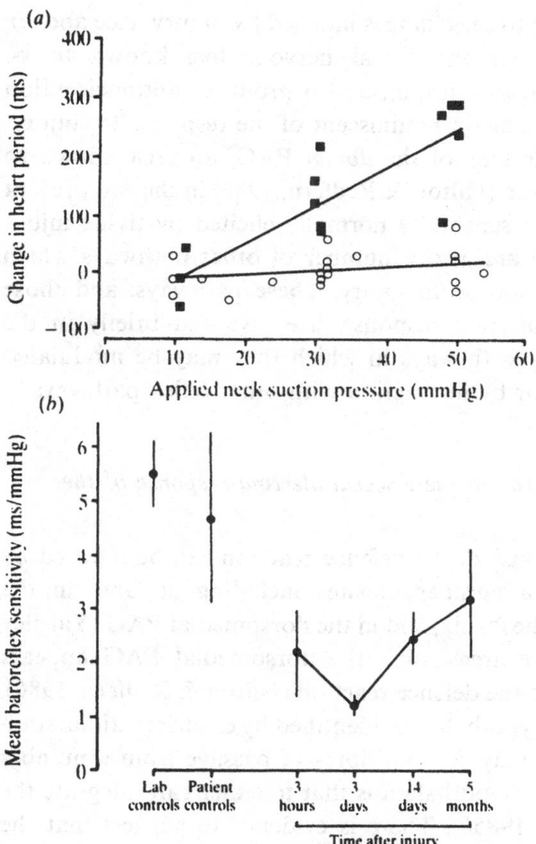


Figure 9.6. (*a*) The relationship between changes in heart period and negative pressure applied to the carotid sinus region of the neck in an injured patient. (○) 2 h after fracture of the right tibia and fibula; (■) 10 days later. The relationships shown are the lines of best fit calculated by the technique of least mean squares. (*b*) Baroreflex sensitivity (the gradient of the line relating change in heart period to applied neck suction pressure) in control groups and in patients tested at different times after injury (Injury Severity Score range 9–17; median 9). Values are shown as mean ± standard error.

that can modulate both cardiovascular function and nociception. One group of central nervous pathways that produce such changes are those involved in the visceral alerting response of the defence reaction (Lovick, 1985*a*), which, in turn, has been implicated in the response to 'injury' (see above).

Activation of the visceral alerting response produces a simultaneous increase in heart rate and blood pressure, and an attenuation of the baroreceptor reflex, similar to the changes induced by 'injury' (see above). Furthermore, stimulation within central nervous loci known to be involved in the visceral alerting response also produces antinociception (Duggan & Morton, 1983), again reminiscent of the response to 'injury' (Beecher, 1945). Finally, lesions of the *dorsal* PAG, an area known to integrate the defence reaction (Hilton & Redfern, 1986) in the rat, prevent the reduction in baroreflex sensitivity normally elicited by tissue injury (Jones *et al.*, 1990). There are also a number of other pathways which may play a role in the response to injury. These pathways, and those involved in the visceral alerting response, are reviewed briefly in the following section, together with ways in which they may be modulated either pharmacologically or by interaction with other reflex pathways.

*Pathways involved in integrating the visceral alerting response of the defence reaction*

The visceral alerting response of the defence reaction can be induced by electrical stimulation at a number of sites including an area in the hypothalamus ventral to the fornix, and in the dorsomedial PAG (Yardley & Hilton, 1986). Of these areas, only the dorsomedial PAG appears capable of fully integrating the defence reaction (Hilton & Redfern, 1986), whereas the region in the hypothalamus identified by electrical stimulation (Yardley & Hilton, 1986) may contain fibres of passage from a number of more rostral sites in the hypothalamus that together can integrate the defence reaction (Lovick, 1985*b*). There is evidence to suggest that the dorsal PAG may be involved in the response to 'injury' (see above). This area is known to process afferent nociceptive information (Basbaum & Fields, 1978), and was shown to display increased neuronal activity following 'injury' (Jones, 1989; Porro *et al.*, 1991).

The cardiovascular response to 'injury' involves a modulation of two efferent autonomic pathways – the vagal control of heart rate (involved in the baroreceptor reflex, see above), and the sympathetic control of the heart and vasculature. For reasons of clarity, the effects of the 'defence pathways' on these two efferent pathways are discussed separately in the following sections, although it must be stressed that the control of the two efferent limbs of the autonomic nervous system are intimately linked.

*Modulation of vagal efferent activity to the heart* The cell bodies of the vagal preganglionic motor neurones that supply the heart are found in two brainstem nuclei – the nucleus ambiguus and the dorsal vagal motor nucleus (see above). When the baroreceptors are stimulated, activity in the vagal cardiac motor neurones is increased via two main excitatory pathways: from the NTS there is both a 'segmental' pathway within the medulla and a pathway ascending to relay in the anterior hypothalamus before descending again to the vagal nuclei (see above, Figure 9.3*a*). Activity in the 'defence pathways' can inhibit vagal efferent activity by at least three mechanisms. Firstly, there are inhibitory GABA-ergic projections from the defence areas onto the vagal cardiac motor neurones (Jordan *et al.*, 1980). Secondly, activation of the defence reaction can cause an inhibition within the NTS (McAllen, 1976; Mifflin *et al.*, 1988), where GABA has recently been shown to act as an inhibitory transmitter (Bennett *et al.*, 1987). Thirdly, activation of the defence reaction can lead to an excitation of inspiratory neurones within the nucleus ambiguus (Spyer, 1984) which again will inhibit the vagal cardiac preganglionic motor neurones (see above). These pathways are summarised in Figure 9.7. The inhibition by the defence reaction may not be restricted to an attenuation of baroreflex-elicited vagal efferent activity, but may also affect vagal activity generated by other reflexes, e.g. by activation of cardiac C-fibre afferents.

*Modulation of sympathetic efferent activity* The increase in arterial blood pressure during the visceral alerting response is mediated partly by a sympathetically induced increase in total peripheral resistance. However, the increase in total peripheral resistance is not the result of an indiscriminate vasoconstriction, but rather of a highly organised pattern involving increased resistance in vascular beds such as the renal and mesenteric, and a reduction in skeletal muscle vascular resistance. There is sufficient differentiation within the PAG to organise these changes, since it contains groups of cells that are viscerotopically organised with respect to their control over various vascular beds (Carrive *et al.*, 1989).

In addition to the cardiovascular effects, stimulation within the dorsomedial PAG produces an antinociceptive effect (Duggan & Morton, 1983). The efferent pathways mediating the cardiovascular and antinociceptive effects relay in the nucleus paragigantocellularis lateralis (PGL) in the ventrolateral medulla (Hilton *et al.*, 1983; Lovick, 1985*a*, 1986*a*).

The PGL appears to integrate the efferent activity of a number of cardiovascular reflexes and response patterns (Lovick, 1987*a*, 1988*a*), since it receives inputs from a number of sites that are known to be involved in cardiovascular and somatosensory control. These sites include the hypothalamic and PAG defence areas, the lateral hypothalamus, the NTS,

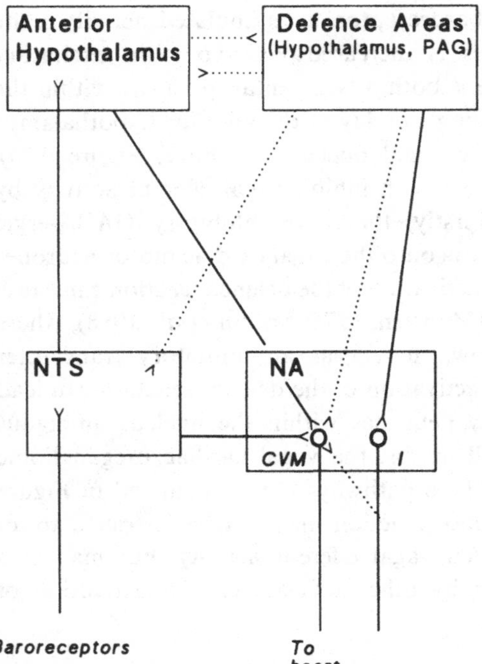


Figure 9.7. Schematic diagram indicating some of the pathways whereby activity in the defence areas (stimulated following injury?) can modify the baroreflex control of vagal efferent activity to the heart. Excitatory pathways are shown as solid lines, inhibitory pathways as broken lines. PAG, periaqueductal grey; NTS, nucleus tractus solitarius; NA, nucleus ambiguus; CVM, cardiac vagal motor neurone; I, inspiratory neurone. See text for details. (Modified from Spyer, 1984.)

the CVLM, nucleus raphe magnus (NRM) and obscurus (NRO) and the nucleus parabrachialis (NPB) (Andrezik *et al.*, 1981; Lovick, 1986*b*, 1988*a*), many of which converge onto the same neurone in the PGL (Lovick, 1988*a*). The PGL, in turn, sends an efferent output to the intermediolateral column (sympathetic preganglionic motor neurones, see above) and to the dorsal horn (Martin *et al.*, 1979; modulation of nociception) of the spinal cord. Stimulation within the PGL therefore produces sympathoexcitation (see above) and antinociception (Lovick, 1987*b*). However, the sympathoexcitatory and antinociceptive effects are not mediated by the same pool of neurones within the PGL (Lovick, 1987*b*; Siddall & Dampney, 1989). Indeed, in animals such as the cat, the cardiovascular sympathoexcitatory drive originates from a specialised subnucleus, the subretrofacial nucleus (Siddall & Dampney, 1989), where

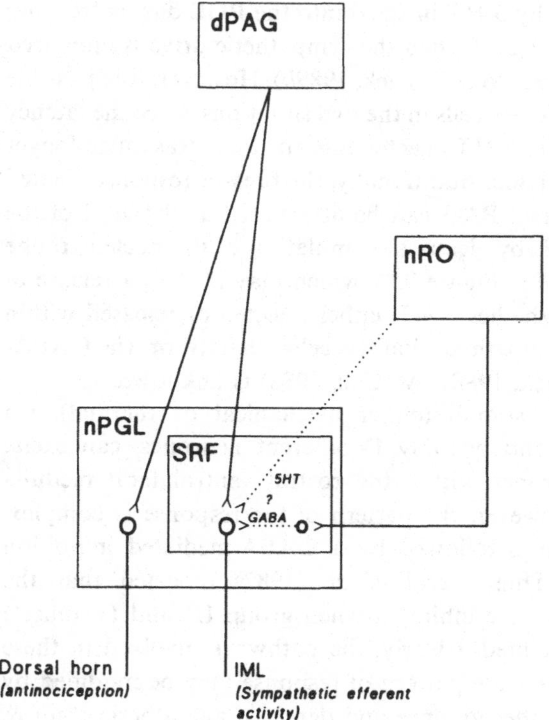


Figure 9.8. Schematic diagram showing some of the possible pathways whereby activity in the dorsal periaqueductal grey may produce sympathoexcitation and antinociception, and how these pathways may be modulated by activation of the raphe. Excitatory pathways are shown as solid lines, inhibitory pathways as broken lines. dPAG, dorsal periaqueductal grey; nRO, nucleus raphe obscurus; nPGL, nucleus paragigantocellularis lateralis; SRF, subretrofacial nucleus; IML, intermediolateral cell column of spinal cord. See text for details.

the neurones are arranged topographically according to the type of vascular bed that they control (McAllen & Dampney, 1990), and receive an equally well-organised projection from equivalent areas within the PAG (Carrive *et al.*, 1989) (see above, and Figure 9.8).

Both the cardiovascular and antinociceptive neurones (at least in the rat) are subject to a tonic GABA-ergic inhibition (Lovick, 1987*b*). However, since different neurones mediate the cardiovascular and antinociceptive effects, there is a possibility of differentially modulating the two effects. Thus the sympathoexcitatory but not the antinociceptive drive from the PGL is subject to a tonic cholinergic inhibition (Lovick, 1987*b*), and can also be inhibited by 5-HT injected into the PGL during 'resting' conditions (Lovick, 1989*a*), and when the sympathetic drive is enhanced by stimulation of the dorsal PAG (Lovick, 1989*b*). However, it is possible that 5-HT is acting on different cells in the two situations, since the latency of the depressor response to 5-HT injected into the PGL was much longer when the PAG was stimulated. Additionally, the pressor response elicited by stimulation of the dorsal PAG can be attenuated at the level of the synaptic relay in the PGL by electrical stimulation of the nucleus raphe obscurus (Gong & Li, 1989; Figure 9.8), which may lead to a release of 5-HT within the PGL. Whether 5-HT, either injected or released within the PGL, inhibits the sympathoexcitatory cells directly or via GABA-ergic interneurones (Lovick, 1988*b*; McCall, 1988) is unknown.

Cutaneous nociceptive stimuli (either mechanical or thermal), via activation of group III and possibly IV afferent neurones, can excite sympathoexcitatory neurones within the rostral ventrolateral medulla (Sun & Spyer, 1991). However, the pattern of the response is complex, and the initial excitation is followed by a GABA-mediated inhibition (Sun & Spyer, 1991). Thus, Terui *et al.* (1987) reported that the sympathoexcitatory cells were inhibited when group III and IV muscle afferent fibres were stimulated. Clearly, the pathways involved in these responses are complex, and the pattern of response may be modified by a number of factors, e.g. the presence and depth of anaesthesia (Sun & Spyer, 1991).

### *Involvement of the raphe pathways in the response to injury*

There is evidence that peripheral 'injury' also induces increased neuronal activity within the NRM (Jones, 1989; Porro *et al.*, 1991). This nucleus has been implicated in modulating sympathetic output to the cardiovascular system and in antinociception. Thus, the NRM is thought to act as a relay in antinociceptive pathways originating in both the lateral hypothalamus (Amione & Gebhart, 1988) and ventral (but not dorsal) PAG (Praag & Frenk, 1990; Figure 9.9). Electrical stimulation within the NRM can produce both increases and decreases in blood pressure, the pressor and depressor areas being organised topographically (Adair *et al.*, 1977). The NRM has been shown to send projections to both the PGL (which are inhibitory; Lovick, 1988*a*) and to the spinal cord (inhibitory and excitatory; McCall, 1984), and can modulate cardiovascular activity and nociception (Figure 9.9). It has therefore been suggested that there are two parallel systems in the medulla, each of which

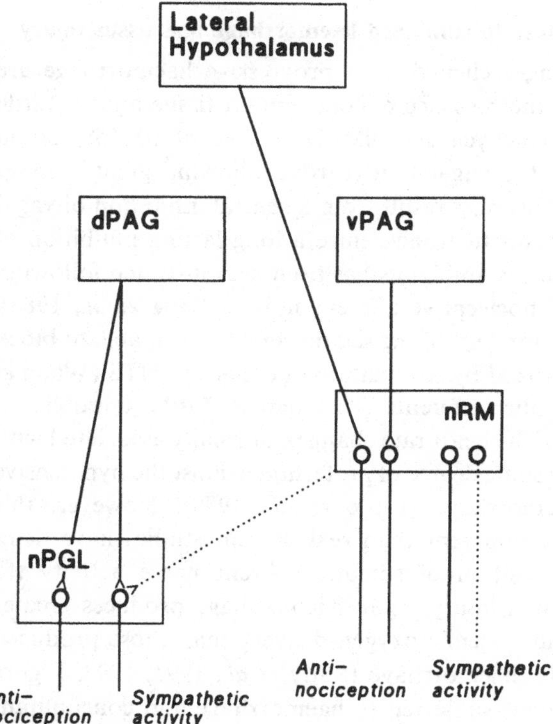


Figure 9.9. Schematic diagram showing possible pathways involving the raphe magnus in modulating sympathetic efferent activity and nociception. Excitatory pathways are shown as solid lines, inhibitory pathways as broken lines. dPAG, dorsal periaqueductal grey; vPAG, ventral periaqueductal grey; nRM, nucleus raphe magnus; nPGL, nucleus paragigantocellularis lateralis. See text for details.

controls cardiovascular and somatosensory activity (Lovick, 1988*a*). When cells in the NRM are activated, they may attenuate activity in the PGL pathway, possibly via a GABA-ergic mechanism (Lovick, 1988*b*; McCall, 1988) to allow the action of the raphe system to predominate (Lovick, 1988*a*), as shown in Figure 9.9.

There are therefore a number of central nervous pathways that *may* be involved in the cardiovascular response to injury. Further studies, both of these central pathways and of the precise haemodynamic response to 'injury', are required to determine which, if any, are involved in the response to injury.

## The cardiovascular response to combined haemorrhage and tissue injury

The cardiovascular changes elicited by a progressive haemorrhage are markedly attenuated by the presence of concomitant tissue injury (Little *et al.*, 1989). The initial tachycardia following a loss of 10–15% blood volume is reduced, and the vagal bradycardia following greater losses prevented (Figure 9.2). This may result from a central inhibition of vagal cardiac preganglionic motor neurones, since a long-lasting inhibition of such neurones in the nucleus ambiguus has been demonstrated following electrical stimulation of nociceptive afferent fibres (Wang *et al.*, 1988). Somatic afferent stimulation (e.g. of the sciatic nerve) is also able to block the vagal bradycardia evoked by stimulation of either the NTS (Wang *et al.*, 1988) or cardiac C-fibre afferents (Kirkman & Little, unpublished data). This attenuation of the heart rate changes, normally associated with blood loss, seems to offer some degree of protection against the hypotensive effects of a severe haemorrhage (Little *et al.*, 1989). However, this protection may be more apparent than real. Recent studies have demonstrated that superimposition of somatic afferent nerve activity (to simulate 'injury'), or a real injury, upon haemorrhage produces greater falls in cardiac index and systemic oxygen delivery than those produced by an equivalent 'simple' haemorrhage (Rady *et al.*, 1991, 1993; Figure 9.10). Furthermore, animals subjected to haemorrhage and concomitant electrical stimulation of the sciatic nerve (to simulate 'injury') demonstrate a lower survival rate compared to animals subjected to haemorrhage alone (Overman & Wang, 1947). It is possible that the better maintenance of blood pressure is achieved at the expense of intense peripheral vasoconstriction leading to ischaemic organ damage, which will exacerbate the severity of injury. It is tempting to speculate that the sphlanchnic circulation may be selectively vulnerable to such ischaemic damage, leading to the release of blood-borne factors, which may impair cardiovascular function. Intestinal permeability may also be increased, leading to enhanced translocation of bacteria and endotoxin (for example, see Wilmore *et al.*, 1988; Deitch, 1990), a suggestion that is reminiscent of Fine's (1961) endotoxin theory of shock.

## Neurotransmitters involved in the response to haemorrhage and injury, and potential pharmacological manipulations

The involvement of a number of neurotransmitters, e.g. the excitatory and inhibitory amino acids, in various aspects of the response to haemorrhage

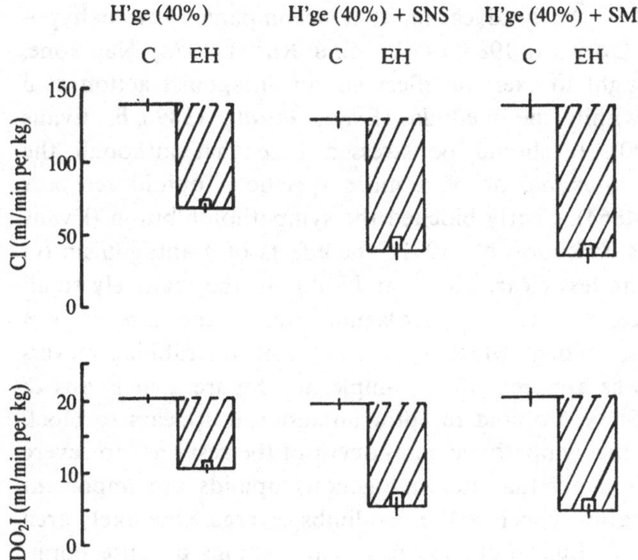


Figure 9.10. Effects of somatic afferent nerve stimulation (SNS) and skeletal muscle injury (SMI) on the changes in cardiac output (expressed as cardiac index, CI) and oxygen delivery index ($DO_2I$) produced by a haemorrhage (H'ge) of 40% of estimated blood volume in pigs anaesthetised with isoflurane. C, values recorded before haemorrhage; EH, values recorded at the end of haemorrhage.

and injury has already been discussed (see above). Unfortunately, pharmacological interference with these amino acid neurotransmitters is unlikely to be useful clinically, since they are major transmitters in a large number of other (unrelated) control systems. However, there are a number of other neurotransmitters that may be involved in the response to haemorrhage and injury, the manipulation of which could be useful in formulating new treatment regimens.

### *The endogenous opioids*

There is a strong body of evidence suggesting that the endogenous opioid system may be involved in the response to severe hypovolaemia. Most of the evidence suggests a role for the opioid system in the sympathoinhibitory response. However, there is also some, albeit weaker, evidence suggesting their role in the bradycardic response. Thus, the opioid antagonist naloxone, when given intravenously, was shown to attenuate the reduction in sympathetic efferent activity and the associated hypotension, and possibly the bradycardia that accompanies severe hypovolaemia (Burke & Dorward, 1988; Ludbrook & Rutter, 1988). Naloxone, in this case, is thought to exert its effect via an antagonist action at $\delta$ opioid receptors within the medulla (Evans *et al.*, 1989*a*, *b*; Evans & Ludbrook, 1990). It should be stressed here that although the administration of naloxone, or of a more specific $\delta$ opioid receptor antagonist (ICI 174864), clearly blocked the sympathoinhibition (Evans *et al.*, 1989*b*; Evans & Ludbrook, 1991), the effects of $\delta$ antagonism on the bradycardia were less clear. This may be due to the relatively small bradycardic response to severe hypovolaemia even in the absence of $\delta$ antagonism in these studies, which were conducted on rabbits. Nevertheless, the trend was apparent (for example, see Figure 2 in Evans & Ludbrook, 1991). Since $\delta$ opioid receptor antagonism appears to block *both* the vagal and the sympathetic component of the response to severe hypovolaemia, it is likely that the endogenous opioids are important early in the reflex pathway, before the two limbs diverge. One likely area is the NTS (Evans & Ludbrook, 1990), which contains a dense population of $\delta$ opioid receptors (Dashwood *et al.*, 1988; May *et al.*, 1989).

In addition to the $\delta$ opioid receptors, the $\mu$ and the $\kappa$ receptors also appear to be capable of modifying the response to severe hypovolaemia. Thus, $\mu$ and $\kappa$ receptor *agonists* can also prevent the reflex sympathoinhibition (and possibly the bradycardia) seen during severe hypovolaemia (Evans *et al.*, 1989*b*; Evans & Ludbrook, 1990, 1991). However, it is unlikely that the $\mu$ opioid receptor participates in the normal 'physiological' response to severe haemorrhage (Evans & Ludbrook, 1990), although the use of $\mu$ receptor agonists, e.g. the anaesthetics fentanyl and alfentanil (Schadt & Ludbrook, 1991) may provide a pharmacological means of inhibiting the depressor effect of a severe haemorrhage. Whether this would be beneficial or detrimental (bearing in mind the potential protective effects of this depressor reflex, and the consequences of blocking it), remains to be seen.

Since 'injury' is also known to activate the endogenous opioid system, and cell bodies that synthesise and release enkephalins are found in the PAG (Uhl *et al.*, 1979; an area known to be involved in the cardiovascular response to 'injury', see above), it is not surprising to learn that naloxone can modify the response to 'injury'. Thus, it has been demonstrated in experimental studies that the administration of naloxone, either centrally or intravenously, can prevent or reverse the reduction in baroreflex sensitivity produced by 'injury' (Eltrafi *et al.*, 1989). Conversely, some of the effects of 'injury' on the baroreflex can be mimicked by the central administration of a long-lasting analogue of met-enkephalin (D-Ala$^2$-Met$^5$-enkephalinamide) (Little *et al.*, 1988).

Therefore, it can be seen that both opioid agonists and antagonists can modify the cardiovascular response to haemorrhage and 'injury'. Clearly, the effects are complex, emphasising the complexity of the underlying neural control mechanisms. Further studies are required to evaluate the role of individual opioid receptor subtypes in these responses, and the resultant haemodynamic changes and their consequences, before any attempts at treatment are made with these agents.

### *5-Hydroxytryptamine*

The role of 5-HT in the central nervous pathways involved in the response to injury has already been described. There have been suggestions that this agent may also be involved in the central nervous pathways mediating the response to severe haemorrhage. Bogle *et al.* (1990) demonstrated that a response that included the 'cardiac reflex' elicited by activation of cardiac–vagal C-fibre afferents could be blocked by methiothepin (a 5-HT receptor antagonist) given centrally (see p. 209 for control of vagal efferent activity). Furthermore, blockade of the 5-HT system, either with *p*-chlorophenylalanine (PCPA, which blocks the synthesis of 5-HT), or with the 5-HT receptor antagonist, methysergide, has been reported to prevent or reverse both the sympathoinhibitory and the bradycardic response to severe blood loss, while leaving baroreflex control intact (Morgan *et al.*, 1988). Although the 5-HT 'blocking' agents were given intravenously in this study, their sites of action were likely to be central, since any effects of 5-HT on the ventricular receptors is mediated via 5-$HT_3$ receptors (Kay & Armstrong, 1990), where methysergide has little activity (Peroutka, 1988).

However, the effects of 5-HT 'blockade' on the response to severe blood loss are equivocal, since other studies have failed to show that PCPA blocks the depressor response to severe haemorrhage (Evans *et al.*, 1992), and have suggested that the action of agents, e.g. methysergide, are not due to blockade of 5-HT but rather to *agonism* at 5-$HT_{1A}$ receptors (Evans *et al.*, 1993). Evans *et al.* (1993) concluded, therefore, that there was no evidence of a physiological role for 5-HT in the depressor response to severe haemorrhage. Recent data from our own laboratories indicate that the 5-$HT_{1A}$ receptor antagonist methiothepin was unable to attenuate the reflex bradycardia that accompanies severe haemorrhage (Kirkman

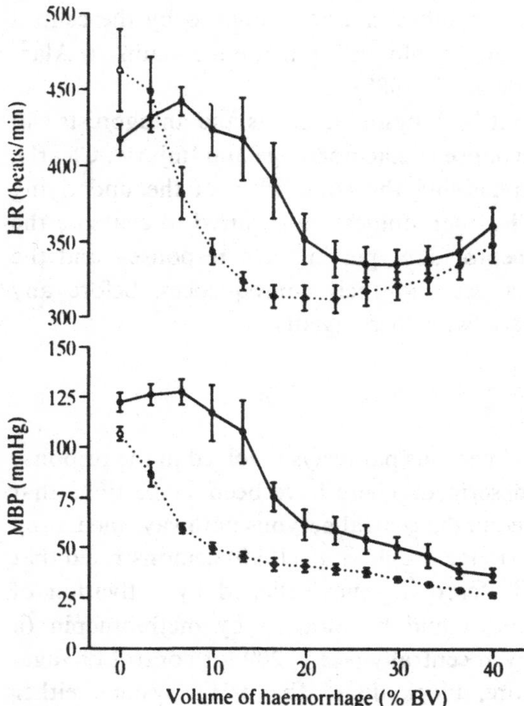


Figure 9.11. Effects of a progressive 'simple' haemorrhage expressed as percentage of estimated total blood volume (BV) on heart rate (HR) and mean arterial blood pressure (MBP) in two groups of six rats anaesthetised with alphadolone/alphaxolone. Animals pretreated with 0.9% w/v saline (●) (5 μl into the IVth cerebral ventricle), or methiothepin (○) (200 μg/kg in 5 μl via the same route). Values are shown as mean ± standard error for dependent and independent variables. Where the error bar is not shown, it is smaller than the size of the symbol.

*et al.*, 1944*b*; Figure 9.11), unlike its effects on the 'cardiac reflex' (see above), suggesting that the two responses may be mediated via different central nervous pathways. Indeed, our studies indicate that 5-HT antagonism may potentiate the depressor response to severe haemorrhage, and therefore our findings support and extend those of Evans *et al.* (1993). Activation of central 5-HT receptors does not appear necessary for the mediation of the depressor response associated with the severe haemorrhage; however, 5-HT may have a 'physiological' role in providing a tonic inhibition of this response.

Thus, 5-HT and its receptors may provide another avenue for pharmacological manipulation of the response to haemorrhage and injury, although, due to the complexity of the system, this possibility lies some way ahead.

### *Effects of ethanol*

Ethanol is a drug taken socially, often preceding events, e.g. an automobile accident, that lead to trauma. The effects of ethanol on the cardiovascular response to haemorrhage and 'injury' are therefore of interest. Recent studies have shown that moderately raised blood levels of ethanol (100–200 mg/100 ml) can exacerbate the 'injury'-induced reduction in baroreflex sensitivity (Kirkman *et al.*, 1994*a*; Figure 9.12). The explanation of the action of ethanol on the cardiovascular response to injury is potentially simple. It has been reported that ethanol may potentiate the effects of endogenous GABA at both the NTS and the vagal outflow nuclei (Varga & Kunos, 1990). Since the response to injury is thought to inhibit the baroreflex via a GABA-ergic mechanism within the brainstem nuclei, it is hardly surprising that ethanol augments the baroreflex-inhibitory effects of injury.

## Conclusions

The organisation of the central nervous pathways involved in the cardiovascular response to haemorrhage and 'injury', i.e. trauma, are very complicated. A better understanding of how these central pathways function and interact, together with a knowledge of the neutrotransmitters and pharmacological receptors involved, is needed to further our understanding of how pharmacological agents may modify the responses, and to allow the development of new treatment regimes. There is evidence that the endogenous opioids have an important role to play, but it is important that the receptor subtypes involved are identified if the cardiovascular changes are to be modified whilst maintaining analgesia. It may be possible to manipulate the cardiovascular and antinociceptive responses to 'injury' using 5-HT agonists and antagonists, but such a possibility lies some way ahead. However, before these new regimes are developed, it is important to determine which of the responses to trauma are beneficial and which are detrimental to the victim. Only then will we be able to decide which aspects of the response to modify and which to leave alone.

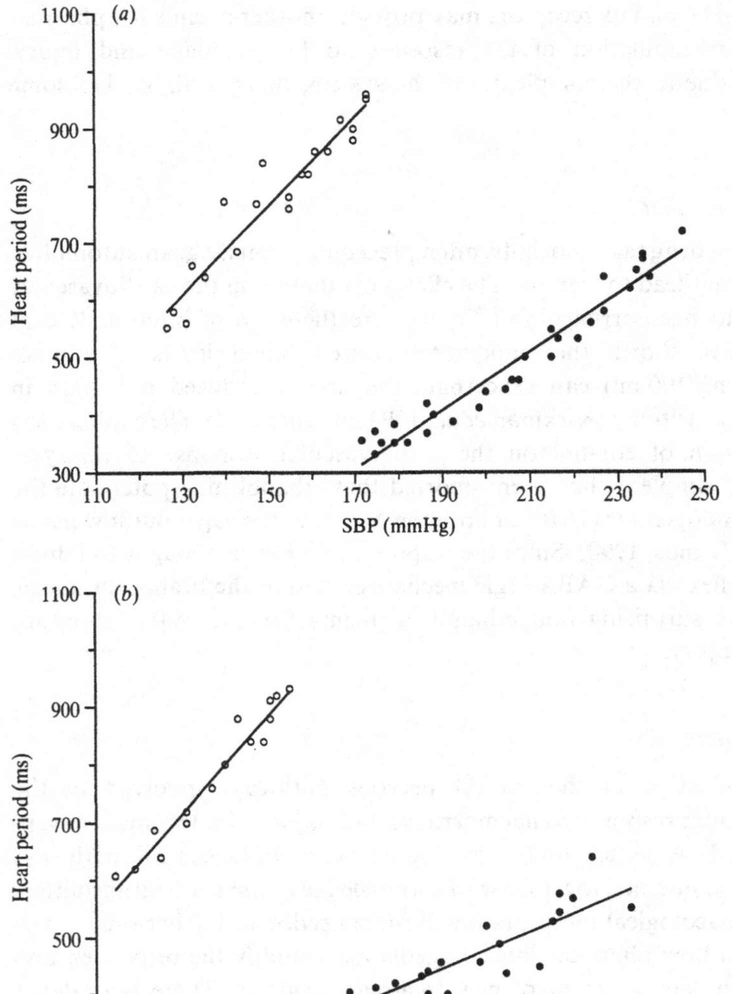


Figure 9.12. The effects of electrically stimulating the central cut end of the sciatic nerve to mimic injury, on the relationship between systolic arterial blood pressure (SBP) and heart period in a dog anaesthetised with propofol. The slope of this relationship is an index of baroreflex sensitivity, while a lateral displacement indicates a resetting of the reflex. Assessment (*a*) during 'control' conditions and (*b*) during the intravenous infusion of ethanol sufficient to produce a blood ethanol level of 152.1 mg/100 ml in the same animal. Data recorded in the absence (○), and in the presence (●) of sciatic nerve stimulation.

## References

Abraham, A. (1967). The structure of baroreceptors in pathological conditions in man. In *Baroreceptors and Hypertension*, ed. P. Kezdi, p. 273. Oxford: Pergamon.

Acker, H. & O'Regan, R. G. (1981). The effects of stimulation of autonomic nerves on carotid body blood flow in the cat. *J. Physiol.*, **315**, 99.

Adair, J. R., Hamilton, B. L., Scappaticci, K. A., Helke, C. J. & Gillis, R. A. (1977). Cardiovascular responses to electrical stimulation of the medullary raphe area of the cat. *Brain Res.*, **128**, 141.

Agarwal, S. K. & Calaresu, F. R. (1992). Electrical stimulation of nucleus tractus solitarius excites vagal preganglionic cardiomotor neurons of the nucleus ambiguus in rats. *Brain Res.*, **574**, 320.

Alam, M. & Smirk, F. H. (1937). Observations in man upon a blood pressure raising reflex arising from the voluntary muscles. *J. Physiol.*, **89**, 372.

Alam, M. & Smirk, F. H. (1938). Observations in man upon a pulse accelerating reflex from the voluntary muscles of the legs. *J. Physiol.*, **92**, 167.

Amione, L. D. & Gebhart, G. F. (1988). Serotonin and/or an excitatory amino acid mediates stimulation produced antinociception from the lateral hypothalamus in the rat. *Brain Res.*, **450**, 170.

Anderson, I. D., Little, R. A. & Irving, M. H. (1990). An effect of trauma on human cardiovascular control: baroreflex suppression. *J. Trauma*, **30**, 974.

Andrezik, J. A., Chan-Palay, V. & Palay, S. L. (1981). The nucleus paragigantocellularis lateralis in the rat. Demonstration of afferents by retrograde transport of horseradish peroxidase. *Anat. Embryol.*, **161**, 373.

Angell-James, J. E. (1971). The effects of changes in extramural, 'intrathoracic', pressure on aortic-arch baroreceptors. *J. Physiol.*, **214**, 84.

Angell-James, J. E. & Daly, M. de B. (1970). Comparison of the reflex vasomotor responses to separate and combined stimulation of the carotid sinus and aortic arch baroreceptors by pulsatile and non-pulsatile pressures in the dog. *J. Physiol.*, **209**, 257.

Angell-James, J. E. & Daly, M. de B. (1975). Some aspects of upper respiratory tract reflexes. *Acta Otolaryngol.*, **79**, 242.

Badoer, E., McKinley, M. J., Oldfield, B. J. & McAllen, R. M. (1992). Distribution of hypothalamic, medullary and lamina terminalis neurones expressing Fos after haemorrhage in conscious rats. *Brain Res.*, **582**, 323.

Baker, D. G., Coleridge, H. M. & Coleridge, J. C. G. (1979). Vagal afferent C-fibres from the ventricle. In *Cardiac Receptors*, ed. R. Hainsworth, C. Kidd & R. J. Linden, p. 117. Cambridge: Cambridge University Press.

Barcroft, H., Edholm, O. G., McMichael, J. & Sharpey-Schafer, E. P. (1944). Posthaemorrhagic fainting. Study by cardiac output and forearm flow. *Lancet*, **i**, 489.

Barriot, P., Riou, B. & Buffat, J.-J. (1987). Pre-hospital management of severe haemorrhagic shock. In *Update in Intensive Care and Emergency Medicine*, vol. 3, ed. J. L. Vincent, p. 377. Berlin: Springer-Verlag.

Basbaum, A. I. & Fields, H. L. (1978). Endogenous pain control mechanisms: review and hypothesis. *Ann. Neurol.*, **4**, 451.

Beecher, H. K. (1945). Pain in men wounded in battle. *Ann. Surg.*, **123**, 96.

Bennett, J. A., Ford, T. W., Kidd, C. & McWilliam, P. N. (1984). Potentiation of carotid sinus baroreceptor and cardiac and pulmonary vagal receptor reflexes in the anaesthetized, decerebrate cat by bicuculline. *J. Physiol.*, **350**, 37P.

Bennett, J. A., Goodchild, C. S., Kidd, C. & McWilliam, P. N. (1985). Neurones in the brain stem of the cat excited by vagal afferent fibres from the heart and lungs. *J. Physiol.*, **369**, 1.

Bennett, J. A., McWilliam, P. N. & Shepheard, S. L. (1987). A gamma-aminobutyric-acid-mediated inhibition of neurones in the nucleus tractus solitarius of the cat. *J. Physiol.*, **392**, 417.

Biscoe, T. J., Purves, M. J. & Sampson, S. R. (1970). The frequency of nerve impulses in single carotid body chemoreceptor afferent fibres recorded *in vivo* with intact circulation. *J. Physiol.*, **208**, 121.

Bogle, R. G., Pires, J. G. & Ramage, A. G. (1990). Evidence that central 5-HT1A-receptors play a role in the von Bezold–Jarisch reflex in the rat. *Br. J. Pharmacol.*, **100**, 757.

Bronk, D. W. & Stella, G. (1935). The response to steady pressures of single end organs in the isolated carotid sinus. *Am. J. Physiol.*, **110**, 708.

Brown, D. L. & Guyenet, P. G. (1984). Cardiovascular neurons of brain stem with projections to spinal cord. *Am. J. Physiol.*, **247**, R1009.

Burke, S. L. & Dorward, P. K. (1988). Influence of endogenous opiates and cardiac baroreceptors on renal nerve activity during haemorrhage in conscious rabbits. *J. Physiol.*, **402**, 9.

Carrive, P., Bandler, R. & Dampney, R. A. (1989). Viscerotopic control of regional vascular beds by discrete groups of neurons within the midbrain periaqueductal gray. *Brain Res.*, **493**, 385.

Chalmers, J. P. & Pilowsky, P. M. (1991). Brainstem and bulbospinal neurotransmitter systems in the control of blood pressure. *J. Hypertens.*, **9**, 675.

Cohen, M. I., Piercey, M. F., Gootman, P. M. & Wolotsky, P. (1974). Synaptic connections between medullary inspiratory neurons and phrenic motoneurons as revealed by cross correlation. *Brain Res.*, **81**, 319.

Cowley, A. W., Liard, J. F. & Guyton, A. C. (1973). Role of baroreceptor reflex in daily control of arterial blood pressure and other variables in dogs. *Circ. Res.*, **32**, 564.

Cowley, A. W., Merril, D., Osborn, J. & Barber, B. J. (1984). Influence of vasopressin and angiotensin on baroreflexes in the dog. *Circ. Res.*, **54**, 163.

D'Silva, J. L., Gill, D. & Mendel, D. (1966). The effects of acute haemorrhage on respiration in the cat. *J. Physiol.*, **187**, 369.

Daly, M. de B. (1983) Peripheral arterial chemoreceptors and the cardiovascular system. In *Physiology of the Peripheral Arterial Chemoreceptors*, ed. H. Acker & R. G. O'Regan, p. 325. Amsterdam: Elsevier Science Publishers.

Daly, M. de B., Kirkman, E. & Wood, L. M. (1988). Cardiovascular responses to stimulation of cardiac receptors in the cat and their modification by changes in respiration. *J. Physiol.*, **407**, 349.

Daly, M. de B., Lambertsen, C. J. & Schweitzer, A. (1954). Observations on the volume of blood flow and oxygen utilization of the carotid body in the cat. *J. Physiol.*, **125**, 67.

Dashwood, M. R., Muddle, J. R. & Spyer, K. M. (1988). Opiate receptor subtypes in the nucleus tractus solitarii of the cat: the effect of vagal section. *Eur. J. Pharmacol.*, **155**, 85–92.

Deitch, E. A. (1990). Intestinal permeability is increased in burn patients shortly after injury. *Surgery*, **107**, 411.

Duggan, A. W. & Morton, C. R. (1983). Periaqueductal grey stimulation: an association between selective inhibition of dorsal horn neurones and changes in peripheral circulation. *Pain*, **15**, 237.

Ellenberger, H. H. & Feldman, J. L. (1988). Monosynaptic transmission of respiratory drive to phrenic motoneurons from brainstem bulbospinal neurons in rats. *J. Comp. Neurol.*, **269**, 47.

Eltrafi, A., Kirkman, E. & Little, R. A. (1989). Reversal of the injury induced reduction in baroreflex sensitivity by naloxone in the conscious rat. *Br. J. Pharmacol.*, **96**, 145.

Evans, R. G., Haynes, J. M. & Ludbrook, J. (1993). Effects of 5-HT-receptor and $\alpha_2$-adrenoceptor ligands on the haemodynamic response to acute central hypovolaemia in conscious rabbits. *Br. J. Pharmacol.*, **109**, 37–47.

Evans, R. G., Kapoor, V. & Ludbrook, J. (1992). A CNS serotonergic mechanism in acute central hypovolaemia in conscious rabbits? *J. Cardiovasc. Pharmacol.*, **19**, 1009–17.

Evans, R. G. & Ludbrook, J. (1990). Effects of mu-opioid receptor agonists on circulatory responses to simulated haemorrhage in conscious rabbits. *Br. J. Pharmacol.*, **100**, 421.

Evans, R. G. & Ludbrook, J. (1991). Chemosensitive cardiopulmonary afferents and the haemodynamic response to simulated haemorrhage in conscious rabbits. *Br. J. Pharmacol.*, **102**, 533.

Evans, R. G., Ludbrook, J. & Potocnik, S. J. (1989*a*). Intracisternal naloxone and cardiac nerve blockade prevent vasodilatation during simulated haemorrhage in awake rabbits. *J. Physiol.*, **409**, 1.

Evans, R. G., Ludbrook, J. & van Leeuwen, A. F. (1989*b*). Role of central opiate receptor subtypes in the circulatory responses of awake rabbits to graded caval occlusions. *J. Physiol.*, **419**, 15.

Evans, R. G., Ludbrook, J., Woods, R. L. & Casley, D. (1991). Influence of higher brain centres and vasopressin on the haemodynamic response to acute central hypovolaemia in rabbits. *J. Autonom. Nerv. Syst.*, **35**, 1.

Fine, J. (1961). Endotoxins in traumatic shock. *Fed. Proc.*, **20** (Suppl. 9), 166.

Fulwiler, C. E. & Saper, C. B. (1984). Subnuclear organization of the efferent connections of the parabrachial nucleus in the rat. *Brain Res. Rev.*, **7**, 229.

Garcia, M., Jordan, D. & Spyer, K. M. (1978). Studies on the properties of cardiac vagal neurones. *Neurosci. Lett.*, **1** (Suppl.), S16.

Gong, Q. L. & Li, P. (1989). Inhibitory effect of nucleus raphe obscurus on the pressor response to stimulation of the hypothalamic and midbrain defence areas in the anaesthetized rabbit. *J. Physiol.*, **418**, 85P.

Hayes, I. P., Evans, R. G. & Ludbrook, J. (1992). Presumptive pulmonary neural blockade following intrapericardial procaine in conscious rabbits. *Proc. Austr. Physiol. Soc.*, **23**, 66P.

Haywood, J. R., Fink, G. D., Buggy, J. Phillips, M. I. & Brody, M. J. (1980). The area postrema plays no role in the pressor action of angiotensin in the rat. *Am. J. Physiol.*, **239**, H108.

Henry, J. L. & Calaresu, F. R. (1972). Topography and numerical distribution of neurons of the thoraco-lumbar intermediolateral nucleus in the cat. *J. Comp. Neurol.*, **144**, 205.

Heymans, C. & Neil, E. (1958). *Reflexogenic Areas of the Cardiovascular System.* London: Churchill.

Hilton, S. M., Marshall, J. M. & Timms, R. J. (1983). Ventral medullary relay neurones in the pathway from the defence areas of the cat and their effect on blood pressure. *J. Physiol.*, **345**, 149.

Hilton, S. M. & Redfern, W. S. (1986). A search for brain stem cell groups integrating the defence reaction in the rat. *J. Physiol.*, **378**, 213.

Howard, J. M., Artz, C. P. & Stahl, R. R. (1955). The hypertensive response to injury. *Ann. Surg.*, **141**, 327.
Jones, R. O. (1989). The identification of the brain areas involved in the interaction between peripheral injuries and baroreceptor reflex activity in the rat. Ph.D. thesis, University of Manchester.
Jones, R. O., Kirkman, E. & Little, R. A. (1990). The involvement of the midbrain periaqueductal grey in the cardiovascular response to injury in the conscious and anaesthetized rat. *Exp. Physiol.*, **75**, 483.
Jordan, D., Khalid, M. E. M., Scheiderman, N. & Spyer, K. M. (1980). The inhibitory control of vagal cardiomotor neurones. *J. Physiol.*, **301**, 54P.
Jordan, D., Khalid, M. E. M., Schneiderman, N. & Spyer, K. M. (1982). The location and properties of preganglionic vagal cardiomotor neurones in rabbit. *Pflügers Arch.*, **395**, 244.
Jung, R., Bruce, E. N. & Katona, P. G. (1991). Cardiorespiratory responses to glutamatergic antagonists in the caudal ventrolateral medulla of rats. *Brain Res.*, **564**, 286.
Kadekaro, M., Summy-Long, J. Y., Terrell, M. L., Lekan, H., Gary, H. E. & Eisenberg, H. M. (1990). Cerebral metabolic and hormonal activations during hemorrhage in sinoaortic-denervated rats. *Am. J. Physiol.*, **259**, R305.
Kapoor, V., Minson, J. & Chalmers, J. (1992). Ventral medulla stimulation increases blood pressure and spinal cord amino acid release. *Neuropeptides*, **3**, 55.
Katic, F., Joy, M. D., Lavery, H., Lowe, R. D. & Scroop, G. C. (1971). Role of central effects of angiotensin in the response to haemorrhage in the dog. *Lancet*, **ii**, 1354.
Kay, I. S. & Armstrong, D. J. (1990). Phenylbiguanide not phenyldiguanide is used to evoke the pulmonary chemoreflex in anaesthetized rabbits. *Exp. Physiol.*, **75**, 383–9.
Kenney, R. A. & Neil, E. (1951). The contribution of aortic chemoreceptor mechanisms to the maintenance of arterial blood pressure of cats and dogs after haemorrhage. *J. Physiol.*, **112**, 223.
Kirchheim, H. (1976). Systemic arterial baroreceptor reflexes. *Physiol. Rev.*, **56**, 100.
Kirkman, E., Marshall, H. W., Banks, J. R. & Little, R. A. (1994*a*). Ethanol augments the baroreflex-inhibitory effects of sciatic nerve stimulation in the anaesthetized dog. *Exp. Physiol.*, **79**, 81–91.
Kirkman, E. & Scott, E. M. (1983). The effect of changes in plasma renin activity on the baroreceptor reflex arc in the cat. *J. Physiol.*, **342**, 73P.
Kirkman, E., Shiozaki, T. & Little, R. A. (1994*b*). Methiothepin does not attenuate the bradycardia associated with severe haemorrhage in the anaesthetized rat. *Br. J. Pharmacol.*, in press.
Knoche, H. & Addicks, K. (1976). Electron microscopic studies of the pressorreceptor fields of the carotid sinus in the dog. *Cell Tiss. Res.*, **173**, 77.
Krauss, J. M. (1979). Structure of the rat aortic baroreceptors and their relationship to connective tissue. *J. Neurocytol.*, **8**, 401.
Lewis, S. J., Machado, B. H., Ohta, H. & Talman, W. T. (1991). Processing of cardiopulmonary afferent input within the nucleus tractus solitarii involves activation of soluble guanylate cyclase. *Eur. J. Pharmacol.*, **203**, 327.
Lewis, T. (1932). Vasovagal syncope and the carotid sinus mechanism. *Br. Med. J.*, **i**, 873.
Little, R. A., Jones, R. O. & Eltraifi, A. E. (1988). Cardiovascular reflex function

after injury. In *Perspectives in Shock Research,* Progress in Clinical and Biological Research, vol. 264, ed. R. F. Bond, H. R. Adams & I. H. Chaudry, pp. 191–200. New York: Liss.

Little, R. A. Marshall, H. W. & Kirkman, E. (1989). Attenuation of the acute cardiovascular responses to haemorrhage by tissue injury in the conscious rat. *Q. J. Exp. Physiol.,* **74**, 825.

Little, R. A., Randall, P. E., Redfern, W. S., Stoner, H. B. & Marshall, H. W. (1984). Components of injury (haemorrhage and tissue ischaemia) affecting cardiovascular reflexes in man and rat. *Q. J. Exp. Physiol.,* **69**, 753.

Loewy, A. D. & Burton, H. (1978). Nuclei of the solitary tract: efferent projections to the lower brain stem and spinal cord of the cat. *J. Comp. Neurol.,* **181**, 421.

Lovick, T. A. (1985*a*). Ventrolateral medullary lesions block the antinociceptive and cardiovascular responses elicited by stimulating the dorsal periaqueductal grey matter in rats. *Pain,* **21**, 241.

Lovick, T. A. (1985*b*). Projections from the diencephalon and mesencephalon to nucleus paragigantocellularis lateralis in the cat. *Neuroscience,* **14**, 853.

Lovick, T. A. (1986*a*). Analgesia and the cardiovascular changes evoked by stimulating neurones in the ventrolateral medulla in rats. *Pain,* **25**, 259.

Lovick, T. A. (1986*b*). Projections from brainstem nuclei to the nucleus paragigantocellularis lateralis in the cat. *J. Auton. Nerv. Syst.,* **16**, 1.

Lovick, T. A. (1987*a*). Differential control of cardiac and vasomotor activity by neurones in nucleus paragigantocellularis lateralis in the cat. *J. Physiol.,* **389**, 23.

Lovick, T. A. (1987*b*). Tonic GABAergic and cholinergic influences on pain control and cardiovascular control neurones in nucleus paragigantocellularis lateralis in the rat. *Pain,* **31**, 401.

Lovick, T. A. (1988*a*). Convergent afferent imports to neurones in nucleus paragigantocellularis lateralis in the cat. *Brain Res.,* **456**, 183.

Lovick, T. A. (1988*b*). GABA-mediated inhibition in nucleus paragigantocellularis lateralis in the cat. *Neurosci. Lett.,* **92**, 182.

Lovick, T. A. (1989*a*). Cardiovascular response to 5HT in the ventrolateral medulla of the rat. *J. Auton. Nerv. Syst.,* **28**, 35.

Lovick, T. A. (1989*b*). Effect of 5HT in the ventrolateral medulla on the pressor response and analgesia evoked by stimulation of the dorsal periaqueductal grey matter in anaesthetized rats. *J. Physiol.,* **418**, 84P.

Lovinger, D. M. & White, G. (1991). Ethanol potentiation of 5-hydroxytryptamine-3 receptor-mediated ion current in neuroblastoma cells and isolated adult mammalian neurons. *Mol. Pharmacol.,* **40**, 263.

Lowe, R. D. & Scroop, G. C. (1969). The cardiovascular response to vertebral artery infusions of angiotensin in the dog. *Clin Sci.,* **37**, 593.

Ludbrook, J. & Rutter, P. C. (1988). Effect of naloxone on haemodynamic responses to acute blood loss in unanaesthetized rabbits. *J. Physiol.,* **400**, 1.

Martin, G. F., Humbertson, A. O., Laxon, C. & Panneton, W. M. (1979). Evidence for direct bulbospinal projections to laminae IX, X and the intermediolateral cell column. Studies using axonal transport techniques in the North American opossum. *Brain Res.,* **170**, 165.

May, C. N., Dashwood, M. R., Whitehead, C. J. & Mathias, C. J. (1989). Differential cardiovascular and respiratory responses to central administration of selective opioid agonists in conscious rabbits: correlation with receptor distribution. *Br. J. Pharmacol.,* **98**, 903.

McAllen, R. M. (1976). Inhibition of the baroreceptor input to the medulla by stimulation of the hypothalamic defence area. *J. Physiol.*, **257**, 45P.
McAllen, R. M., Badoer, E., Shafton, A. D., Oldfield, B. J. & McKinley, M. J. (1992). Haemorrhage induces c-*fos* immunoreactivity in spinally projecting neurones of the cat subretrofacial nucleus. *Brain Res.*, **575**, 329.
McAllen, R. M. & Dampney, R. A. (1990). Vasomotor neurons in the rostral ventrolateral medulla are organized topographically with respect to type of vascular bed but not body region. *Neurosci. Lett.*, **110**, 91.
McAllen, R. M. & Spyer, K. M. (1976). Two types of vagal preganglionic motoneurones projecting to the heart and lungs. *J. Physiol.*, **282**, 353.
McCall, R. B. (1984). Evidence for a serotonergically mediated sympathoexcitatory response to stimulation of medullary raphe nuclei. *Brain Res.*, **311**, 131.
McCall, R. B. (1988). GABA-mediated inhibition of sympatho-excitatory neurons by midline medullary stimulation. *Am. J. Physiol.*, **255**, R605.
McMahon, S. E., McWilliam, P. N., Robertson, J. & Kaye, J. C. (1992). Inhibition of carotid sinus baroreceptor neurones in the nucleus tractus solitarius of the anaesthetized cat by electrical stimulation of hindlimb afferent fibres. *J. Physiol.*, **452**, 224P.
Mifflin, S. W., Spyer, K. M. & Withington-Wray, D. J. (1988). Baroreceptor inputs to the nucleus tractus solitarius in the cat: modulation by the hypothalamus. *J. Physiol.*, **399**, 369.
Morgan, D. A., Thorén, P., Wilczynski, E. A., Victor, R. G. & Mark, A. L. (1988). Serotonergic mechanisms mediate renal sympathoinhibition during severe haemorrhage in rats. *Am. J. Physiol.*, **255**, H496.
Morilak, D. A., Somogyi, P., McIlhinney, R. A. J. & Chalmers, J. (1989). An enkephalin-containing pathway from nucleus tractus solitarius to the pressor area of the rostral ventrolateral medulla of the rabbit. *Neuroscience*, **31**, 187.
Morrison, S. F., Callaway, J., Milner, T. A. & Reis, D. J. (1991). Rostral ventrolateral medulla: a source of the glutamatergic innervation of the sympathetic intermediolateral nucleus. *Brain Res.*, **562**, 126.
Öberg, B. & Thorén, P. (1972). Increased activity in left ventricular receptors during haemorrhage on occlusion of the caval veins in the cat. A possible cause of the vasovagal reaction. *Acta Physiol. Scand.*, **85**, 164.
Öberg, B. & Thorén, P. (1973). Circulatory response to stimulation of left ventricular receptors in the cat. *Acta Physiol. Scand.*, **88**, 8.
Overman, R. R. & Wang, S. C. (1947). The contributory role of the afferent nervous factor in experimental shock: sublethal haemorrhage and sciatic nerve stimulation. *Am. J. Physiol.*, **148**, 289.
Peroutka, S. J. (1988). 5-Hydroxytryptamine receptor sub types: molecular, biochemical and physiological characterization. *Trends Neurosci.*, **11**, 496.
Porro, C. A., Cavazzuti, M., Galetti, A. & Sassatelli, L. (1991). Functional activity mapping of the rat brainstem during formalin-induced noxious stimulation. *Neuroscience*, **41**, 667.
Potter, E. K. & McCloskey, D. I. (1987). Excitation of carotid body chemoreceptors by neuropeptide-Y. *Resp. Physiol.*, **67**, 357.
Praag, H. & Frenk, H. (1990). The role of glutamate in opiate descending inhibition of nociceptive spinal reflexes. *Brain Res.*, **524**, 101.
Quest, J. A. & Gebber, G. L. (1972). Modulation of baroreceptor reflexes by somatic afferent nerve stimulation. *Am. J. Physiol.*, **222**, 1251.

Rady, M. Y. A., Kirkman, E., Cranley, J. J. & Little, R. A. (1993). A comparison of the effects of skeletal muscle injury and somatic afferent nerve stimulation on the response to hemorrhage in anesthetized pigs. *J. Trauma*, in press.

Rady, M. Y. A., Little, R. A., Edwards, J. D., Kirkman, E. & Faithfull, S. (1991). The effect of nociceptive stimulation on the changes in hemodynamics and oxygen transport induced by hemorrhage in anesthetized pigs. *J. Trauma*, **31**, 617.

Redfern, W. S. (1981). Effects of limb ischaemia on the cardiac component of the baroreceptor reflex in the unanaesthetized rat – afferent, central and efferent mechanisms, Ph.D. Thesis, University of Manchester.

Redfern, W. S., Little, R. A., Stoner, H. B. & Marshall, H. W. (1984). Effect of limb ischaemia on blood pressure and the blood pressure–heart rate reflex in the rat. *Q. J. Exp. Physiol.*, **69**, 763.

Ross, C. A., Ruggiero, D. A., Joh, T. H., Park, D. H. & Reis, D. J. (1984). Rostral ventrolateral medulla: selective projections to the thoracic autonomic cell column from the region containing $C_1$ adrenaline neurons. *J. Comp. Neurol.*, **228**, 168.

Schadt, J. C. & Ludbrook, J. (1991). Hemodynamic and neurohumoral responses to acute hypovolemia in conscious mammals. *Am. J. Physiol.*, **260**, H305.

Scherrer, U., Vissing, S., Morgan, B., Hanson, P. & Victor, R. G. (1990). Vasovagal syncope after infusion of a vasodilator in a heart-transplant recipient. *N. Engl. J. Med.*, **322**, 602–4.

Scroop, G. C. & Lowe, R. D. (1969). Efferent pathways of the cardiovascular response to vertebral artery infusions of angiotensin in the dog. *Clin. Sci.*, **37**, 605.

Secher, N. H. & Bie, P. (1985). Bradycardia during reversible haemorrhagic shock – a forgotten observation? *Clin. Physiol.*, **5**, 315.

Seller, H. (1991). Central baroreceptor reflex pathways. In *Baroreceptor Reflexes: Integrative Functions and Clinical Aspects*, ed. H. R. Kirchheim & P. B. Persson, p. 45. Berlin: Springer-Verlag.

Shapiro, R. E. & Miselis, R. R. (1985). The central nervous connections of the area postrema in the rat. *J. Comp. Neurol.*, **234**, 344.

Shen, Y. T., Cowley, A. W. & Vatner, S. F. (1991). Relative roles of cardiac and arterial baroreceptors in vasopressin regulation during haemorrhage in conscious dogs. *Circ. Res.*, **68**, 1422–36.

Shen, Y. T., Knight, D. R., Thomas, J. X. & Vatner, S. F. (1990). Relative roles of cardiac receptors and arterial baroreceptors during haemorrhage in conscious dogs. *Circ. Res.*, **66**, 397–405.

Siddall, P. J. & Dampney, R. A. (1989). Relationship between cardiovascular neurones and descending antinociceptive pathways in the rostral ventrolateral medulla of the cat. *Pain*, **37**, 347.

Skoog, K. M., Blair, M. L., Sladek, C. D., Williams, W. M. & Mangiapane, M. L. (1990). Area postrema: essential for support of arterial pressure after hemorrhage in rats. *Am. J. Physiol.*, **258**, R1472.

Sporton, S. C., Shepheard, S. L., Jordan, D. & Ramage, A. G. (1991). Microinjections of 5-HT1A agonists into the dorsal motor vagal nucleus produce a bradycardia in the atenolol-pretreated anaesthetized rat. *Br. J. Pharmacol.*, **104**, 466.

Spyer, K. M. (1984). Central control of the cardiovascular system. *Recent Adv. Physiol.*, **10**, 163.

Sun, M. K. & Spyer, K. M. (1991). Nociceptive inputs into rostral ventrolateral
medulla-spinal vasomotor neurones in rats. *J. Physiol.*, **436**, 685.
Terui, N., Saeki, Y. & Kumada, M. (1987). Confluence of barosensory and nonbarosensory inputs at neurons in the ventrolateral medulla in rabbits. *Can. J. Physiol. Pharmacol.*, **65**, 1584.
Uhl, G. R., Goodman, R. R., Kuhar, M. J., Childers, S. R. & Snyder, S. H. (1979). Immunohistochemical mapping of enkephalin containing cell bodies, fibres and nerve terminals in the brain stem of the rat. *Brain Res.*, **166**, 75.
Varga, K. & Kunos, G. (1990). Ethanol inhibition of baroreflex bradycardia: role of brainstem GABA receptors. *Br. J. Pharmacol.*, **101**, 773.
Verberne, A. J., Beart, P. M. & Louis, W. J. (1989). Excitatory amino acid receptors in the caudal ventrolateral medulla mediate a vagal cardiopulmonary reflex in the rat. *Exp. Brain Res.*, **78**, 185.
Wang, Q., Guo, X.-Q. & Li, P. (1988). The inhibitory effects of somatic input on the excitatory responses of vagal cardiomotor neurones to stimulation of the nucleus tractus solitarius in rabbits. *Brain Res.*, **439**, 350.
Ward, D. G. (1989). Neurons in the parabrachial nuclei respond to hemorrhage. *Brain Res.*, **491**, 80.
Ward, D. G. & Darlington, D. N. (1987). Lesions of the caudal periaqueductal gray prevent compensation of arterial pressure during haemorrhage. *Brain Res.*, **407**, 369.
Wilmore, D. W., Smith, R. J., O'Dwyer, S. T., Jackobs, D. O., Ziegler, T. R. & Wang, X.-D. (1988). The gut: a central organ after surgical stress. *Surgery*, **104**, 917.
Yardley, C. P. & Hilton, S. M. (1986). The hypothalamic and brainstem areas from which the cardiovascular and behavioural components of the defence reaction are elicited in the rat. *J. Auton. Nerv. Syst.*, **15**, 227.

# 10

# Neuroendocrine responses to physical trauma

FRANK BERKENBOSCH

Major trauma can provoke a neuroendocrine response that is characterized by activation of the sympathetic–adrenomedullary system and by stimulation of neurohypophysial neurones in the hypothalamus, resulting in alterations in synthesis and secretion of various pituitary hormones and subsequent changes in secretion of adrenal, pancreatic and thyroid hormones. This complex response has been well described after a variety of physical injuries, including long-bone fractures, multiple injuries and burns. The neuroendocrine response to physical injury is accompanied by and possibly causally linked to a number of metabolic and immunological disturbances in patients. These include negative nitrogen balance as a consequence of increased protein breakdown, changes in thermoregulation, metabolic acidosis and immunosuppression as evidenced by the high mortality caused by sepsis in traumatized patients. The neuroendocrine response to physical injury is thought to be initiated by three main factors: emotionality caused by perception, fluid loss and tissue damage. The temporal integration of a sequence of neuroendocrine and metabolic reactions has led to a division of the response to injury into two phases, which have been named the 'ebb' and 'flow' phase (Cuthbertson, 1930; Frayn, 1986).

The ebb phase, which lasts up to 12–24 h after injury, represents a coordinated response by the brain, and is characterized by mobilization of energy stores together with apparent restraints on energy utilization. Early studies have reported that the ebb phase is characterized by a fall in metabolic heat production. However, subsequent studies, in particular in humans, have demonstrated that heat production is usually raised soon after injury, with a magnitude dependent on the type and severity of the insult (Little, 1988).

The flow phase or catabolic phase is characterized by a rise in metabolic rate, roughly coincident with an increase in urinary nitrogen secretion, which lasts up to 10 days after the injury. This phase of the response resembles a state that has been denoted the acute phase response, which is known to be largely regulated by cytokines, such as interleukin-1 (IL-1), interleukin-6 (IL-6) and tumor necrosis factor (TNF) (Dinarello, 1984; Kaplan *et al.*, 1989; Heinrich *et al.*, 1990).

The main emphasis of this chapter is to review the nature and cause of changes in hormone concentrations that occur after physical injuries. A brief description of the possible effects is added, to promote a more adequate understanding of the regulatory role of the neurohormonal response to injury.

## Pathways to initiate neuroendocrine responses to injury

### *Brain corticotropin-releasing factor and the coordination of endocrine responses*

Various brain areas are involved in the adaptation reaction to stressors such as physical injury. Their coordinated action is translated in neuroendocrine responses as part of the defensive manoeuvre to fight the consequences of the physical injury. The specific ways by which injury affects neuroendocrine responses is not well understood. Some years ago, a 41-amino acid residue peptide was characterized and named corticotrophin-releasing factor (CRF) (Vale *et al.*, 1983). Various lines of evidence indicate that CRF is the predominant regulator of adrenocorticotrophic hormone (ACTH) and related peptides (e.g. endorphin) from the pituitary gland (Vale *et al.*, 1983; Tilders *et al.*, 1985). Moreover, CRF is additionally involved in controlling the release of other pituitary hormones such as the gonadotrophins, by interfering with the release of other hypophysiotrophic factors such as luteinizing hormone releasing factor (LHRH) (Rivier & Vale, 1984). The CRF involved in regulation of ACTH secretion (and other pituitary hormones) is produced mainly in the hypothalamus – in the paraventricular nucleus (PVN). In addition to this well-studied integrative nucleus, other CRF systems have been described in the brain. Some of these are located in the limbic structures such as the septum and amygdala, and project to the nuclei in the brainstem that are involved in regulation of sympathetic outflow. Particularly, the CRF input to the locus coeruleus deserves attention, since this nucleus is the main source of noradrenergic terminals in the forebrain and is well known to be associated with behavioural and physiological factors (Aston-Jones *et al.*, 1984). CRF administration in the brain activates the sympathoadrenomedullary system, increases metabolic heat production and elevates plasma glucose and glucagon levels, while reducing insulin concentrations elicit a number of behavioural reactions that also occur during physical and/or emotional stresses (Brown & Fisher, 1985; Koob & Britton, 1990). The observation that an α-helical CRF receptor antagonist can suppress stress-induced behavioural, autonomic and neuroendocrine responses (Brown & Fisher, 1985; Rivier & Plotsky, 1986; Tazi *et al.*, 1987; Berridge & Dunn, 1989) has led to the hypothesis that brain CRF systems may play a coordinating role in response to emotional and possibly physical stressors.

### *Perception*

Emotions are now well recognized as activating the hypothalamic defence systems, leading to release of several pituitary hormones (ACTH, growth hormone (GH), thyroid stimulating hormone (TSH), prolactin, endorphins) and to activation of the sympathetic–adrenomedullary system (adrenaline, noradrenaline) (Tilders *et al.*, 1985; Berkenbosch, 1992). This emergency response is thought to serve its goal of rapidly mobilizing energy in order to prepare the organism to encounter the threatening danger by increased physical activity. When the danger has been successfully encountered, the endocrine response fades to resting levels.

It has been recognized for some time that limbic structures of the telencephalon (septal, amygdalar and hippocampal regions) control pituitary hormone release. These limbic influences are thought to be relayed via the bed nucleus of the stria terminalis, which is known to receive inputs from both the hippocampal formation and the amygdala, and which project to the hypothalamus, in particular to the PVN (Sawchenko & Swanson, 1985). These limbic structures, in particular the amygdala, have also been found to be associated with the central control of autonomic functions (Gray, 1989), providing the basis of the integrated responses of the pituitary and sympathetic nervous system to emotional stimuli.

### *Fluid loss and pain*

The neuroendocrine response to the encountered danger will be reinforced and modified once the physical injury has occurred. Most of the physical injuries are accompanied by considerable fluid loss leading to hypovolaemia and osmolarity changes. The pathways to the areas of the hypothalamus and brainstem involved in conveying signals from the cardiovascular system are well studied, in particular in animals such as the rat or dog, and appear to be organized in a so-called homeostatic reflex (Gann *et al.*, 1978).

Baroreceptors in the right atrium and high-pressure receptors in the carotid arteries respond to hypovolaemia. Information is conveyed via the vagus and glossopharyngeal nerves to the nucleus of the tractus solitarius, medullary reticular formation and locus coeruleus. Each of these nuclei projects mainly via noradrenergic fibres to specific parts of the hypothalamus, in particular to the PVN (Sawchenko & Swanson, 1985). Since these brainstem nuclei are also involved in autonomic regulation, these pathways may provide a means of integrating the activity of hypophysial outputs with complementary autonomic outputs. Also worthy of attention in this respect is the hypothalamic input from the subfornical organ (Miseles, 1981), one of the circumventricular organs that is known as a probable site of action of angiotensin II, to elicit drinking responses and the release of arginine vasopressin (AVP) (Simpson, 1981). This pathway seems especially well suited to integrate adenohypophysial (ACTH-induced mineralo- and glucocorticoid release), neurohypophysial (AVP-induced water retention) and behavioural responses (drinking) to reduction in blood volume.

In addition to these pathways, glucose receptors respond to changes in the composition of the blood, contributing by unknown pathways to the neuroendocrine response. The importance of the nociceptive afferents from the damaged tissue has also been demonstrated (Stoner, 1976), but again it is not clear how the impulses are directed to the neuroendocrine centres. Neuroendocrine responses occur in surgical patients under anaesthesia, implying that conscious perception of pain is not the only requirement for the neuroendocrine responses to occur.

### *Tissue factors*

It is well recognized that the cytokine IL-1 is induced after tissue damage. IL-1 exists in several molecular forms, called IL-1$\alpha$ and IL-1$\beta$, coded for by separate genes (Oppenheim *et al.*, 1986). Despite the low sequence similarity between these two forms, they have virtually identical biological action. IL-1$\alpha$ is thought to be a local hormone involved in cell signalling, whereas IL-1$\beta$ has been shown to be a secretory product. Nevertheless, circulating IL-1$\beta$ concentrations during trauma are difficult to detect with the current sensitivities of the assays, even under conditions of severe trauma and sepsis. The recently cloned IL-1 receptor antagonist, which is coproduced with IL-1 by macrophages, has been shown to be a potent therapeutic agent to prevent septic shock in animals and humans (Dinarello, 1991*a*; Dinarello, communication at the Philip Laudat Meeting, Strasbourg, 1992). There are several possible ways by which IL-1 may be generated during trauma. Cleavage products of the complement system have been shown to be early mediators after trauma (Gelfand *et al.*, 1982), and to induce the release of IL-1 from monocytes and macrophages (Goodman *et al.*, 1982; Okusawa *et al.*, 1987). Keratinocytes contain IL-1 and their injury results in release of IL-1 (Sauder *et al.*, 1986).

Additionally, bacterial contamination with endotoxins and exotoxins of wounds may trigger the release of IL-1 from peripheral macrophages (DeRijk & Berkenbosch, 1992) and from macrophages in the brain (van Dam *et al.*, 1992). Both systemic and local actions of IL-1 have been described in detail elsewhere (Dinarello, 1984; Kaplan *et al.*, 1989). These effects indicate that IL-1 plays a role as a signal in the response to trauma.

As described above, trauma patients exhibit alterations in metabolism such as muscle proteolysis, associated with increases in urine nitrogen excretion and increased plasma levels of acute-phase proteins that are produced by the liver. Moreover, during trauma there are marked changes in glucose and lipid metabolism and utilization resulting either from the direct effects of the injury or from the altered activity of the neuroendocrine systems. IL-1 increases muscle proteolysis, stimulates hepatic functions leading to synthesis and secretion of acute phase proteins, alters cation distribution, causes a decrease in lipoprotein lipase activity leading to increased lipolysis and changes the glucose formation and utilization by altering plasma levels of glucagon and insulin (Dinarello, 1984; Kaplan *et al.*, 1989). Moreover, IL-1 administration can mimic the effects of trauma on neuroendocrine functions (Table 10.1). IL-1 increases pituitary–adrenal activity and sympathoadrenomedullary activity, increases AVP plasma concentrations, affects GH release, and lowers plasma levels of LH and testosterone and of TSH, triiodothyronine ($T_3$) and thyroxine ($T_4$). In some instances, the actions of IL-1 may involve the brain, as has been demonstrated most clearly for the development of CRF in the pituitary adrenal response (Berkenbosh *et al.*, 1987; Sapolsky *et al.*, 1987), but IL-1 may additionally act at other levels, as has been demonstrated for the pituitary gland (Bernton *et al.*, 1987), adrenal gland (Andreis *et al.*, 1991) and gonads (Rivier, 1990).

Many of the stimuli that cause synthesis of IL-1 also induce TNF and

Table 10.1. *Neuroendocrine effects of IL-1*

| Action | Effect | Reference |
|---|---|---|
| *In vitro* | | |
| Hypothalamus | | |
| CRF | s | Tsagarakis *et al.*, 1989 |
| SS, GH | s | Honegger *et al.*, 1991 |
| AVP | s | Nakatsura *et al.*, 1991 |
| Pituitary | | |
| ACTH, LH, GH, TSH | s | Bernton *et al.*, 1987 |
| PRL | i | Bernton *et al.*, 1987 |
| AVP | s | Christensen *et al.*, 1989 |
| Adrenal | | |
| CORT | s | Andreis *et al.*, 1991 |
| *In vivo* | | |
| Peripheral administration | | |
| PRL | – | Berkenbosch *et al.*, 1989 |
| ACTH; CORT | s | Berkenbosch *et al.*, 1989; Berkenbosch *et al.*, 1987; Sapolsky *et al.*, 1987; Besedovsky *et al.*, 1986 |
| A, NA | s | Berkenbosch *et al.*, 1989; Rivier *et al.*, 1989 |
| TSH, $T_3$, $T_4$ | i | Dubius *et al.*, 1988; Hermes *et al.*, 1992; Berkenbosch *et al.*, 1992*b* |
| CRF | s | Berkenbosch *et al.*, 1987; Sapolsky *et al.*, 1987 |
| Glucagon | s | del Rey *et al.*, 1987 |
| Insulin | s/– | del Rey *et al.*, 1987; Berkenbosch *et al.*, 1990 |
| Testosterone | i | Rivier, 1990 |
| Central administration | | |
| ACTH, CORT | s | Berkenbosch *et al.*, 1990 |
| PRL | – | Payne *et al.*, 1992 |
| LH | i | Rivier, 1990 |
| GH, GRH | s/i | Payne *et al.*, 1992 |

s, Stimulation; i, inhibition; –, no effects; CRF, corticotrophin-releasing factor; SS, somatostatin; GH, growth hormone; AVP, arginine vasopressin; ACTH, adrenocorticotrophic hormone; LH, luteinizing hormone; TSH, thyroid-stimulating hormone; PRL, prolactin; CORT, corticosterone; A, adrenaline; NA, noradrenaline; $T_3$, triiodothyronine; $T_4$, thyroxine; GRH, growth hormone releasing hormone.

IL-6. In addition, TNF can cause release of IL-1 (Nawroth *et al.*, 1986; Dinarello *et al.*, 1986), and IL-1 can stimulate IL-6 release (Heinrich *et al.*, 1990; Berkenbosch *et al.*, 1992*b*). Elevated plasma levels of TNF and IL-6 have been detected in sera of patients with sepsis or major trauma such as burns (Nijsten *et al.*, 1987; Brown & Grosso, 1989). IL-1, TNF and IL-6 share many biological activities, including those on the neuroendocrine system. For instance, TNF and IL-6 are both potent activators of the pituitary–adrenal system (Berkenbosch *et al.*, 1992*a*) and are recognized to be potent pyrogens (Kluger, 1991; Rothwell, 1992). Moreover, it has been clearly demonstrated that, for some of their biological activities, these cytokines act in a synergistic fashion. For instance, effects of IL-1 on pituitary–adrenal activity are potentiated by IL-6 (Perlstein *et al.*, 1991), while the cytotoxic effects on pancreatic islet cells are exposed only after combined treatment with IL-1 and TNF (Pukel *et al.*, 1988). Such observations suggest that cytokines released under conditions of trauma are involved in a web of regulatory control that acts between individual tissues and cells.

## Pituitary and secondary hormone responses during trauma

### *ACTH and glucocorticoids*

The increase in circulating glucocorticoid concentrations is probably the most extensively described endocrine effect of trauma. There is little doubt that, in most types of trauma, the increase in cortisol is mediated by ACTH released by the pituitary gland (Newsome & Rose, 1971; Barton *et al.*, 1987). ACTH is formed as part of a large precursor molecule called proopiomelanocortin, which also gives rise to the opiate receptor ligand endorphin (Berkenbosch, 1992). Not well understood are the observations that the initial magnitude of the cortisol response relates inversely to the severity of trauma, i.e. plasma cortisol levels increase after minor and moderate injuries, but are low in patients with severe injuries (Carey *et al.*, 1971; Shirani *et al.*, 1983; Barton *et al.*, 1987). However, unlike its initial magnitude, the duration of the cortisol response seems to increase fairly consistently with the severity of the injury and can span the ebb as well as the flow phase. After moderate-to-severe accidental injuries, plasma cortisol concentrations are increased for over a week (Barton & Passingham, 1981; Frayn *et al.*, 1983); however, during burns, elevated circulating cortisol concentrations persist for more than 2 weeks (Vaughan *et al.*, 1982; Balogh *et al.*, 1984). The chronic elevation of cortisol levels suggests that feedback inhibition by persistently increased cortisol levels is overridden. It is worth noting, in this respect, that during sepsis glucocorticoid receptors are downregulated, explaining the well-known glucocorticoid resistance of these patients (Zonghai *et al.*, 1987). Recent studies show that glucocorticoid receptors in the brain (hippocampus) are rapidly downregulated by administration of cytokines such as IL-1, suggesting that glucocorticoid resistance may be caused by the actions of cytokines at the level of cytosolic glucocorticoid receptors (Weidenfeld *et al.*, 1989). In addition, cytokines such as IL-1 have been shown to stimulate glucocorticoid secretion at the levels of the adrenal (Andreis *et al.*, 1991). This observation may not only explain the persistently increased cortisol levels, but also relate to the fact that plasma cortisol levels are often poorly correlated with plasma ACTH concentrations after trauma (Barton *et al.*, 1987).

### *Vasopressin*

AVP levels are generally increased after accidental injuries such as burns or surgery. The increased plasma concentrations of AVP tend to decline during the first few days after burns (Hauben *et al.*, 1980; Morgan *et al.*, 1980), although some reports have noted inappropriately high AVP levels for several weeks in this condition (Shirani *et al.*, 1983). This difference in the duration of the AVP response to burns may be related to prolonged activation of the renin–angiotensin system as has been reported to occur frequently after severe burns (see below). AVP plasma concentrations determined by bioassay or immunoassay rise rapidly during various types of surgery but usually return to normal levels between 2 and 3 days after surgery (Haas & Click, 1978). The increase in AVP plasma concentrations is not due to general anaesthesia (Philbin, 1983), and nociceptive afferents rather than changes in osmolarity or blood volume are thought to mediate the AVP response (Le Quesne *et al.*, 1985). The AVP response can therefore be considered as an ebb-phase response, but may extend to the flow phase probably depending on the duration of the activation of the renin–angiotensin system.

### *TSH and thyroid hormones*

During trauma profound changes in thyroid function occur both in human patients and in animals. Whereas basal TSH plasma concentrations are usually normal or may be decreased, marked reductions in plasma levels of 3, 5, 3-triiodothyronine ($T_3$) occur independently of the type of trauma, whereas plasma concentrations of reverse $T_3$ ($rT_3$) are reciprocally increased (Popp *et al.*, 1977; Adami *et al.*, 1978; Becker *et al.*, 1982; Balogh *et al.*, 1984; Philips *et al.*, 1984). The low $T_3$ and high $rT_3$ levels are probably due to inhibition of peripheral conversion of thyroxine ($T_4$) to $T_3$ and a reduction in $rT_3$ catabolism because of a reduction in hepatic

5-deiodinase activity. Plasma $T_4$ concentrations may vary, depending on the severity of the trauma and subsequent illness, being lowest in patients with poor prognosis (Kaptein, 1986). The marked changes in plasma concentration of $T_3$ and $rT_3$ start immediately after trauma, and can persist for a few days after moderate injury or for 2 weeks or longer after accidental injury or burns, respectively. Thyroid hormone disturbances can thus be considered as features of the flow phase. Although mechanisms underlying changes in plasma thyroid hormones are probably multifactorial, experiments involving bolus injections of infusions with cytokines in animals and humans suggest that these soluble factors play a major role in changes in plasma thyroid concentrations after trauma. In humans, a single bolus injection of TNF induces significant decreases in $T_3$ and TSH levels and a significant increase in $rT_3$ levels (van der Poll *et al.*, 1990), whereas in rats, similar observations have been described with bolus injections and infusions of IL-1 or TNF (Dubius *et al.*, 1988; Berkenbosch *et al.*, 1992*a*; Hermes *et al.*, 1992; Sweep *et al.*, 1992).

### *Gonadotrophins and gonadal steroids*

Little is known about the effects of trauma on plasma gonadotrophin and gonadal steroid levels in females; most of the observations on the effects of trauma have been performed in males. In general, there seems to be little disturbance of the hypothalamic–pituitary–testicular axis during the ebb phase after trauma. During the flow phase, there is a consistent fall in plasma testosterone concentrations, with little change in plasma levels of LH (Wang *et al.*, 1978; Dolecek *et al.*, 1979; Brizio-Molteni *et al.*, 1984). Although this observation is unexplained, peripheral administration of IL-1 in rats lowers plasma testosterone concentrations without any effect on plasma LH concentrations; IL-1 has been suggested to reduce the responsiveness of the Leydig cells to LH stimulation (Rivier, 1990). In contrast to LH plasma levels, follicle stimulating hormone (FSH) concentrations are a sensitive indicator of burn trauma, in both males and females (Dolecek *et al.*, 1979; Balogh *et al.*, 1984; Brizio-Molteni *et al.*, 1984). Its low levels may persist for many weeks after burns, corresponding with the low plasma testosterone level, and this response may therefore be considered as a feature of the flow phase. Amenorrhoea is often seen in burned females, and is not caused by a lack of oestrogens, since plasma levels are normal or even elevated for many weeks after burn trauma (Dolecek, 1989).

### *Growth hormone*

Plasma GH concentrations readily rise during various types of trauma including accidental injury, surgery and burns (Noel *et al.*, 1972; Sowers *et al.*, 1977; Hagen *et al.*, 1980), but in general do not stay elevated for longer than 2 days after trauma (Popp *et al.*, 1977; Dolecek *et al.*, 1979; Balogh *et al.*, 1984). The available data indicate that the GH response is limited to the first few hours after trauma and can therefore be considered as a feature of the ebb phase.

### *Prolactin*

As for GH, the plasma prolactin response to trauma appears to be restricted to the ebb phase and does not continue in the flow phase. Modestly increased plasma prolactin levels have been reported in male patients on admission to hospital for chest injuries or burns (MacFarlane & Rosin, 1980). A number of studies have demonstrated a rapid increase in plasma prolactin concentrations during surgery in both males and females (Noel *et al.*, 1972; Sowers *et al.*, 1977; Yasuda & Greer, 1978; MacFarlane & Rosin, 1980; Adams & Hamilton, 1984), but it has been doubted whether this response is related directly to surgery rather than to general anaesthesia (Sowers *et al.*, 1977).

## The sympathetic–adrenomedullary system in trauma

### *Adrenaline and noradrenaline*

Plasma adrenaline and noradrenaline increase rapidly during various types of injury. The magnitude and the duration of this response appears to be related to severity of the injury, i.e. very high circulating adrenaline levels are observed in critically injured patients (Frayn, 1986). The duration of the response usually corresponds with the time interval of the ebb phase; only in patients who are critically ill after their injuries, do high concentration of circulating catecholamine persist within the flow phase (Hamberger *et al.*, 1980). Correlation studies suggest that the increases in circulating noradrenaline and adrenaline are independently regulated (Frayn, 1986); this is in line with the evidence that circulating adrenaline originates largely from the chromaffin cells of the adrenal medulla, whereas most of the circulating noradrenaline is secreted as spill-over from direct sympathetic innervation of the tissues (Kvetnansky *et al.*, 1979).

### *Glucagon*

The rise in plasma glucagon concentrations after trauma may be considered as characteristic of the early flow phase, although increased values have been reported at the later stages of the ebb phase as well. Patients with burns generally show similar response characteristics to those with non-thermal injury; there is a delay of approximately 12 h before the rise in plasma glucagon concentration starts, and if the trauma is classified as moderate or severe, the increase can persist for up to 2 weeks (Frayn, 1986). Although $\beta$-adrenergic mechanisms participate in the glucagon response to injury (Porte & Robertson, 1973; Lindsey *et al.*, 1975), the divergence in the time-courses of catecholamine and glucagon responses may indicate that other mediators also participate in the increase in glucagon concentrations. Cytokines such as IL-1 and TNF are potent stimulators of glucagon secretion, and therefore may be considered as potential mediators of this response during trauma (del Rey & Besedovsky, 1987; Evans *et al.*, 1991). In addition, it has been suggested that alterations in circulating amino acid concentrations that occur during trauma may contribute to the increased plasma glucagon levels (Frayn, 1986; Barton, 1987).

### *Insulin*

Plasma insulin concentrations are generally depressed in relation to elevated plasma glucose concentrations in the ebb phase after injury (Frayn, 1986) and are not stimulated in response to glucose infusion (Allison *et al.*, 1968). The blunted insulin response to elevated levels of glucose may be caused by the inhibitory effects of adrenaline on insulin secretion (Frayn, 1986). The depressed insulin concentrations result in diminished glucose utilization. It is as if the body tries to conserve the fuel mobilized for the initial attempt to encounter the endangering situation preceding the trauma. In the flow phase, several days after trauma, plasma insulin concentrations are raised above normal, irrespective of whether the trauma was caused by accidental injury, burns or surgery (Barton, 1987). Moreover, the plasma insulin response to glucose infusion is dramatically enhanced (Allison *et al.*, 1968). The elevation of the insulin concentrations during the flow phase is probably subject to multifactorial controls, and it may be the result of the removal of the adrenergic restraint to respond normally to increased glucose levels. However, it is worth noting that insulin concentrations during the flow phase are usually inappropriately high for the glucose levels.

This super-increased insulin concentration may be a reflection of the stimulatory actions of cytokines, as reported in experimental animals (del Rey & Besedovsky, 1987; Evans *et al.*, 1991), in addition to elevated levels of amino acids including arginine, a potent stimulator of insulin secretion (Fajans *et al.*, 1967). Insulin resistance has also been noted to occur early during the flow phase (Frayn, 1986), thus preventing the anabolic actions of insulin. However, the underlying nature of the insulin remains unclear.

### *Renin–angiotensin–aldosterone hormones*

The renin–angiotensin system plays an important role in the regulation of the aldosterone secretion, whereas ACTH appears to be less important in the control of this mineraloglucocorticoid. Angiotensin II is also an important regulator of AVP secretion by actions involving the subfornical organ (see above). The activities of aldosterone and renin (the enzyme that converts angiotensinogen to angiotensin I) are greatly increased throughout the first two weeks after burning (Dolecek, 1989). Variable renin responses have been described after surgery, but all reports show increased aldosterone secretion, irrespective of the presence or absence of changes in the plasma concentrations of renin (Barton, 1987). Although the available data are not conclusive, changes in the renin–angiotensin–aldosterone system may be characteristic of both the ebb and flow phase.

## Adaptive and maladaptive features of the neuroendocrine response to injury

### *Ebb phase*

Mobilization of body fuels is a prominent feature of the ebb phase in response to injury. There is little doubt that the neuroendocrine response is the most important trigger for this metabolic change, although the contribution of each specific hormone appears difficult to evaluate. Since the neuroendocrine response is in large part regulated by the brain and, as discussed above, may involve central CRF neuronal systems, the response can therefore be considered as a means by which the brain initiates compensatory mechanisms needed to withstand the effects of injury.

The posttraumatic ebb phase is predominantly characterized by hyperglycaemia and increased glucose turnover (Frayn, 1986; Barton, 1987; Douglas & Shaw, 1989). The increased glucose turnover during this stage is thought to provide essential fuel for inflammatory and reparative tissue, which optimizes host defence and ensures wound repair. Increased sympathetic activity is likely to initiate hepatic glycogenolysis and glucagon release, while simultaneously inhibiting insulin release from the endocrine pancreas (Frayn, 1986). Cytokines and glucocorticoids probably play a facilitatory role in the posttraumatic changes in glucose turnover and utilization either directly (Kaplan *et al.*, 1989; Evans *et al.*, 1991) or indirectly, by affecting the release of other neuroendocrine hormones (Table 10.1).

The hyperglycaemic response to injury is accompanied by increased lipolysis, which paradoxically is only sometimes associated with increased plasma levels of fatty acids (Frayn, 1986; Douglas & Shaw, 1989). Lipolysis may provide an additional source of oxidative fuel to counteract the consequences of injury. However, it is worth noting that the preference for fat as an energy substrate is more pronounced in patients with sepsis than in those with trauma. Several hormonal factors are likely to act simultaneously to stimulate lipolysis in adipose tissue, i.e. breakdown of triacylglycerol to free fatty acids and glycerol. Raised plasma levels of catecholamines, glucagon, glucocorticoids and cytokines may all contribute to this response, whereas low insulin levels allow this process to proceed without counteregulation (Frayn, 1986; Douglas & Shaw, 1989; Kaplan *et al.*, 1989; Evans *et al.*, 1991).

Another important facet of the ebb phase is the haemodynamic changes as a result of injury. Changes in the cardiovascular system (i.e. precapillary vasoconstriction and increase in heart rate and myocardial contractility) are likely to be regulated by sympathetic discharge in response to injury, whereby vasoconstriction will help to limit blood loss from the wounds. The increase in plasma AVP levels and activation of the renin–angiotensin system contribute to the restoration of fluid balance in the injured, by increasing water retention (AVP) and drinking (angiotensin II). Irrespective of peripheral vasoconstriction, trauma patients are frequently hypotensive, partly due to hypovolaemia after severe blood loss.

Evidence has also been presented that cytokines, in particular IL-1, may act as mediators of this response (Kaplan *et al.*, 1989). The haemodynamic effects of cytokines such as IL-1 may be caused by stimulation of L-arginine-dependent induction of nitric oxide, known to act as a physiological regulator of smooth muscle contraction mediated by guanylate cyclase (Bealey, 1990). The hypotensive response to injury may be viewed as a maladaptive response, which deserves correction by pharmacological manipulations. Cytokine receptor antagonists, purified soluble cytokine receptors or nitric oxide synthesis inhibitors are likely candidates for such a purpose (Dinarello, 1991*b*; Moncada *et al.*, 1991).

In addition, to haemodynamic and metabolic changes, trauma is often accompanied by an immediate depression of the immune response; in particular, cell-mediated immunity appears to be affected (Munster, 1984). Recent evidence indicates that immune cells are exposed to extensive neuroendocrine control, and immunity appears to be balanced by immunopermissive hormones such as GH and PRL and immunosuppressive hormones such as catecholamines and glucocorticoids (Berczi & Nagy, 1987; Berkenbosch, 1992; DeRijk & Berkenbosch, 1993). Their integrated effects result in trauma-induced changes in immunity. The observations so far are too limited to draw conclusions on the adaptive or maladaptive consequences of the injury-induced immunosuppression, although it has been suggested that this effect may contribute to induction of septic symptoms.

### *Flow phase*

The hallmarks of the flow phase are an increase in metabolic rate and net protein breakdown (Cuthbertson, 1930; Frayn, 1986; Douglas & Shaw, 1989), but the role of the hormonal changes in these processes has not been resolved. The increased metabolic rate is likely to be a reflection of cytokine secretion during this stage after trauma (Rothwell, 1992), but the mechanisms of protein catabolism are not clearly understood. Although increased body temperature has been shown to be of considerable advantage for the organism (Kluger, 1991), the body wasting accompanying the increased metabolic rate is clearly detrimental, especially after prolonged duration and when accompanied by a reduced food intake. Skeletal muscle is the major site at which protein breakdown is accelerated during the flow phase (Douglas & Shaw, 1989). However, the increased rate of protein release from skeletal muscles is not simply due to degradation of damaged tissue. Glucocorticoids are well known for their permissive role in protein catabolism. They do not act as a stimulus directly, but facilitate the actions of other catabolic agents. Glucocorticoids have been shown to upregulate IL-1 receptor expression in a variety of cells (Akahoshi *et al.*, 1988; Spriggs *et al.*, 1990), and such effects may underlie facilitation of muscle proteolysis by IL-1. *In vitro*, IL-1 causes proteolysis by a prostaglandin-mediated mechanism (Baracos *et al.*, 1983). However, it is worthy of note that prostaglandin synthesis inhibitors do not affect proteolysis in traumatized animals (Hasselgren *et al.*, 1985). The teleological explanation for catabolism of muscle protein reserves, as provision of substrate for increased hepatic protein synthesis to defend against infection and to promote wound healing, is an appealing explanation of the changes in protein metabolism during the flow phase after injury. The fact that hepatic protein synthesis is profoundly stimulated by the combination of cytokines and glucocorticoids is in line with this notion (Fey & Gauldie, 1991). However, the loss of protein can eventually pose a serious threat to survival by causing severe body wasting (cachexia), resulting in the maladaptive reactions such as pulmonary and cardiovascular insufficiency, and impaired wound healing and immune functions. At present, various attempts are being undertaken to reduce the consequences of severe autocannibalism, by selective inhibition of the effect of cytokines, or by treatment with anabolic hormones (insulin, anabolic steroids, GH; Douglas & Shaw, 1989). However, the therapeutic role of these interventions in catabolic patients must await further evaluation.

## Acknowledgement

I thank Jek Persoons for his help with the literature research.

## References

Adami, H. O., Johansson, H., Thoren, L., Wide, L. & Akerstrom, G. (1978). Serum levels of TSH, $T_3$, $rT_3$, $T_4$ and $T_3$-resin uptake in surgical trauma. *Acta Endocrinol.*, **88**, 482–9.

Adams, D. O. & Hamilton, T. (1984). The cell biology of macrophage activation. *Ann. Rev. Immunol.*, **2**, 283–318.

Akahoshi, T., Oppenheim, J. J. & Matsushima, K. (1988). Interleukin-1 stimulates its own receptor expression on human fibroblast through the endogenous production of prostaglandins. *J. Clin. Invest.*, **82**, 1219–24.

Allison, S. P., Hinton, P. & Chamberlain, M. J. (1968). Intravenous glucose-tolerance, insulin and free-fatty acid levels in burned patients. *Lancet*, **ii**, 1113–16.

Andreis, P. G., Neri, G., Belloni, A. S., Mazzocchi, G., Kasprzak, A. & Nussdorfer, G. G. (1991). Interleukin-1 beta enhances corticosterone secretion by acting directly on the rat adrenal gland. *Endocrinology*, **129**, 53–7.

Aston-Jones, G., Foote, S. L. & Bloom, F. E. (1984). Anatomy and physiology of locus coeruleus neurons: functional implications. In *Norepinephrine*, M. G. Ziegle & G. R. Lake, pp. 92–116. Baltimore: Williams and Wilkins.

Balogh, D., Moncayo, R. & Baurer, M. (1984). Hormonal dysregulation in severe burns. *Burns*, **10**, 257–63.

Baracos, V., Rodemann, P., Dinarello, C. A. & Goldberg, A. L. (1983). Stimulation of muscle protein degradation and prostacyclin E2 by leucocyte pyrogen (interleukin-1). *N. Engl. J. Med.*, **308**, 553–8.

Barton, R. N. (1987). The neuroendocrinology of physical injury. *Balliere's Clin. Endocrinol.*, **355**, 374.
Barton, R. N. & Passingham, B. J. (1981). Effect of binding to plasma proteins on the interpretation of plasma cortisol concentrations after accidental injury. *Clin. Sci.*, **61**, 399–405.
Barton, R. N., Stoner, H. B. & Watson, S. M. (1987). Relationships among plasma cortisol, adrenocorticotrophin, and severity of injury in recently injured patients. *J. Trauma*, **27**, 384–92.
Bealey, D. (1990). Interleukin-1 and endotoxin activate soluble guanylate cyclase in vascular smooth muscle. *Am. J. Physiol.*, **259**, R38–R44.
Becker, R. A., Vaughan, G. M., Ziegler, M. G., Seraile, L. G., Goldfarb, I. W., Mansour, E. H., McManus, W. F., Pruitt, B. A. & Mason, A. D. (1982). Hypermetabolic low triiodothyronine syndrome after burn injury. *Crit. Care Med.*, **10**, 870–5.
Berczi, I. & Nagy, E. (1987). The effect of prolactin and growth hormone on hemolymphopoietic tissue and immune function. In *Hormones and Immunity*, ed. I. Berczi & Kovacs, F., pp. 145–71.
Berkenbosch, F. (1992). Corticotropin releasing factor and catecholamines: a study on their role in stress-induced immunomodulation. In *Perspectives in Behavioral Medicine; Stress and Disease Processes*, ed. N. Schneiderman, P. McCabe & A. Baum, pp. 73–91.New Jersey: Lawrence Erlbaum Associates.
Berkenbosch, F., de Goey, D. C. E., Del Rey, A. & Besedovsky, H. O. (1989). Neuroendocrine, sympathetic and metabolic responses induced by interleukin-1. *Neuroendocrinology*, **50**, 570–6.
Berkenbosch, F., DeRijk, R., Schotanus, K., Wolvers, D. & van Dam, A.-M. (1992*a*). The immune–hypothalamo–pituitary–adrenal axis: its role in immunoregulation and tolerance to self antigens. In *Interleukin-1 and the Brain*, ed. N. J. Rothwell & R. D. Dantzer, pp. 75–91. Oxford: Pergamon Press.
Berkenbosch, F., Rijk, R., Del Rey, A. & Besedovsky, H. O. (1990). Neuroendocrinology of interleukin-1. In *Circulating Regulatory Factors and Neuroendocrine Function*, ed. J. C. Porter & D. Jezova, pp. 303–14. New York: Plenum Press.
Berkenbosch, F., van Dam, A.-M., DeRijk, R. & Schotanus, K. (1992*b*). Role of the immune hormone interleukin-1 in brain controlled adaptive responses to infection. In *Stress: Neuroendocrine and Molecular Approaches*, ed. R. Kvetnansky, R. McCarthy & J. Axelrod, pp. 623–40. New York: Gordon and Breach.
Berkenbosch, F., van Oers, J., Del Rey, A., Tilders, F. & Besedovsky, H. (1987). Corticotropin-releasing factor-producing neurons in the rat activated by interleukin-1. *Science*, **238**, 524–6.
Bernton, E. W., Beach, J. E., Holaday, J. W., Smallridge, R. C. & Fein, H. C. (1987). Release of multiple hormones by a direct action of interleukin-1 on pituitary cells. *Science*, **238**, 519–21.
Berridge, C. W. & Dunn, A. J. (1989). CRF and restraint-stress decrease exploratory behavior in hypophysectomized mice. *Pharmacol. Biochem. Behav.*, **34**, 517–19.
Besedovsky, H. O., Del Rey, A., Sorkin, E. & Dinarello, C. A. (1986). Immunoregulatory feedback between interleukin-1 and glucocorticoid hormones. *Science*, **233**, 652–4.
Brizio-Molteni, L., Molteni, A., Warpeha, R. L. , Angelats, J., Lewis, N. & Fors,

E. M. (1984). Prolactin, corticotropin and gonadotropin concentrations following thermal injury in adults. *J. Trauma*, **24**, 1–9.

Brown, J. M. & Grosso, M. A. (1989). Cytokines, sepsis and the surgeon. *Surg. Gynecol. Obstet.* **169**, 568–75.

Brown, M. R. & Fisher, L. A. (1985). Corticotropin releasing factor: effects on the autonomic nervous system and visceral systems. *Fed. Proc.*, **44**, 243–8.

Carey, L. C., Cloutier, C. T. & Lowery, B. D. (1971). Growth hormone and adrenal cortical response to shock and trauma in human. *Ann. Surgery*, **174**, 451–8.

Christensen, J. D., Hansen, E. W. & Fjalland, B. (1989). Interleukin-1 beta stimulates the release of vasopressin from rat neurohypophysis. *Eur. J. Pharm.*, **171**, 233–5.

Cuthbertson, D. P. (1930). The disturbance of metabolism produced by bone injury, with notes in certain abnormal conditions of bone. *Biochem. J.*, **24**, 1244–63.

del Rey, A. & Besedovsky, H. (1987). Interleukin-1 affects glucose homeostasis. *Am. J. Physiol.*, **253**, R794–R798.

DeRijk, R. & Berkenbosch, F. (1992). Development and application of a radioimmunoassay to detect interleukin-1 in rat peripheral plasma. *Am. J. Physiol.*, **26**, E1–E7.

DeRijk, R. & Berkenbosch, F. (1993). Suppressive and permissive actions of glucocorticosteroids: a way to control innate immunity and to facilitate specificity of adaptive immunity? In *Hormones and Immunity: Bilateral Communication between the Endocrine and Immune Systems*, ed. C. J. Grossman. New York: Springer-Verlag, in press.

Dinarello, C. A. (1984). Interleukin-1 and the pathogenesis of the acute-phase-response. *N. Eng. J. Med.*, **311**, 1413–18.

Dinarello, C. A. (1991*a*). The proinflammatory cytokines interleukin-1 and tumour necrosis factor and treatment of the septic shock syndrome. *J. Infect. Dis.*, **163**, 1177–84.

Dinarello, C. A. (1991*b*). The proinflammatory cytokines interleukin-1 and tumour necrosis factor and treatment of the septic shock syndrome. *J. Infect. Dis.*, **163**, 1177–84.

Dinarello, C. A., Cannon, J. G., Wolff, S. M., Bernheim, H. A., Beutler, J., Cerami, A., Figari, I. S., Palladin, M. A. & O'Connor, J. V. (1986). Tumor necrosis factor (cachectin) is an endogenous pyrogen and induced production of interleukin-1. *J. Exp. Med.*, **163**, 1433–50.

Dolecek, R. (1989). Endocrine changes after burn trauma – a review. *Keio J. Med.*, **38**, 262–76.

Dolecek, R., Adamkova, M., Sotornikova, T., Zavada, M. & Kracmar, P. (1979). Endocrine responses after burn. *Scand. J. Plast. Reconstr. Surg.*, **13**, 9–16.

Douglas, R. G. & Shaw, J. H. F. (1989). Metabolic response to sepsis and trauma. *Br. J. Surg.*, **76**, 115–22.

Dubius, J. M., Dayer, J. M., Siegrist-Kaiser, C. A. & Burger, A. G. (1988). Human recombinant interleukin-1 beta decreases plasma thyroid hormone and thyroid stimulating hormone levels. *Endocrinology*, **123**, 2175–81.

Evans, R. D., Argiles, J. M. & Williamson, D. H. (1991). Metabolic effects of tumor necrosis factor alpha (cachectin) and interleukin-1. *Clin. Sci.*, **1989**, 357–64.

Fajans, S. S., Floyd, J. C., Knopf, R. F. & Conn, J. W. (1967). Effect of amino acids and proteins on insulin secretion in man. *Recent Prog. Horm. Res.*, **23**, 617–62.

Fey, G. & Gauldie, J. (1991). The acute phase response of the liver in inflammation. In *Progress in Liver Disease*, ed. H. Popper & F. Schnaffner. Orlando, FL: Grune and Stratton.

Frayn, K. N. (1986). Hormonal control of metabolism in trauma and sepsis. *Clin. Endocrinol.*, **24**, 577–99.

Frayn, K. N., Stoner, H. B., Barton, R. N., Heath, D. F. & Galasko, C. S. B. (1983). Persistence of high plasma glucose, insulin and cortisol concentrations in elderly patients with proximal femoral fractures. *Age Aging*, **12**, 70–6.

Gann, D. S., Ward, D. G. & Carlson, D. E. (1978). Neural control of ACTH: a homeostatic reflex. *Recent Prog. Horm. Res.*, **34**, 357–96.

Gelfand, J. A., Doneland, M. B., Hawinger, A. & Burk, J. F. (1982). Alternative complement pathway activation increases mortality in a model burn after injury in mice. *J. Clin. Invest.*, **70**, 1170–6.

Goodman, M. G., Chenoweth, D. E. & Weigle, W. D. (1982). Induction of interleukin-1 secretion and enhancement of humoral immunity by binding of human C5a to macrophage surface C5a receptors. *J. Exp. Med.*, **156**, 912–17.

Gray, T. S. (1989). Autonomic neuropeptide connections of the amygdala. In *Neuropeptides and Stress*, ed. Y. Tahe, J. E. Morley & M. R. Brown, pp. 92–105. Berlin: Springer-Verlag.

Haas, M. & Click, S. M. (1978). Radioimmunoassayable plasma vasopressin associated with surgery. *Arch. Surg.*, **113**, 597–600.

Hagen, C., Brandt, M. R. & Kehlet, H. (1980). Prolactin, LJ, FSH, GH and cortisol response to surgery and the effect of epidural analgesia. *Acta Endocrinol.*, **94**, 151–4.

Hamberger, B., Franebo, L. O. & Liljedahl, S. O. (1980). Plasma noradrenaline and dopamine in burn patients. *Burns*, **7**, 20–4.

Hasselgren, P., Talmini, M., LaFrance, R., James, J. H., Peters.. J. C. & Fisher, J. E. (1985). Effect of indomethacin on proteolysis in septic muscle. *Ann. Surg.*, **202**, 557–62.

Hauben, D. J., Le Roith, D., Click, S. M. & Mahler, D. (1980). Nonoliguric vasopressin oversecretion in severely burned patients. *Israel J. Sci.*, **16**, 101–5.

Heinrich, P. C., Castell, J. V. & Andus, T. (1990). Interleukin-6 and the acute phase response. *Biochem. J.*, **265**, 621–36.

Hermes, A. R. M. M., Sweep, C. G. J., Ross, A., Smals, A. G. H., Benraad, T. J. & Kloppenborg, P. W. C. (1992). Continuous infusion of interleukin-1 beta induces a nonthyroid illness syndrome in the rat. *Endocrinology*, **131**, 1–9.

Honegger, J., Spagnoli, A., D'Urso, R., Navarra, P., Tsagarakos, S., Besser, G. M. & Grossman, A. B. (1991). Interleukin-1 beta modulates the acute release of growth hormone releasing hormone and somatostatin from rat hypothalamus *in vitro*, whereas tumor necrosis factor and interleukin-6 have no effect. *Endocrinology*, **129**, 1275–82.

Kaplan, E., Dinarello, C. A. & Gelfand, J. A. (1989). Interleukin-1 and the response to injury. *Immunol. Res.*, **8**, 118–29.

Kaptein, E. M. (1986). Thyroid hormone metabolism in illness. In *Thyroid Hormone Metabolism*, ed. G. Hennemann, pp. 297–333. New York: Dekker.

Kluger, M. J. (1991). Fever: role of pyrogens and cryogens. *Physiol. Rev.*, **71**, 93–127.

Koob, G. F. & Britton, K. T. (1990). Behavioral effects of corticotropin releasing factor. In *Corticotropin Releasing Factor: Basic and Clinical Studies of Neuropeptide*, ed. E. B. De Souza & C. B. Nemeroff, pp. 253–74. Boca Raton: CRF Press.

Kvetnansky, R., Weise, V. K., Thoa, N. B. & Kopin, I. J. (1979). Effect of chronic guanethidine treatment and adrenalectomy on plasma levels of catecholamines and corticosterone in forcibly immobilized rats. *J. Pharmacol. Exp. Ther.*, **209**, 287–93.

Le Quesne, L. P., Cochrane, J. P. S. & Fieldman, N. P. (1985). Fluid and electrolyte disturbances after trauma: the role of adrenocortical and pituitary hormones. *Br. Med. Bull.*, **41**, 212–17.

Lindsey, C. A., Faloona, G. R. & Unger, R. H. (1975). Plasma glucagon levels during rapid exsanguination with and without adrenergic blockade. *Diabetes*, **24**, 313–16.

Little, R. A. (1988). Metabolic rate and thermoregulation after injury. In *Recent Advances in Critical Care Medicine*, ed. I. Ledingham. London: Churchill.

MacFarlane, I. A. & Rosin, M. D. (1980). Galactorrhea following surgical procedures to the chest wall: the role of prolactin. *Postgrad. Med. J.*, **23**, 5.

Miseles, R. (1981). The efferent projections of the subfornical organ of the rat: a circumventricular organ with neural network subserving water balance. *Brain Res.*, **230**, 1–23.

Moncada, S., Palmer, R. M. J. & Higgs, E. A. (1991). Nitric oxide: physiology, pathophysiology and pharmacology. *Pharmacol. Rev.*, **43**, 109–42.

Morgan, R. J., Martyn, J. A. J., Philbin, D. M., Coggins, G. H. & Burke, J. F. (1980). Water metabolism and antidiuretic hormone (ADH) response following thermal injury. *J. Trauma*, **20**, 468–72.

Munster, A. M. (1984). Immunological response of trauma and burns: an overview. *J. Am. Med. Assoc.*, **76**, 142–5.

Nakatsura, K., Ohgo, S., Oki, Y. & Matsukura, S. (1991). Interleukin-1 (IL-1) stimulates arginine vasopressin (AVP) release from superfused rat hypothalamo-neurohypophyseal complexes independently of a cholinergic mechanism. *Brain Res.*, **554**, 38–45.

Nawroth, P. P., Bank, I., Handley, D., Cassimir, J., Chess, L. & Stern, D. (1986). Tumor necrosis factor/cachectin interacts with endothelial cell receptors to induce release of interleukin-1. *J. Exp. Med.*, **163**, 1363–75.

Newsome, H. H. & Rose, J. C. (1971). The response of human adrenocorticotrophic hormone and growth hormone to surgical stress. *J. Clin. Endocrinol. Metab.*, **33**, 481–7.

Nijsten, M. W. N., De Groot, E. R., ten Duis, H. J., Klasen, H. J., Hack, E. & Aarden, L. A. (1987). Serum levels of interleukin-6 and acute phase responses. *Lancet*, **ii**, 921.

Noel, G. L., Suh, H. K., Stone, J. G. & Frantz, A. G. (1972). Human prolactin and growth hormone release during surgery and other conditions of stress. *J. Clin. Endocrinol. Metab.*, **35**, 840–51.

Okusawa, S., Dinarello, C. A., Yancey, K. B. Endres, S., Lawley, T. J., Frank, M. M., Burke, J. F. & Gefland, J. A. (1987). C5a induction of human interleukin-1; synergistic effect with endotoxin and interferon. *J. Immunol.*, **139**, 2634–40.

Oppenheim, J. J., Kovacs, E. J., Matsushima, K. & Durum, S. K. (1986). There is more than one interleukin-1. *Immunol. Today*, **7**, 45–56.

Payne, L. C., Obal, F., Opp, M. R. & Krueger, J. M. (1992). Stimulation and inhibition of growth hormone secretion by interleukin-1 beta: the involvement of growth hormone releasing hormone. *Neuroendocrinology*, **56**, 118–23.

Perlstein, R. S., Mougey, E. H., Jackson, W. E. & Neta, R. (1991). Interleukin-1 and interleukin-6 act synergistically to stimulate the release of adrenocorticotropic hormone *in vivo*. *Lymphokine Cytokine Res.*, **10**, 141–6.

Philbin, D. M. (1983). Vasopressin and anesthesia. In *Endocrinology and the Anaesthetist*, ed. T. Oyama, pp. 81–94. Amsterdam: Elsevier.

Philips, R. H., Valente, W. A., Caplan, E. S., Connor, T. B. & Viswell, J. G. (1984). Circulating thyroid hormone changes in acute trauma: prognostic implications for clinical outcome. *J. Trauma*, **24**, 116–19.

Popp, M. B., Srivastava, L. S., Knowles, H. C. Jr & MacMillan, B. G. (1977). Anterior pituitary function in thermally injured children and young adults. *Surg. Gynecol. Obstet.*, **145**, 517–24.

Porte, D. & Robertson, R. P. (1973). Control of insulin secretion by catecholamines, stress, and sympathetic nervous system. *Fed. Proc.*, **32**, 1792–6.

Pukel, C., Baquerizo, H. & Rabinovitch, A. (1988). Destruction of rat islet cell monolayers by cytokines. Synergistic interaction of interferon gamma, tumor necrosis factor, lymphotoxin and interleukin-1. *Diabetes*, **37**, 133–6.

Rivier, C. (1990). Role of endotoxin and interleukin-1 in modulating ACTH, LH and sex steroid secretion. *Ad. Exp. Med. Biol.*, **274**, 295–301.

Rivier, C. J. & Plotsky, P. M. (1986). Mediation of corticotropin releasing factor (CRF) on adenohypophyseal hormone secretion. *Annu. Rev. Physiol.*, **48**, 475–94.

Rivier, C. & Vale, W. (1984). Influence of corticotropin releasing factor (CRF) on reproductive functions in the rat. *Endocrinology*, **114**, 914–21.

Rivier, C., Vale, W. & Brown, M. (1989). In the rat, interleukin-1 alpha and beta stimulate adrenocorticotropin and catecholamine release. *Endocrinology*, **125**, 3096–112.

Rothwell, N. J. (1992). Metabolic responses to IL-1. In *Interleukin-1 in the Brain*, ed. N. J. Rothwell & R. D. Dantzer, pp. 115–34.

Sapolsky, R. M., Rivier, C., Yamamoto, P., Plotsky, P. & Vale, W. (1987). Interleukin-1 stimulates the secretion of hypothalamic corticotropin releasing factor. *Science*, **238**, 522–4.

Sauder, D. N., Semple, J., Truscotte, D., George, B. & Clowes, G. H. A. (1986). Stimulation of muscle protein degradation by murine and human epidermal cytokines: relationship to thermal injury. *J. Invest. Dermatol.*, **87**, 711–14.

Sawchenko, P. E. & Swanson, L. W. (1985). Localization, colocalization and plasticity of corticotropin releasing factor immunoreactivity in rat brain. *Fed. Proc.*, **44**, 221–7.

Shirani, K. Z., Vaughan, G. M., Robertson, G. L., Pruitt, B. A., McManus, W. F., Stallings, R. J. & Mason, A. D. (1983). Inappropriate vasopressin secretion (SIADH) in burned patients. *J. Trauma*, **23**, 217–24.

Simpson, J. B. (1981). The circumventricular organs and the central actions of angiotensin. *Neuroendocrinology*, **33**, 248–56.

Sowers, J. R., Raj, R. P., Hershman, J. M., Carlson, H. E. & McCallum, R. W. (1977). The effect of stressful diagnostic studies and surgery on anterior pituitary hormone release in man. *Acta Endocrinol.*, **86**, 25–32.

Spriggs, M. K., Lioubin, P. J., Slack, J., Dower, S. K., Jones, U., Cosman, D., Sims, J. E. & Bauer, J. (1990). Induction of an interleukin-1 receptor (IL-IR) on monocytic cells. *J. Biol. Chem.*, **265**, 22499–505.

Stoner, H. B. (1976). Causative factors and afferent stimuli involved in the metabolic response to injury. In *Metabolism and Response to Injury*, ed. A. W. Wilkinson & D. P. Cuthbertson, pp. 202–14. London: Pitman Medical.

Sweep, C. G. J., van der Meer, M., Ross, A., Vranckx, R., Visser, T. J. & Hermes, A. R. M. M. (1992). Chronic infusion of TNF alpha reduces plasma T4 binding without affecting pituitary thyroid activity in rats. *Am. J. Physiol.*, **263**, E1–7.

Tazi, A., Dantzer, R., Le Moal, M., Rivier, J., Vale, W. & Koob, G. F. (1987). Corticotropin releasing factor antagonist blocks stress induced fighting in rats. *Regul. Pept.*, **18**, 37–42.

Tilders, F. J. H., Berkenbosch, F. & Smelik, P. G. (1985). Control of secretion of peptides related to adrenocorticotropin, melanocyte stimulating hormone and endorphin. *Front. Horm. Res.*, **14**, 161–96.

Tsagarakis, S., Gillies, G., Ress, L. H., Besser, M. & Grosman, A. (1989). Interleukin-1 directly stimulates the release of corticotropin releasing factor from rat hypothalamus. *Neuroendocrinology*, **49**, 98–101.

Vale, W., Rivier, C., Brown, M. R., Spiess, J., Koob, G., Swanson, L., Bilezikjian, L., Bloom, F. & Rivier, J. (1983). Chemical and biological characterization of corticotropin releasing factor. *Recent Prog. Horm. Res.*, **39**, 245–70.

van Dam, A.-M., Brouns, M., Louisse, S. & Berkenbosch, F. (1992). Appearance of interleukin-1 in macrophages and in ramified microglia in the brain of endotoxin-treated rats: a pathway for the induction of non-specific symptoms of sickness? *Brain Res.*, **588**, 291–6.

van der Poll, T., Romijn, J. A., Wiersinga, W. R. & Sauerwein, H. P. (1990). Tumor necrosis factor: a putative mediator of the sick euthyroid syndrome in man. *J. Clin. Endocrinol. Metab.*, **71**, 1567–72.

Vaughan, G. M., Becker, R. A., Allan, J. P., Goodwin, C. V., Pruitt, B. A. & Mason, A. D. (1982). Cortisol and corticotropin in burned patients. *J. Trauma*, **22**, 263–73

Wang, C., Chan, V. & Yeung, R. T. T. (1978). Effect of surgical stress on pituitary–testicular function. *Clin. Endocrinol.*, **9**, 255–66.

Weidenfeld, J., Abramsky, O. & Ovadia, H. (1989). Effect of interleukin-1 on ACTH and corticosterone secretion in dexamethane and adrenalectomized pretreated rats. *Neuroendocrinology*, **50**, 650–4.

Yasuda, N. & Greer, M. A. (1978). Evidence that the hypothalamus mediates the endotoxin stimulation of adrenocorticotropic hormone secretion. *Endocrinology*, **102**, 947–53.

Zonghai, H., Han, G. & Renbao, X. (1987). Study on glucocorticoid receptors during intestinal ischemia shock and septic shock. *Circ. Shock*, **23**, 27–36.

# 11

# Central control of metabolic and thermoregulatory responses to injury

ANGELA L. COOPER and NANCY J. ROTHWELL

## Introduction

Changes in body temperature and metabolism (energy and substrate metabolism) are common features of many disease states, and have been well documented following various forms of tissue injury. Body temperature is a precisely regulated phenomenon such that core temperature (most probably brain temperature) is normally maintained within a narrow range by physiological controls operating on heat loss and heat production (metabolic rate). In contrast, energy metabolism is highly variable, depending on the balance between energy intake and expenditure (heat production and physical work). Nevertheless, there is extensive evidence that this balance between energy input and output remains remarkably constant over long periods of time in many organisms, including humans. Thus total body energy content, mainly in the form of fat and protein, can be stable for months or even years. The physiological regulation of body temperature and energy metabolism, which are both under direct control of the central nervous system (CNS), are closely related. The regulation of core temperature is achieved by controls operating on heat loss and heat production, with the latter predominating in many situations. Thus, development of fever is almost always associated with increased rates of heat production and, if sustained, these will lead to depletion of body energy stores and weight loss which are confounded by reduced levels of food intake. In contrast, increased heat production, if not fully compensated by enhanced heat loss, will lead to a rise in body temperature, although this does not necessarily manifest itself as 'fever' according to strict physiological definition.

For these reasons, the central control of body temperature and the metabolic rate response to injury will be considered in parallel. Alterations in specific nutrient metabolism (e.g. protein and lipid metabolism) following injury are numerous and complex, and will therefore not be reviewed in detail, although it is obvious that these both influence and are directly dependent on variations in core temperature and metabolic rate.

### Basic aspects of thermoregulation and metabolic rate – definitions and measurement

Body temperature is most reliably determined from measurements of deep core temperature, i.e. gut or brain temperature. Rectal temperature can provide a reliable index of this parameter but is sometimes inconvenient, while oral temperature may be unreliable. In experimental animals, core temperature is usually determined by insertion of a thermocouple beyond the rectal sphincter into the colon. Obvious disadvantages of this technique are that it may cause stress, so that it is preferable to adapt animals to the procedure, and it prohibits continuous measurements in free-moving animals. Remote telemetry achieved by implantation of a temperature-sensitive probe (usually into the peritoneum), circumvents these problems, but does require surgical intervention prior to experimentation. Telemetry has also proven valuable for continuous monitoring of core temperature in humans (usually gut temperature, as the transmitter is swallowed), but the costs of equipment and transmitter pills are high.

Variations in core temperature may result from passive changes in body heat content due to gain or loss from the environment, such as hyperthermia caused by heat stress. In contrast, fever is a regulated increase in body temperature, which is dependent on an elevation in the central set-point and is achieved by simultaneous increased heat production and reduced heat loss. This distinction between fever and secondary hyperthermia is particularly important when considering thermoregulatory responses to injury, where there is often doubt whether raised body temperatures represent 'true fever' (see below). Furthermore, a raised body temperature is widely used as a clinical index of infection, although this may not be a valid assumption.

Physiological variations in metabolic rate commonly occur in response to changes in the amount or type of food consumed, or reduced environmental temperatures. These regulatory changes in heat production, usually referred to as thermogenesis, appear to be under direct control by the CNS, and have been ascribed to activation of the sympathetic nervous system and increased heat production in brown adipose tissue (Rothwell *et al.*, 1983) at least in experimental animals. In humans, active brown adipose tissue is present and is stimulated in response to disease states (Bianchi *et al.*, 1989; Bruce *et al.*, 1990) but its quantitative importance is unknown. Such variations in metabolic rate occur in normal resting subjects and animals, and may be critically important in obtaining reliable estimates of heat production, even in resting or sleeping conditions. While it is widely recognised that small changes in physical activity or even muscle tone exert marked effects on metabolic rate, the importance of defined and constant conditions of environmental temperature and nutritional state are sometimes ignored. Consideration of nutritional state is particularly difficult in comparisons of patients who are fasting with those who are feeding voluntarily (i.e. in discrete meals) or receiving intravenous nutrition, which is usually administered continuously.

Metabolic rate is most commonly determined by indirect calorimetry, i.e. measurements of oxygen consumption ($V_{O_2}$), and often carbon dioxide production ($V_{CO_2}$). Direct calorimetry, which necessitates measuring all forms of heat loss, is expensive and often impractical, particularly for clinical studies. Numerous commercially available indirect calorimeters, many of which are portable, are now available for small experimental animals and for human subjects, and provide simple, reliable estimates of $V_{O_2}$, $V_{CO_2}$ and respiratory quotient (RQ). However, while the practical problems of assessing metabolic rate in the clinical setting can now be quite readily overcome, those of interpretation of the data remain to be considered. It is usually not possible to obtain continuous, 24 h values for metabolic rate. Highly questionable is the validity of extrapolation of 'sample' measurements, usually taken over 1–2 h, to total energy expenditure, which depends on the normal physical activity, state of consciousness, stressful interventions (e.g. surgery) and feeding patterns of the subject, patient or animal.

Further difficulties may be encountered in attempts to compare values for metabolic rates with those of healthy individuals, which vary considerably. Results obtained on patients may be artificially low, because of loss of body mass (particularly when lean tissue is wasted), and it is usually advantageous to express data both as absolute values and, where possible, as corrected for body size or lean body mass.

In spite of these difficulties in interpretation, there is a considerable literature on the effects of various forms of injury on metabolic rate and body temperature in the human (see below). Nevertheless, understanding the brain mechanisms controlling these parameters requires intervention studies, which are clearly not possible in humans, even under experimental conditions. This has necessitated the use of experimental animals, which have provided much of our current understanding of this subject. Where it has been possible to compare the results of research on animals with clinical or experimental data in humans, it appears that this approach is clinically relevant. A detailed discussion of the validity and limitations of research on animal models of injury is provided in Chapter 3.

## Effects of injury on metabolic rate and body temperature in humans

The thermoregulatory and metabolic changes that occur following injury have been well documented, although it is often difficult to compare data from different studies, and the mechanisms involved in their development and maintenance still remain to be fully elucidated. These responses vary in magnitude and time-course; however, even relatively small but prolonged increases in energy expenditure cause a significant energy deficit, which necessitates the mobilization of energy stores and loss of body weight (see Rothwell, 1990*a*). Body wasting (cachexia) may actually prove to be detrimental to recovery of the patient, and in young children may attenuate subsequent growth (Childs *et al.*, 1990).

Classically, the thermoregulatory and metabolic responses to injury have been divided into two phases: the early, transient 'ebb' phase and the subsequent 'flow' phase (Cuthbertson, 1932). The ebb phase is due to inhibition of thermoregulation and is characterised by hypothermia and hypometabolism, whilst the flow phase is associated with hypermetabolism and often with a raised body temperature.

Evidence for the ebb phase is controversial. Studies in experimental animals have demonstrated that following scald injury and hindlimb ischaemia in the rat, injured animals exhibit hypothermia and also hypometabolism (Stoner, 1961; Threlfall *et al.*, 1980; and see below). Injured patients may also present with a reduced body temperature soon after injury, although there is no evidence to suggest the presence of hypometabolism (Little & Stoner, 1981). More recent data, however, obtained from both experimental animals and humans, have failed to reveal an ebb phase immediately following injury. In patients, early hypermetabolic responses have been documented in burn injury (Childs, 1988, 1993), trauma (Winthrop *et al.*, 1987), severe injury (Edwards *et al.*, 1988) and surgery Carli & Aber, 1987).

The flow phase of injury is well recognised and is characterised not only by hypermetabolism, but also fever, anorexia, muscle proteolysis, acute-phase protein synthesis, altered endocrine status and intermediary metabolism.

The hypermetabolic response to injury has been studied extensively, both in experimental animals and in patients. In humans, this response is proportional to the severity of the injury. For example, relatively minor insults such as surgery and bone fracure cause 10–20% increases in energy expenditure in adults (Frayn *et al.*, 1984; Carli & Aber, 1987), although in postoperative paediatric patients this response is absent (Groner *et al.*, 1989). Greater increases in energy expenditure (20–100%) are observed following multiple trauma (Ott *et al.*, 1987), but in paediatric patients (Winthrop *et al.*, 1987) the magnitude of this response is smaller than predicted. Head injury also causes large increases in energy expenditure (Clifton *et al.*, 1989; Moore *et al.*, 1989) even though a relatively small amount of tissue is damaged compared to multiple peripheral injuries. Recent evidence also suggests that the type of head injury affects the hypermetabolic response (Hadfield, 1990), since diffuse injury causes greater and more sustained increases in energy expenditure than a focal area of ischaemic damage. Infection of wounds and the development of sepsis exacerbates the hypermetabolic responses to injury even further (Long, 1977; Elwyn *et al.*, 1981).

The largest increases in energy expenditure are generally observed following thermal injury, and a curvilinear relationship exists between burn size and the extent of hypermetabolism. This relationship is maintained not only immediately after the injury is incurred, but also throughout the healing process (Matsuda *et al.*, 1987). Recent evidence from burn-injured children has also demonstrated a hypermetabolic response, although again the magnitude appears to be smaller than observed in adults (Childs, 1993).

Severe injury, particularly head injury and burns, is associated with a raised body temperature, which is often termed a fever, although this may be an inaccurate description. As a 'true' fever represents an upward resetting of the set-point for body temperature, the increase in body temperature observed in injured patients may actually represent hyperthermia resulting from an imbalance of heat production and heat loss. For example, during febrile infection, there is a linear relationship between the rise in body temperature and an increase in energy expenditure (13% increase for every degree Celsius rise in body temperature). Following severe injury, however, the rise in metabolic rate is greater than that predicted by the rise in body temperature (i.e. increases in energy expenditure of 100% should cause a 10 deg.C rise in body temperature). During burn injury, it has been demonstrated that hypermetabolism has a fever-dependent and fever-independent component. In the former case the raised body temperature is defended over a range of environmental temperatures (Wilmore *et al.*, 1975), indicating an upward resetting of the set-point. However, the magnitude of this fever accounts for only about 20% of the observed hypermetabolism (Aulick & Wilmore, 1983), indicating a fever-independent component. This relationship is probably also true for other injuries such as multiple trauma and head injury.

## Experimentally induced changes in metabolic rate and thermoregulation in humans

Because of ethical considerations, which limit the study of injury in patients, experimental approaches to investigate the metabolic and thermoregulatory responses to injury have concentrated on the development of protocols in healthy human volunteers. In addition, there are further problems associated with the study of spontaneous injuries, such as variations in the time-course, magnitude and severity of responses, and also the preexisting condition of the patient, thus making results from such studies difficult to interpret. In view of these problems, several protocols mimicking the pyrogenic and thermogenic responses to injury have been developed. However, these models are somewhat compromised, since no wound or inflammatory focus is present, and they may more accurately reflect host responses to infection rather than injury.

One procedure used to study the responses to injury is co-infusion of the hormones adrenaline, glucagon and hydrocortisone (Bessey *et al.*, 1985). Intravenous infusion of these hormones over a 72-h period induced a sustained hypermetabolism (30% above controls), and elicited a number of other responses associated with the flow phase of injury (e.g. negative nitrogen balance), although fever was not apparent. Subsequent studies combining triple hormone infusion and repeated injection of the naturally occurring steroid, etiocholanolone (Watters *et al.*, 1986), resulted in fever and acute-phase protein synthesis, in addition to the previously observed responses. Thus, the combined protocol induces the thermoregulatory and metabolic responses characteristic of injury as well as other acute phase responses.

Fever and hypermetabolism have also been induced in human volunteers by injection or infusion of endotoxin. Intravenous administration of this bacterial pyrogen caused marked fever, hypermetabolism and endocrinological changes consistent with those observed following injury and infection in patients (Wolff *et al.*, 1965; Michie *et al.*, 1988; Revhaug *et al.*, 1988). However, the magnitude of the hypermetabolism following endotoxin administration was proportional to the rise in body temperature and this is often found not to be the case following injury in humans. Also, the time-course of action of endotoxin is relatively short (approximately 5 h), and therefore only mechanisms involved in the development of these responses can be studied. Another problem with intravenous injection of pyrogens is that this model does not represent the pathophysiological responses to injury, since there is no inflammatory focus, and the population of the immune cells encountered (principally macrophages) are entirely different from those activated following tissue injury. These problems can be partly overcome by using intramuscular injection of typhoid vaccine as a protocol to induce fever and hypermetabolism (Cooper *et al.*, 1992). Responses to type and variance develop following local inflammation around the site of injection and are maintained for approximately 24 h.

**Experimentally induced injury in laboratory animals**

The vast majority of studies in injury have been undertaken on laboratory rodents, because of the cost and ethical objections to using larger or higher mammals, and because of our extensive understanding of the normal physiology of rodents. Various experimental procedures have been used to induce injury in animals, including bone fracture, brain injury (mechanical, ischaemic), scald or burn injury, local inflammation (e.g. sterile abscess), and limb ischaemia. The effects of these manipulations (as with clinical observations) on metabolic rate and body temperature vary, depending on factors such as the severity of the insult, the age, species and strain of animals used and the environmental conditions under which they are maintained. However, where detailed information exists, it appears that injury usually results in increases in energy expenditure and temperature, as well as in changes in food intake and body weight (see Table 11.1 for summary). The time-course of such alterations is, however, highly dependent on the specific intervention. For example, scald injury in the rat induces a transient ($\approx$24 h) reduction in $V_{O_2}$ and colonic temperature, which is followed by a later (at least 3 days) increase in both parameters (Rothwell *et al.*, 1991), which may be sustained for several days, although this may be influenced by subsequent infection of the wound. In contrast, hindlimb inflammation, resulting from a sterile abscess caused by intramuscular injection of turpentine in the rat, elicits a rapid rise in $V_{O_2}$ and the body temperature within 1 h, which is sustained for at least 24 h (Cooper & Rothwell, 1991). Investigation into the mediators of the hypermetabolic response to sterile abscess indicates that mechanisms underlying the early

Table 11.1. *Changes in body weight, food intake, metabolic rate and body temperature after hindlimb inflammation (intramuscular turpentine), scald injury (20% bovine serum albumen), focal cerebral ischaemia, chronic infusion of bacterial endotoxin in the rat, infection with* Legionella pneumophilia *in the guinea-pig or malarial infection in the mouse*

| | Body weight | Food intake | Metabolic rate | Body temperature |
|---|---|---|---|---|
| *Injury* | | | | |
| Hind limb inflammation | ↓ | ↓ 20% | ↑ 25% | +1.5 °C |
| Scald injury | ↓↓ | ↓ 20% | ↑ 16% | +1.0 °C |
| Cerebral ischaemia | ↓ | ↓ 10% | ↑ 20% | – |
| *Infection* | | | | |
| Endotoxin infusion | ↓ | ↓ 20% | ↑ 15% | +0.8 °C |
| *Legionella* | ↓↓ | ↓ 30% | ↑ 33% | +1.5 °C |
| Malaria | ↓↓↓ | ↓ 30% | ↑ 30% | – |

–, No change.

phase (0–4 h) differ from those responsible for the later response (8–24 h) (see below).

Extensive studies have been undertaken to investigate mechanisms and potential treatments for neuronal damage resulting from various forms of brain injury in animals. These have employed techniques such as percussive or rotational injury, focal or global ischaemia usually induced by temporary or permanent occlusion of the carotid arteries or middle cerebral artery, respectively, or injection of autologous blood or neurotoxic agents onto or into the brain. The relevance of these procedures to head injury, stroke, cerebral haemorrhage, subdural haematoma, etc. has been argued extensively (Meldrum, 1990), but very few studies have investigated the effects on metabolic rate or body temperature. When maintained under general anaesthesia, animals subjected to cerebral ischaemia show variable temperature responses, exhibiting either hyper- or hypothermia. Rats allowed to recover consciousness following ischaemia induced by middle cerebral artery occlusion (MCAO) exhibit a delayed (6–24 h) increase in metabolic rate (O'Shaughnessy *et al.*, 1990), which more closely mimics the observations on head injury in humans (see above). Temporary global ischaemia, for example induced by carotid artery occlusion, usually induces marked increases in body temperature, which may have severely detrimental effects on neuronal outcome (Busto *et al.*, 1989).

Effects of bacterial infection, or the administration of pyrogens such as endotoxin or cytokines, on metabolic rate and body temperature have been widely studied in experimental animals, and usually provoke marked increases in thermogenesis and body temperature. These studies have generally been directed towards understanding febrile and metabolic responses to pathogenic infections. However, since many of the mechanisms underlying the effects of injury and infection on metabolism and thermoregulation may be similar or closely related, and because of the frequent complication of infection in injured patients, the results may nevertheless be relevant to the present topic.

## Mechanisms of metabolic and thermoregulatory responses to injury

There is now extensive evidence to indicate that thermoregulatory and metabolic responses to injury are under direct control by the CNS. The brain receives both the neural and humoral afferent signals and subsequently activates peripheral effector mechanisms leading to changes in heat production and heat loss and thus to alterations in body temperature.

### *Peripheral effector mechanisms*

Sympathetic activation of non-shivering thermogenesis is an important effector pathway involved in the generation of fever and hypermetabolism following both injury and infection. In experimental animals, hypermetabolic responses can be reduced, although often not abolished, by β-adrenergic blockade following endotoxin-induced fever (Jepson *et al.*, 1988), inflammation (Cooper & Rothwell, 1991), cerebral ischaemia (O'Shaughnessy *et al.*, 1990) and burn injury (Wolfe & Durkot, 1982). In humans, the hypermetabolic response to experimentally induced fever can also be abolished (Cooper *et al.*, 1992) and the responses to burn injury attenuated (Wilmore *et al.*, 1974; Breitenstein *et al.*, 1990) by administration of the β-adrenoceptor antagonist propranolol. In addition, propranolol also attenuates the weight loss observed following thermal injury (Szabo, 1979). These data therefore indicate a significant β-adrenergic component of the hypermetabolic responses to injury.

Although inhibition of the sympathetic nervous system reduces hypermetabolic responses, it has little effect on body temperature. This probably signifies the presence of a 'true' fever (i.e. an upward resetting of the hypothalamic set-point), as the febrile host will attempt to maintain an elevated body temperature, despite inhibition of non-shivering thermogenesis. In these circumstances, the host therefore recruits other mechanisms of non-sympathetic heat conservation (e.g. shivering or reduced heat loss) to maintain an elevated body temperature.

The principal effector organ for sympathetically mediated increases in thermogenesis, at least in small mammals, is brown adipose tissue (BAT). Heat production in BAT is activated by $\beta_3$ adrenoceptors (Arch *et al.*, 1984), and is due to the presence of a unique proton conductance pathway which allows the uncoupling of oxidative phosphorylation across the inner mitochondrial membrane (Nicholls & Locke, 1984). An increase in BAT activity has been observed in a number of experimental models of hypermetabolism associated with disease. Increased activity of the tissue (as assessed by guanosine bisphosphate binding to the uncoupling site) has been observed during fever (Cooper *et al.*, 1989; Dascombe *et al.*, 1989; Cooper & Rothwell, 1991; Scarpace *et al.*, 1991) and following scald injury (Rothwell *et al.*, 1991).

The role of BAT in humans is, however, controversial. Although it is an important site of heat production in the human neonate, its activity is thought to decline with age (Lean & James, 1986). Preliminary evidence of functional BAT in young children has , however, suggested that activity of the tissue may be increased in disease states associated with hypermetabolism. BAT activity of perirenal tissue excised from children with malignant disease and cachexia and from victims of severe burn injury is 100% greater than that found in age-matched controls (Bianchi *et al.*, 1989; Bruce *et al.*, 1990). Whether the increased heat production in this tissue contributes to the rise in whole body energy expenditure, however, remains to be determined.

Other potential effector tissues activated in hypermetabolic responses to injury are skeletal muscle, liver, adipose tissue and the wound itself. Studies investigating the contribution of the wound in thermal injury have concluded that it is not a major site of energy expenditure as the wound functions anaerobically, although its requirements for protein and carbohydrate substrates may necessitate hypermetabolism in other tissues. Increases in intermediary metabolism, particularly in protein turnover and substrate cycles in carbohydrate and lipid metabolism, have been postulated in possible effector sites for hypermetabolism. Increased protein turnover in muscle would not, however, appear to be a major site of heat production, since only a small percentage of the hypermetabolism can be accounted for by the increase in protein turnover, and no relationship has been observed between the two variables (Duke *et al.*, 1970; Winthrop *et al.*, 1987; Jahoor *et al.*, 1988). Sympathetically mediated increases in glucose and triglyceride cycling have been observed following burn injury in humans (Wolfe *et al.*, 1987). The quantitative importance of this substrate cycling in the hypermetabolic response has not, however, been determined.

## Afferent pathways

The afferent signal for fever and hypermetabolism may be of either a neural or humoral nature (detailed descriptions of afferent pain pathways are included in Chapter 9). These two types of signal may act independently or synergistically to initiate or maintain these responses. Recent evidence suggests that both types of signal may be involved sequentially in fever and hypermetabolism (Cooper & Rothwell, 1991).

Where pain is incurred following injury and inflammation, neural pathways may play a significant role in activating pyrogenic and thermogenic responses. The initial activation of thermoregulatory and metabolic responses after tissue injury have been attributed to the activation of nociceptor afferents (C-fibre afferents) since depletion of these fibres abolishes both the fall in body temperature following hindlimb ischaemia (Redfern *et al.*, 1984) and also the fever and hypermetabolism associated with inflammation in the rat (Cooper & Rothwell, 1991). Sustained responses to injury, however, have neurally dependent components which differ according to the injury. For example, fever and hypermetabolism persist despite denervation of the wound or inhibition of sensory input into the brain in patients (Wilmore, 1976), and during inflammation and endotoxin administration in experimental animals (Szekely & Scolcsanyi, 1979; Cooper & Rothwell, 1991). Normal febrile responses are observed in quadriplegic patients (Schmidt & Chan, 1990), although the hypermetabolic response is abolished in paraplegic head-injured patients (Clifton *et al.*, 1989), suggesting that spinally injured patients increase body temperature by changes in heat loss.

Afferent neural pathways that are activated by changes in cardiovascular functions (e.g. hypotension resulting from haemorrhage) or local pressure, such as that caused by tissue inflammation, are well defined (see Chapter 9). However, their precise effects on metabolic rate are largely unknown, although modest haemorrhage does lead to increased thermogenesis, whereas severe blood loss usually elicits a fall in metabolic rate and body temperature, probably because of impaired tissue perfusion (Rady *et al.*, 1991).

A number of circulating factors that are increased after injury may act as afferent signals. These include inflammatory mediators, usually released at the site of damage, such as prostaglandins, catecholamines and kinins. However, great interest and investigation has recently focused on the role of cytokines as mediators of many aspects of the acute phase response and as activators of fever and thermogenesis.

### *Cytokines*

The cytokines are a large and diverse group of polypeptides comprising the interleukins, interferons (IFN), tumour necrosis factors and various growth- and cell-stimulating factors. Cytokines exert pleiotropic actions and are particularly important in activation of peripheral immune cells and inflammation. Of the large and rapidly growing number of cytokines, interleukin-1 (IL-1), IL-6 and tumour necrosis factor-$\alpha$ (TNF$\alpha$) have been shown to play important roles in control of systemic host defence responses, although the involvement of other members of this family (e.g. IL-8, IFN-$\gamma$) is now becoming apparent. In addition to local (autocrine or paracrine) actions, these cytokines may be released into the circulation with actions at distant sites including the brain (see Rothwell, 1990*d*, 1991*b*).

Numerous reports have described circulating concentrations of cytokines (usually IL-1, IL-6 and TNF$\alpha$) in animals or human volunteers in response to experimental interventions or in clinical conditions of injury, infection, inflammation and malignant disease (e.g. Moldawer *et al.*, 1987; LeMay *et al.*, 1990*a*, *b*; Dinarello, 1991; Dinarello & Thompson, 1991). The variability in results of these studies is due largely to experimental problems of cytokine assays such as the presence of endogenous inhibitors, circulating receptors, binding proteins and biologically inactive (but often immunoreactive) precursor or breakdown products (see Whicher & Ingham, 1990).

Increases in plasma concentrations of IL-1 have been observed following injury. In humans, a transient rise has been observed during, but not following, surgery (Baigrie *et al.*, 1991), and, following thermal injury, plasma IL-1 is elevated (Cannon *et al.*, 1990*a*) but quickly returns to control values. During experimentally induced fever in human volunteers, elevated plasma concentrations of IL-1 have been observed (Hesse *et al.*, 1988; Cannon *et al.*, 1990*b*), although other studies have failed to demonstrate a significant increase in plasma IL-1 (Horan *et al.*, 1989). In addition, the rise in plasma IL-1 did not correlate with the magnitude or the time-course of the temperature responses (Cannon *et al.*, 1990*b*).

During sepsis or septic shock, plasma IL-1 was also increased (Calandra *et al.*, 1990; Waage *et al.*, 1989), albeit only in the patients who subsequently died from shock (Waage *et al.*, 1989), and a significant relationship between IL-1 appearance and mortality has been observed in these patients (Cannon *et al.*, 1990*b*).

These data therefore do not support the hypothesis that IL-1 is the major circulating endogenous cytokine. However, studies in experimental animals using antibodies or antagonists to IL-1 have observed reduced febrile and hypermetabolic responses (Long *et al.*, 1990; Rothwell *et al.*, 1990) and increased survival following lethal endotoxaemia (Alexander *et al.*, 1991), indicating that IL-1 has a functional role in injury and infection. Therefore, IL-1 may induce fever by acting either locally at the site of injury and causing secondary release of other endogenous pyrogens, or by acting directly within the central nervous system.

TNF$\alpha$ is another endogenous pyrogen implicated in fever and hypermetabolism. Increased plasma concentrations of TNF are observed following head injury (Goodman *et al.*, 1990) and burn injury (Cannon *et al.*, 1990*a*; Marano *et al.*, 1990) in humans, but not following femur fracture in the rat (Stylianos *et al.*, 1991). During sepsis, in both patients and experimental animals, plasma TNF may be increased (Hesse *et al.*, 1988; deGroot *et al.*, 1989; Calandra *et al.*, 1990; Dofferhoff *et al.*, 1992), although this occurs in only a small proportion of the patients tested (Waage, 1987; deGroot *et al.*, 1989). This may be because of rapid clearance of TNF from plasma, since experimentally induced fever causes only transient increases in plasma TNF (60–90 min following endotoxin administration) that occur before the onset of fever (Michie *et al.*, 1988; Long *et al.*, 1989). Furthermore, the correlation between plasma TNF and fever in these studies is poor. Since TNF is more commonly associated with infection, it may not be a marker of injury but instead indicate the presence of sepsis/infection or shock, as plasma TNF concentrations correlate with both infection and mortality (Waage *et al.*, 1987; Calandra *et al.*, 1990), although Calandra *et al.* (1990) found that other physiological parameters were stronger indicators of outcome than was plasma TNF.

TNF may, however, be an important mediator of host responses to disease, although probably not of fever and hypermetabolism, since antibodies to TNF increase survival from endotoxic and septic shock both in experimental animals and patients (Beutler *et al.*, 1985; Hinshaw *et al.*, 1990; Silva *et al.*, 1990). Recent evidence in experimental animals has suggested that TNF does not mediate fever but acts as an endogenous antipyretic, since administration of an antiserum to TNF enhances febrile responses following LPS injection in the rat (Long *et al.*, 1989), although it does inhibit pyrogenic and thermogenic responses to localised inflammation and injury in the rat (Cooper & Rothwell, unpublished data).

IL-6 can be induced by both IL-1 and TNF *in vivo* (Helle *et al.*, 1988; Broukaert *et al.*, 1989; Shalaby *et al.*, 1989; Gershenwald *et al.*, 1990). Increased plasma concentrations of IL-6 of up to 100-fold are observed following various types of injuries in patients, including burns (Nijsten *et al.*, 1987), head injury (McClain *et al.*, 1990), septic shock (Waage *et al.*, 1987; Hack *et al.*, 1989; Dofferhoff *et al.*, 1992) and surgery (Shenkin *et al.*, 1989; Pullicino *et al.*, 1990). These studies have shown that plasma IL-6 concentrations, unlike those of IL-1 and TNF, correlate strongly with the magnitude of febrile responses and the severity of the disease or injury, and also with the outcome. However, these may not be causal relationships. Instead, increases in plasma IL-6 may be induced by local release of IL-1 and/or TNF. For example, in experimental animals, neutralisation of endogenous IL-1 reduces fever and plasma IL-6 during LPS-induced fever (LeMay *et al.*, 1990*a*), and neutralisation of TNF attenuates the rise in IL-6 following injury (Cooper & Rothwell, unpublished data).

The ability and mechanisms by which peripherally elaborated cytokines enter and activate the brain have been a subject of long-standing debate and controversy (see Blatteis, 1988, 1992). Several studies have indicated that IL-1, which like other cytokines, is a large molecule ($\approx$17 kDa), does not enter the brain when administered systemically (see Blatteis, 1988; Rothwell, 1991*b*). A transport system for IL-1 has been described in the brain (Banks *et al.*, 1990), but since considerably less than 1% of the circulating cytokine can enter the brain by this route, and circulating concentrations are usually low in non-fatal conditions (see above), the biological relevance of active transport remains to be demonstrated. In contrast, circulating concentrations of IL-6 can increase dramatically (often by three orders of magnitude) in response to injury, but its ability to enter the brain is unknown.

Alternatively, circulating cytokines may influence body temperature and metabolic rate by acting at brain sites that lack a functional blood–brain barrier (BBB). One of these, the organum vasculosum of the lamina terminalis (OVLT), has been proposed as a site of action of IL-1 in pyrogens (see Blatteis, 1988). In situations where endotoxin levels are high, or there is damage to the brain, loss of a functional BBB occurs with resulting entry of large molecules and invasion of immune cells such as macrophages, an important source of cytokines. This situation is further complicated by the demonstration that cytokines are synthesised within the brain itself in response to both local and systemic stimuli (see Koenig, 1991; Rothwell, 1991*a*; Relton & Rothwell, 1992).

## Central mechanisms

### *Brain sites controlling temperature and thermogenesis*

The primary brain region involved in the control of autonomic function including thermoregulation and thermogenesis is the hypothalamus. Extensive research has supported a primary role for the preoptic anterior hypothalamus (POAH) in the regulation of body temperature and the development of fever. Thermosensitive neurones in the POAH respond to many putative endogenous pyrogens such as prostaglandins and cytokines (see Blatteis, 1988, 1992) and increased prostaglandin synthesis occurs in this brain region during pyrogenesis (see Dascombe, 1985; Milton, 1982; Cooper, 1987; Blatteis, 1988). However, reports that destruction of the POAH in experimental animals does not prevent febrile responses (see Blatteis, 1988) questions the primary function of this brain region. The ventromedial hypothalamus (VMH), originally identified as a satiety centre, has now been strongly implicated in the central control of thermogenesis (see Rothwell, 1989*b*). Destruction of the VMH apparently attenuates the development of fever (Blatteis, 1992), while electrical stimulation elicits marked increases in metabolic rate, body temperature and brown-fat activity in laboratory rodents (Perkins *et al.*, 1981; Holt *et al.*, 1987; Iwai *et al.*, 1987). Furthermore, the cytokine IL-1$\beta$ increases the firing rate of glucose-sensitive VMH neurones (Kuriyama *et al.*, 1990). The paraventricular nucleus (PVN) plays an important role in 'stress' responses, and is a primary site of synthesis of corticotrophin releasing factor (CRF) (Dunn & Berridge, 1990; Rothwell, 1990*b*) which is directly involved in CNS responses (including fever and thermogenesis) to pyrogens and injury (see below). Electrical stimulation of the PVN also elicits increases in body temperature and thermogenesis in the rat (Rothwell, 1989*b*), but although lesions of the PVN result in obesity and impaired diet-induced thermogenesis (see Rothwell, 1989*b*), their effects on metabolic and thermoregulatory responses to injury remain to be tested.

Several extrahypothalamic brain regions are likely to influence body temperature and metabolic rate after injury, either directly or indirectly, via synaptic connections with hypothalamic nuclei or release of mediators/modifiers of temperature and thermogenesis. For example, prepontine decerebration causes maximal activation of thermogenesis and dramatic decreases in body temperature and BAT activity (Benzi *et al.*, 1988) in the rat (Rothwell *et al.*, 1983; Shibata *et al.*, 1987), implying that brainstem regions exert tonic stimulation over these parameters. Structures such as the raphe nucleus, the locus coeruleus and Barrington's nucleus (in the pons) all influence autonomic responses, and are responsive to physical stress. The hippocampus is an important site of action of glucocorticoids, and shows the most dense staining for IL-1$\beta$ and its receptors (see Farrar *et al.*, 1987; Haour *et al.*, 1990; Cunningham *et al.*, 1991; and below).

At present, evidence to support a direct role of specific brain regions in the metabolic and thermoregulatory responses to injury are at best circumstantial and often derived from studies on related functions (e.g. fever, diet-induced thermogenesis). There is clearly a requirement for systematic investigation into specific brain regions in such responses, where primary emphasis might be placed on those regions involved in normal regulation of body temperature and autonomic function, or on brain areas implicated in other responses to trauma, e.g. the periaqueductal grey.

## CNS pathways

Current understanding of neurochemical mediators of the CNS control of metabolism and temperature in response to injury is principally derived from studies on normal physiological functions or closely related phenomena (e.g. fever and thermogenic responses to cold or diet). These indicate complex (and often poorly defined) relationships between noradrenergic, cholinergic, glutamatergic, GABA-ergic and serotonergic pathways, and have been reviewed in detail elsewhere (see Rothwell, 1989*b*).

Hypothalamic noradrenergic pathways, particularly the ventral noradrenergic bundle, appear to influence metabolic responses to peripheral injury in rodents (see Little, 1988), and the ratio of noradrenaline to serotonin release or turnover in the hypothalamus is particularly significant in thermoregulation (see Cooper, 1987; Blatteis, 1988). Peripheral administration of IL-1 (see below) markedly influences hypothalamic catecholamine turnover in the rat (see Dunn, 1988), and we have demonstrated that central administration of a 5-$HT_3$ receptor antagonist markedly inhibits the effects of IL-1 on temperature and thermogenesis in the rat (LeFeuvre & Rothwell, unpublished data).

Amir (1990) has demonstrated marked increases in thermogenesis in rats injected centrally with the amino acid glutamate. This excitatory transmitter is released in large quantities in response to many forms of brain damage (see Choi & Rothman, 1990; Meldrum, 1990), and induces release of IL-1 in the brain (see below) indicating a potential role in metabolic responses to brain damage. Inhibition of endogenous arachidonic acid release (and subsequent eicosanoid synthesis) in brain, by dietary modification in the rat, prevents thermogenic actions of glutamate (Cooper & Rothwell, unpublished data), indicating possible movement of eicosanoids in the effects of this amino acid (see below).

Nitric oxide has recently been identified as an endogenous modulator of synaptic activity in the brain and has been proposed as a mediator of ischaemic and excitotoxic brain damage (Beckman, 1991; Dawson *et al.*, 1991). Inhibition of nitric oxide synthase activity in the brain inhibits the pyrogenic and thermogenic responses to endotoxin in the rat, and indirect evidence suggests that nitric oxide may be involved in synthesis of IL-1 in the brain (LeFeuvre & Rothwell, unpublished data).

Research into the central mechanisms of thermogenic and thermoregulatory responses to injury and infection has largely focused on the actions of inflammatory mediators such as eicosanoids and cytokines, both of which act directly in the brain and have been strongly implicated in responses to injury.

### *Eicosanoids*

The importance of eicosanoids (mainly the prostaglandins) in the development of fever was first implied over four centuries ago, and is now supported by an extensive body of experimental and clinical data. Thus cyclooxygenase inhibitors, which prevent synthesis of prostaglandins, abolish or inhibit many forms of fever and associated changes in metabolic rate. Peripheral or central (into the brain or cerebral ventricles) injections of prostaglandins in experimental animals elicit rapid increases in body temperature and metabolic rate, and the concentrations of prostaglandins in the circulating cerebrospinal fluid (CSF) and locally in the brain are markedly increased in response to infection or administration of pyrogens (see Milton, 1982; Dascombe, 1985; Cooper, 1987; Blatteis, 1988).

However, the role of eicosanoids in metabolic and thermoregulatory responses to injury in the absence of associated fever is not as clear. Administration of cyclooxygenase inhibitors reportedly lowers body temperature in patients with various forms of injury (Childs & Little, 1988; Wallace *et al.*, 1992), although in some cases only modest, transient effects have been observed. From these observations it is difficult to distinguish the importance of eicosanoids at the site of injury or inflammation from their role as CNS mediators. An example of this is provided by the results of experiments on animals with localised sterile abscess (hindlimb turpentine). In this situation, the early rise in body temperature and metabolic rate is prevented by peripheral injection of a cyclooxygenase inhibitor (flurbiprofen), but is unaffected by central (intracerebroventricular (i.c.v.)) administration of a dose that blocks many other forms of fever (Cooper & Rothwell, 1991). These data suggest that cyclooxygenase products are released systemically, probably at the site of injury, where they may act as afferent signals, but are not involved in CNS control of early temperature and thermogenic responses. This proposal is supported by findings that inhibition of the cyclooxygenase enzyme is relatively ineffective in cases of brain damage. Children with severe head injury showed marked and sustained increases in body temperature, which are often resistant to treatment with cyclooxygenase inhibitors (C. Childs, personal communication). Similarly, brain trauma induced by focal cerebral ischaemia (MCAO) in the rat results in a delayed (6–8 h) increase in metabolic rate, which is unaffected by administration of cyclooxygenase or lipoxygenase inhibition (Relton, Rothwell & O'Shaughnessy, unpublished data).

In spite of these reservations, eicosanoid synthesis within the brain may be involved in metabolic and temperature responses to some forms of injury, are of undoubted importance in febrile responses to infection, and mediate many actions of cytokines within the CNS.

### *Cytokines*

Several endogenous cytokines have been shown to elicit marked increases in body temperature and metabolic rate, probably by direct actions on the brain (see Kluger, 1989, 1990; Rothwell, 1990*d*, 1991*b*, 1992). IL-1 was originally known as 'endogenous pyrogen', and is the subject of considerable research interest, so much of our current knowledge of cytokine action in the brain relates to IL-1.

Evidence that cytokines influence temperature and thermogenesis by direct effects within the CNS is summarised in Table 11.2. For example, very much lower doses (up to 1000-fold) are required to elicit maximal responses when recombinant cytokines are administered to rodents centrally (i.c.v.) rather than systemically (see Kluger, 1990; Rothwell, 1990*d*). IL-1, IL-6, IL-8, TNF$\alpha$ and IFN-$\gamma$ cause rapid and significant increases in body temperature and metabolic rate when injected into the

Table 11.2. *Experimental evidence for the action of cytokines as endogenous pyrogens in the brains of rodents*

| | IL-1α | IL-1β | IL-6 | TNFα |
|---|---|---|---|---|
| Increased circulating concentration in fever | +/− | +/? | +++ | + |
| Induced in brain during fever | − | ++ | +/? | +/? |
| Induction of fever thermogenesis in rats | | | | |
| Peripheral dose (ng) | 1000 | 1000 | >5000 | >5000 |
| Central dose (ng) | 50 | 5 | 30 | 50–100 |
| Effect on fever of i.c.v. injection of neutralising antibodies | − | ↓ | ↓ | ↓/↑ |

brain of conscious rodents in quantities of only a few picomoles (see Rothwell, 1990*d*). However, it is difficult to relate these doses and effects of recombinant materials to the actions or importance of endogenous brain cytokines. Inhibition of the actions of endogenous IL-1β or IL-6 by i.c.v. injection of neutralising antibodies to these cytokines markedly attenuates the pyrogenic and thermogenic responses to peripherally administered endotoxin in the rat (Rothwell *et al.*, 1990; 1992). In contrast, passive immunoneutralisation of brain IL-1α does not influence these responses to endotoxin (Rothwell *et al.*, 1990). Thus, endogenous brain IL-1β and IL-6 apparently mediate changes in body temperature and metabolic rate induced by systemic pyrogens. Preliminary data further indicate a role for IL-1β in the central control of metabolic and thermoregulatory responses to peripheral sterile inflammation in the rat (Cooper & Rothwell, unpublished data).

The source of these cytokines in the brain is unknown (see above), but IL-1, IL-6 and TNFα are expressed by neurones and glia within the CNS (see Koenig, 1991) and are increased following injury and infection (Table 11.3). Synthesis of IL-1β and its mRNA in the brain is markedly increased in experimental animals in response to peripheral or local administration of pyrogens, brain damage, focal ischaemia or mechanical injury, administration of convulsants or immobilisation stress (Fontana *et al.*, 1984; Giulian & Lachman, 1985; Higgins & Olschowka, 1991; Minami *et al.*, 1990, 1991, 1992; Ban *et al.*, 1992). In patients, CSF concentrations of IL-1 and IL-6 and TNF are reportedly elevated following head injury (McClain *et al.*, 1987, 1990; Goodman *et al.*, 1990),

Table 11.3. *Reported increases in expression of cytokines in the brains of experimental animals and patients*

| | |
|---|---|
| *Experimental* | |
| Pyrogens | IL-1, IL-6 |
| Seizures | IL-1$\beta$ |
| Injury | IL-1$\beta$ |
| Inflammation | IL-1$\beta$, TNF$\alpha$, IL-2 |
| Ischaemia | IL-1$\beta$ |
| *Clinical* | |
| Infection | IL-1, IL-6, TNF$\alpha$ |
| Injury | IL-1 |
| Multiple sclerosis | IL-2, ?IL-1 |
| Down's syndrome | IL-1 |
| Alzheimer's disease | IL-1, IL-6 |

during CNS infections (Frei *et al.*, 1990) or in multiple sclerosis (Merrill & Chen, 1991), and increased expression of IL-1 and IL-6 have been observed in chronic neurological disorders (e.g. AIDS, Alzheimer's disease) (Gallo *et al.*, 1989; Griffin *et al.*, 1989; Merrill & Chen, 1991). The sites of synthesis and action of cytokines in the brain probably vary depending on the stimulus and the response. Thus, brain injury causes increased synthesis locally, whereas stress or pyrogens result in IL-1$\beta$ expression predominantly in the hypothalamus (particularly the ventromedial hypothalamus).

Receptors for IL-1 and IL-6 have been identified in the rodent brain (Farrar *et al.*, 1987; Cunningham *et al.*, 1991; Schobitz *et al.*, 1992). In the case of IL-6, the pattern of localisation in the hypothalamus (Schobitz *et al.*, 1992) is consistent with the likely locus of action on temperature and metabolic rate. However, for IL-1 receptors the picture is more complex. Binding sites that exhibit properties consistent with the type 1 (80 kDa) IL-1 receptor have been identified in the hippocampus and choroid plexus, but contradictory reports exist on the identification of IL-1 receptors in the hypothalamus (Farrar *et al.*, 1987; Katsuura *et al.*, 1988; Haour *et al.*, 1990; Cunningham *et al.*, 1991). In laboratory rodents, the central effects of IL-1$\beta$ on body temperature and metabolic rate appear to depend on interaction with a type II (68 kDa) IL-1 receptor. Central injection of neutralising monoclonal antibody to the type II IL-1 receptor inhibits the effects of IL-1$\beta$ or endotoxin (but not IL-1$\alpha$) on fever and thermogenesis

(Luheshi, Rothwell, Dascombe & Hopkins, unpublished data). However, administration of recombinant interleukin-1 receptor antagonist protein (IL-1ra), which binds predominantly to the type I receptor and effectively inhibits actions in the periphery, does not influence the central effects of IL-1$\beta$ on fever or thermogenesis (Kent *et al.*, 1992). These data indicate that the two forms of IL-1 interact with different brain receptors and that selective inhibition of IL-1 actions in the brain may be possible through development of specific receptor antagonists.

Central effects of many pyrogenic cytokines (IL-1$\alpha$, IL-1$\beta$, TNF$\alpha$, IL-6, IFN-$\gamma$) on temperature and metabolic rate are dependent on prostanoid synthesis (see Blatteis, 1988, 1992; Rothwell, 1990*d*, 1991*a*, 1992), and probably $PGE_2$, although other prostaglandins (e.g. $PGF_2\alpha$) may also be involved. An exception to this are the smaller molecular weight (8 kDa) cytokines such as IL-8 and macrophage inflammatory protein, whose effects on fever are not blocked by cyclooxygenase inhibitors (see Rothwell, 1990*d*). Recent data have indicated that metabolic and pyrogenic effects of some cytokines are also dependent on synthesis of corticotrophin-releasing factor (CRF).

### *Corticotrophin-releasing factor*

CRF is best recognised as a hypothalamic releasing factor that activates the pituitary–adrenal axis. However, this peptide also has a number of direct actions within the brain, including stimulation of body temperature and metabolic rate, which are independent of the pituitary and illustrate the role of CRF as a mediator of many aspects of the stress response (see Rothwell, 1989*b*; Dunn & Berridge, 1990). Synthesis of brain CRF is stimulated by psychological stress, tissue damage or inflammation, and by cytokines and eicosanoids (see Rothwell, 1989*b*; Dunn & Berridge, 1990).

The increases in body temperature and thermogenesis that result from central injection of the cytokines IL-1$\beta$, IL-6 or IL-8 or prostaglandin $F_{2\alpha}$ in rodents are almost completely prevented by pretreatment with a CRF receptor antagonist or neutralizing antibody (Busbridge *et al.*, 1989; Rothwell, 1989*a*). It is now apparent that CRF mediates several actions of cytokines on the brain in addition to thermoregulatory and metabolic actions (e.g. pituitary adrenal activation, peripheral immune function, behavioural alterations). Central injections of CRF receptor antagonist or antibodies also attenuate the increases in metabolic rate and body temperature elicited by focal cerebral ischaemia (Relton & Rothwell, 1993) or sterile abscess in the rat (Cooper & Rothwell, 1991). However, the high cost and poor brain permeability of available CRF antagonists have so far precluded studies to test the involvement of brain CRF in responses to injury in humans.

### *Endogenous brain inhibitors*

Several naturally occurring inhibitors of fever and thermogenesis have been identified or proposed that may facilitate the development of effective therapeutic interventions. Glucocorticoids are potent antiinflammatory agents that inhibit the synthesis and/or actions of molecules such as eicosanoids, cytokines and CRF. Synthetic or natural glucocorticoids markedly inhibit pyrogenic and thermogenic responses to cytokines or peripheral injury in experimental animals, probably by direct actions on the brain. Antiinflammatory actions of glucocorticoids have been ascribed to release of an endogenous protein (or proteins) known as lipocortin-1 (annexin-1) (Flower, 1988). Central injection of recombinant lipocortin-1 markedly inhibits the increases in metabolic rate induced by cytokines or cerebral ischaemia in the rat (Carey *et al.*, 1990; Relton *et al.*, 1991). Lipocortin-1 is present in rodent and human brain (Johnson *et al.*, 1989; Strijbos *et al.*, 1991) and its expression is increased in response to local damage (e.g. brain injury, ischaemia, and inflammation (Johnson *et al.*, 1989; Relton *et al.*, 1991; Strijbos & Rothwell, unpublished data). Central injection of antibodies to neutralise brain lipocortin-1 largely reverses the antipyretic actions of glucocorticoids (Carey *et al.*, 1990) and normalises impaired pyrogenic and thermogenic responses to IL-1 in ageing or genetically obese rats and mice (Strijbos & Rothwell, unpublished data). Thus, lipocortin-1 appears to act as a mediator of glucocorticoid action and an endogenous inhibitor of metabolism and thermoregulatory responses to cytokines. However, lipocortin-1 synthesis in the brain can occur independently of glucocorticoid status, and the mechanism by which it modifies cytokine action appears to depend on inhibition of CRF action on temperature and metabolic rate, rather than on suppression of eicosanoid synthesis (Strijbos *et al.*, 1993).

α-Melanocyte stimulating hormone (α-MSH) and arginine vasopressin (AVP) inhibit actions of cytokines and have been proposed as endogenous inhibitors of fever (Lipton, 1990), although we have failed to observe effects on thermogenesis (Rothwell *et al.*, unpublished data) and their effects on responses to injury have not been tested.

An endogenous IL-1ra has recently been identified that competitively binds to IL-1 receptors and inhibits many biological actions of IL-1

(Eisenberg *et al.*, 1990). This IL-1ra, which shares about 25% sequence homology with IL-1$\alpha$ or IL-1$\beta$, is released into circulation in large quantities in response to inflammatory stimuli such as bacterial endotoxin (see Dinarello & Thompson, 1991). IL-1ra is also present in the brain (Licinio *et al.*, 1991), but its biological importance is unknown. Central administration of IL-1ra in the rat does not inhibit pyrogenic or thermogenic responses to IL-1$\beta$ (Kent *et al.*, 1992), although significant antipyretic effects have been reported in the rabbit (Opp & Kreuger, 1991). This antagonist does, however, potently inhibit neuronal damage induced by cerebral ischaemia in the rat brain (Relton & Rothwell, 1993).

## Clinical relevance and implications for treatment

It is not possible to investigate directly the central control of body temperature and thermogenesis in humans by experimental intervention. Therefore, the relevance of mediators and mechanisms demonstrated from studies on experimental animals remains uncertain (see Chapter 3). Nevertheless, observations in patients, and experiments on human volunteers are generally inconsistent with data obtained in animals. For example, similar patterns of temperature and metabolic responses and circulating concentrations of mediators such as cytokines, eicosanoids and glucocorticoids have been observed in a wide range of species, including humans. Expression of cytokines, prostaglandins, CRF and lipocortin-1 in human brain or CSF parallel those seen in animals subjected to experimental injury or infection. Direct evidence that parallel mechanisms operate in rodents and humans may be provided by the development of selective pharmacological interventions to modify specific points on the pathways that lead to alterations in body temperature and metabolic rate.

Such interventions may also be of therapeutic value in management of the injured patient. However, in order to justify such treatments, the overall value of modifying responses to injury must be critically considered. It has been argued that fever is a beneficial host defence response facilitating the elimination of invading pathogens (Kluger, 1990). Thus, antipyretic agents might be considered of dubious benefit. However, fever, like most aspects of the acute phase response and immune activation, is probably beneficial when activated in a controlled manner for limited duration, usually in response to modest and survivable insults. Excessive or sustained activation of the acute phase response can prove severely detrimental or even fatal. Furthermore, it should be noted that evolutionary advantages of such responses may be invalid with respect to seriously ill or injured patients, who benefit from a vast array of surgical and pharmacological interventions, allowing recovery from insults that would previously have proven fatal. Thus, 'defence response' in these patients may be completely inappropriate.

There is in fact no evidence that increases (or, more rarely encountered, decreases) in body temperature and metabolic rate offer advantages to injured animals or patients, and may be deleterious. For example, increases in temperature severely impair neuronal survival after brain damage (Busto *et al.*, 1989). Elevated temperature and metabolic rate impose additional demands for oxygen and substrates, at a time when both may already be limited, and lead to increased waste products (e.g. in lactacidosis). Sustained increases in metabolic rate, together with reduced food intake, leads to wasting of body energy reserves and the condition of cachexia. Cachexia, which is often associated with loss of body protein, impairs recovery and may be directly fatal, particularly in susceptible groups such as the very young or the very old.

The summary of our current knowledge of the cascade of events leading to increased body temperature and thermogenesis is shown in Figure 11.1 and indicates several potential sites of therapeutic intervention. Inhibition of nociceptive afferents or sensations of pain may limit subsequent responses. Similarly, inhibition of cytokine action either systemically or within the brain may influence many aspects of the acute phase response. Indeed, antibodies to TNF$\alpha$ and IL-1ra are both subjects of clinical trial for conditions such as septic shock, and may also prove effective in limiting thermoregulatory and metabolic responses. Identification of distinct IL-1 receptor subtypes within the brain, which mediate different actions of this cytokine, indicates the potential for selective intervention.

Suppression of eicosanoid synthesis is already used widely to limit fever, but may not be effective in injured patients (see above). Inhibition of actions of endogenous CRF release or action, or activation of endogenous inhibitory factors (e.g. lipocortin, $\alpha$-MSH, AVP) might modify temperature and metabolic responses and limit the extent of tissue damage. For example, lipocortin-1 potently inhibits ischaemic and excitotoxic brain damage in rodents, an effect that is not mimicked by glucocorticoids (Relton & Rothwell, 1993).

The functional importance of BAT in humans remains to be determined, but considerable effort is now being expended by the pharmaceutical industry to develop selective $\beta_3$ adrenoceptor agonists as potential antiobesity agents. $\beta_3$ antagonists might prove successful as inhibitors of hypermetabolic responses to injury, with the possible advantage that

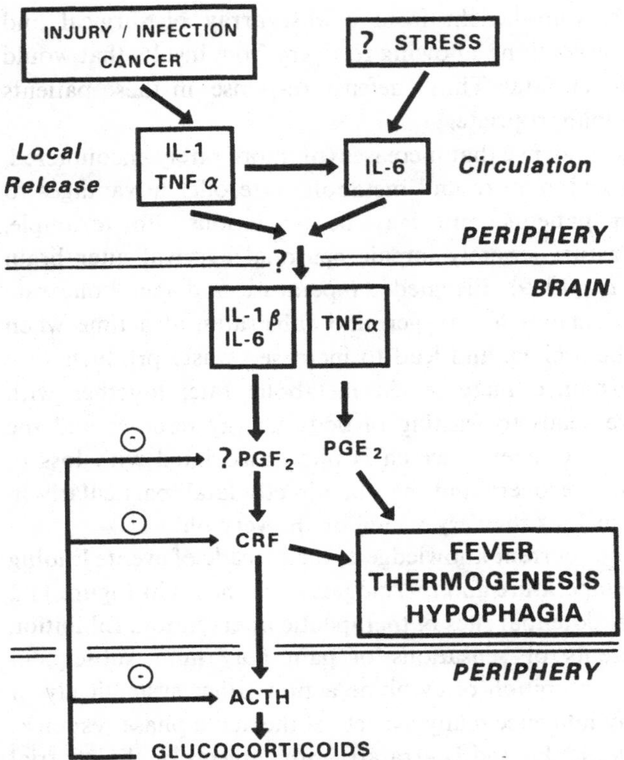


Figure 11.1. Hypothetical scheme of the possible involvement of cytokines and their mechanisms of action on fever, thermogenesis, food intake and the hypothalamic–pituitary–adrenal axis.

febrile responses (i.e. involving increases in set-point) would probably be unaffected, as alternative effector mechanisms are substituted. Dietary intervention, by altering the type of foods consumed voluntarily, or composition of parenteral and enteral feeds, is now emerging as an attractive method of patient care. Substitution or supplementation of diets with fatty acids of the omega-3 series reduces membrane arachidonic acid content, thus inhibiting the synthesis of pro-inflammatory eicosanoids. This treatment has been claimed to offer benefits to patients with chronic inflammatory conditions such as rheumatoid arthritis and psoriasis (Belch *et al.*, 1988; Bittiner *et al.*, 1988).

In rodents, dietary supplementation with eicosapentanoic acid markedly attenuates the increases in body temperature and metabolic rate induced by hindlimb inflammation or cytokine injection (Cooper & Rothwell, unpublished data). After 8–9 weeks of this supplementation, responses to central injection of IL-1 are attenuated, probably reflecting alteration in brain membrane composition, and at this time neurological damage sustained in rats after focal ischaemia or excitotoxic damage is also reduced (Cooper & Rothwell, 1993; Relton *et al.*, 1993). We have further observed that in human volunteers supplemented with 4.5 g omega-3 fatty acids per day for 6 weeks, fever and therogenic responses to intramuscular typhoid injection were reduced (Cooper *et al.*, 1993). Unfortunately, the time required (at least 4–6 weeks) for alterations in membrane composition, severely limits the benefits of dietary intervention in the treatment of acutely injured patients. Nevertheless, dietary modification could prove advantageous prior to elective surgery or in chronically ill patients.

It may be premature at the present time to consider specific therapeutic interventions to limit metabolic and thermoregulatory responses to injury. Nevertheless, within the past few years, research on this topic has led to important advances in our understanding of the mechanisms of such responses, and has provided further support and specific examples of the complex interactions between the immune system and the brain.

## References

Alexander, H. R., Dohert, G. M., Buresh, C. M., Vanzon, D. J. & Norton, J. A. (1991). A recombinant human receptor antagonist to interleukin-1 improves survival after lethal endotoxaemia in mice. *J. Exp. Med.*, **173**, 1029–32.

Amir, S. (1990). Intraventromedial injection of glutamate stimulates BAT thermogenesis. *Brain Res.*, **571**, 341–4.

Arch, J. R. S., Ainsworth, A. T., Cawthorne, M. A., Piercy, M. V., Sennitt, M. V., Thody, V. E. & Wilson, S. (1984) Atypical β-adrenoreceptor on brown adiopocytes: target for antiobesity drugs. *Nature*, **309**, 163–5.

Arnold, J., Rothwell, N. J. & Little, R. A. (1989). Energy balance and brown adipose tissue thermogenesis during chronic endotoxaemia in the rat. *J. Appl. Physiol.*, **66**, 1970–5.

Aulick, L. H. & Wilmore, D. W. (1983). Hypermetabolism in trauma. In *Mammalian Thermogenesis*, ed. L. Girardier & M. J. Stock, pp. 259–304. London: Chapman & Hall.

Baigrie, R. J., Lamont, P. M., Dallman, M. & Morris, P. J. (1991). The release of interleukin-1β (IL-1) precedes that of interleukin-6 (IL-6) in patients undergoing major surgery. *Lymphokine Cytokine Rev.*, **10**, 253–6.

Ban, E., Haour, F. & Leinstra, R. (1992). Brain interleukin 1 gene expression induced by peripheral lipopolysaccharide administration. *Cytokine*, **4**, 48–54.

Banks, W. A., Kastin, A. J. & Durham, D. A. (1990). Bidirectional transport of interleukin-1 alpha across the blood brain barrier. *Brain Res. Bull.*, **23**, 439–42.

Beckman, J. S. (1991). The double edged role of nitric oxide in brain function and superoxide-mediated injury. *J. Develop. Physiol.*, **15**, 53–9.
Belch, J. J. F., Ansell, D., Madhok, R., O'Dowd, A. & Sturrock, R. D. (1988). Effects of altering essential fatty acids on requirements for non-steroidal anti-inflammatory drugs in patients with rheumatoid arthritis: a double blind placebo controlled study. *Ann. Rheum. Dis.*, **47**, 96–104.
Benzi, R. H., Shibata, M., Seydoux, J. & Girardier, L. (1988). Prepontine knife cut induced hyperthermia in the rat. *Pflüers Archiv.*, **411**, 593–9.
Bessey, P. Q., Watters, J. M., Aoki, T. T. & Wilmore, D. W. (1985). Combined hormonal infusion stimulates the metabolic respone to injury. *Ann. Surg.*, **200**, 264–81.
Beutler, B., Milsark, I. W. & Cerami, A. (1985). Passive immunization against cachectin/tumor necrosis factor protects mice from lethal effects of endotoxin. *Science*, **229**, 869–71.
Bianchi, A., Bruce, J., Cooper, A. L., Childs, C., Kohli, M., Morris, I. D., Morris-Jones, P. & Rothwell, N. J. (1989). Increased brown adipose tissue activity in children with malignant diseases. *Horm. Metabol. Res.*, **21**, 587–642.
Bittiner, S. B., Tucker, W. F., Cartwright, I. & Bleehan, S. S. (1988). A double blind randomised placebo controlled trial of fish oil in psoriasis. *Lancet*, **1**, 378–80.
Blatteis, C. M. (1988). Neural mechanisms in the pyrogenic and acute phase responses to interleukin-1. *Int. J. Immunol., Neurosci.*, **38**, 223–32.
Blatteis, C. M. (1992). The pyrogenic actions of cytokines. In *Interleukin-1 in the Brain*, ed. N. J. Rothwell & R. Dantzer, pp. 115–34. London: Pergamon Press.
Breitenstein, E., Chiolero, R. L., Jequier, E., Dayer, P., Krupp, S. & Schutz, Y. (1990). Effects of beta-blockade on energy metabolism following burns. *Burns*, **16**, 259–64.
Broukaert, P., Spriggs, D. R., Demetri, G., Kuffe, D. W. & Fiers, W. (1989). Circulating interleukin-6 during a continuous infusion of tumor necrosis factor and interferon-gamma. *J. Exp. Med.*, **169**, 2257–62.
Bruce, J., Childs, C. C., Cooper, A. L. & Rothwell, N. J. (1990). Brown adipose tissue in relation to disease status. *Proc. Nutr. Soc.*, **49**, 189A.
Busbridge, N. J., Dascombe, M. J., Tilders, F. J. A., van Oers, J. W. A. M., Linton, E. A. & Rothwell, N. J. (1989). Central activation of thermogenesis and fever by interleukin-1$\beta$ and interleukin-1$\alpha$ involves different mechanisms. *Biochem. Biophys. Res. Commun.*, **162**, 591–6.
Busto, R., Dietrich, M. Y. T., Globus, I. & Ginsberg, M. D. (1989). The importance of brain temperature in cerebral ischaemic injury. *Stroke*, **20**, 1113–20.
Calandra, T., Baumgartner, J. D., Grau, G. E., Wu, M. M., Lambert, P. H., Schellekens, J., Vehoef, J., Glauser, M. P. & The Swiss–Dutch JC Immunoglobulin study group. (1990). Prognostic values of tumor necrosis factor/cachectin, interleukin-1, interferon $\alpha$ and interferon-gamma in the serum of patients with septic shock. *J. Infect. Dis.*, **161**, 982–7.
Cannon, J. G., Gelfand, J. A., Tompkins, R. G., Hegarty, M. T., Burke, J. F. & Dinarello, C. A. (1990*a*). Plasma IL-1$\beta$ and TNF$\alpha$ levels in humans following cutaneous injury. In *The Physiological and Pathological Effects of Cytokines*, pp. 301–6. New York: Wiley–Liss Inc.
Cannon, J. G., Tompkins, R. G., Gelfand, J. A., Michie, H. R., Stanford, G. G., van der Meer, J. W., Endres, S., Lonneman, G., Corsetti, J., Chernow, B., Burke, J. F. & Dinarello, C. A. (1990*b*). Circulating interleukin-1 and

tumor necrosis factor in septic shock and experimental endotoxin fever. *J. Infect. Dis.*, **161**, 79–84.
Carey, F., Forder, R., Edge, M. D., Greene, A. R., Horan, M. A., Strijbos, P. J. L. M. & Rothwell, N. J. (1990). Lipocortin 1 fragment modifies the pyrogenic actions of cytokines in the rat. *Am. J. Physiol.*, **259**, R266–R269.
Carli, F. & Aber, V. R. (1987). Thermogenesis after major elective surgical procedures. *Br. J. Surg.*, **74**, 1041–4.
Childs, C. (1988). Fever in burned children. *Burns*, **14**, 1–6.
Childs, C. (1993). Oxygen consumption during the acute phase of burn injury in infants and children. *Proc. Nutr. Soc.*, **52**, 4A.
Childs, C., Hall, T., Davenport, P. & Little, R. A. (1990). Dietary intake and changes in body weight in burned children. *Burns*, **16**, 418–22.
Childs, C. & Little, R. A. (1988). Acetaminophen (paracetamol) in the management of burned children with fever. *Burns*, **14**, 343–8.
Choi, D. W. & Rothman, S. M. (1990). The role of glutamate neurotoxicity in hypoxic ischaemic neuronal death. *Ann. Rev. Neurosci.*, **13**, 171–82.
Clifton, G. L., Robertson, C. S. & Grossman, R. G. (1989). Cardiovascular and metabolic responses to severe head injury. *Neurosurg. Rev.*, **12**, 465–73.
Cooper, A. L., Fitzgeorge, R. B. F., Baskerville, A., Little, R. A. & Rothwell, N. J. (1989). Bacterial infection (*Legionella pneumophila*) stimulates fever, metabolic rate and brown adipose tissue activity in the guinea-pig. *Life Sci.*, **45**, 843–7.
Cooper, A. L., Gibbons, L., Horan, M. A., Little, R. A. & Rothwell, N. J. (1993). Effect of dietary fish oil supplementation on responses to typhoid vaccine and cytokine production in human volunteers. *Clin. Nutr.*, in press.
Cooper, A. L., Horan, M. A., Little, R. A. & Rothwell, N. J. (1992). Metabolic and febrile responses to typhoid vaccine in humans: effect of β-adrenergic blockade. *J. Appl. Physiol.*, **72**, 2322–38.
Cooper, A. L. & Rothwell, N. J. (1991). Mechanisms of the early and late hypermetabolism and fever after localised tissue injury in rats. *Am. J. Physiol.*, **261**, E687–E705.
Cooper, A. L. & Rothwell, N. J. (1993). Inhibition of the thermogenic and pyrogenic responses to interleukin-1β by dietary n-3 fatty acid supplementation. *Prostaglandins, Leukotrienes, Essent. Fatty Acids*, **49**, 615–26.
Cooper, K. E. (1987). The neurobiology of fever: thoughts on recent developments. *Ann. Rev. Neursci.*, **10**, 297–24.
Cunningham, E. T. Jr, Wada, E., Carter, D. B., Tracey, D. E., Battey, J. F. & DeSouza, E. B. (1991). Localization of interleukin-1 receptor messenger in murine hippocampus. *Endocrinology*, **128**, 2666–8.
Cuthbertson, D. P. (1932). Observation in the disturbance of metabolism produced by injury to the limbs. *Q. J. Exp. Med.*, **1**, 233–46.
Dascombe, M. J. (1985). The pharmacology of fever. *Rev. Inf. Dis.*, **6**, 51–95.
Dascombe, M. J., Rothwell, N. J., Sagay, B. O. & Stock, M. J. (1989). Pyrogenic and thermogenic effects of interleukin-1β in the rat. *Am. J. Physiol.*, **256**, E7–E11.
Dawson, V. L., Dawson, T. M., London, E. D., Bredt, D. S. & Snyder, S. H. (1991). Nitric oxide mediates glutamate neurotoxicity in primary cortical cultures. *Proc. Natl. Acad. Sci. USA*, **88**, 6368–77.
deGroot, M. A., Martin, M. A., Densen, P., Pfaller, M. A. & Wenzel, R. P. (1989). Plasma TNF levels in patients with presumed sepsis. *J. Am. Med. Assoc.*, **262**, 249–51.

Dinarello, C. A. (1991). Interleukin-1 and interleukin-1 antagonism. *Blood*, **77**, 1627–52.

Dinarello, C. A. & Thompson, R. C. (1991). Blocking IL-1: interleukin-1 receptor antagonist *in vivo* and *in vitro*. *Immunol. Today*, **12**, 404–10.

Dofferhoff, A. S., Bom, V. J., de Vries-Hospers, H. G., van Ingen, J., van der Meer, J., Hazenberg, B. P., Mulder, P. O. & Weits, J. (1992). Patterns of cytokines, plasma endotoxin, plasminogen activator inhibitor, and acute-phase proteins during the treatment of severe sepsis in humans. *Crit. Care Med.*, **20**, 185–92.

Duke, J. H., Jorgensen, S. B., Broell, J. R., Long, C. L. & Kinney, J. M. (1970). Contribution of protein to caloric expenditure following injury. *Surgery*, **68**, 168–74.

Dunn, A. J. (1988). Systemic interleukin-1 administration stimulates hypothalamic norepinephrine metabolism paralleling the increased plasma corticosterone. *Life Sci.*, **43**, 429–435.

Dunn, A. J. & Berridge, C. W. (1990). Physiological and behavioural responses to corticotrophin releasing factor: is CRF a mediator of anxiety or stress responses? *Brain Res. Rev.*, **15**, 71–100.

Edwards, J. D., Redmond, A. D., Nightengale, P. & Wilkins, R. G. (1988). Oxygen consumption following trauma: a reappraisal in severely injured patients requiring mechanical ventilation. *Br. J. Surg.*, **75**, 690–2.

Eisenberg, S. P., Evans, R. J., Arend, W. P., Verderber, E., Brewer, M. T., Hannum, C. H. & Thompson, R. S. (1990). Interleukin-1 receptor antagonist activity of a human interleukin-1 inhibitor. *Nature*, **343**, 341–6.

Elwyn, D. H., Kinney, J. M. & Askanasi, J. (1981). Energy expenditure in surgical patients. *Surg. Clin. N. Am.*, **61**, 545–56.

Farrar, W. L., Kilian, P. C., Ruff, M. R., Hill, J. M. & Pert, C. B. (1987). Visualization and characterization of interleukin 1 receptors in brain. *J. Immunol.*, **139**, 459–63.

Flower, R. J. (1988). Lipocortin and the mechanisms of action of the glucocorticoids. *Br. J. Pharmacol.*, **65**, 987–1015.

Fontana, A., Weber, E. & Dayer, J.-M. (1984). Synthesis of interleukin-1/endogenous pyrogen in the brain of endotoxin-treated mice: a step in fever induction? *J. Exp. Med.*, **133**, 1696–8.

Frayn, K. N., Little, R. A. & Stoner, H. B. (1984). Metabolic control in non-septic patients with musculoskeletal injuries. *Injury*, **16**, 73–79.

Frei, K., Nadal, D. & Fontana, A. (1990). Intracerebral synthesis of tumour necrosis factor-alpha and interleukin-6 in infectious meningitis. *Ann. NY Acad. Sci.*, **594**, 326–35.

Gallo, P., Frei, K., Rordorf, C., Lazdins, J., Tavolato, B. & Fontana, A. (1989). Human immunodeficiency virus type 1 (HIV-1) infection of the central nervous system: an evaluation of cytokines in cerebrospinal fluid. *J. Neuroimmunol.*, **23**, 109–16.

Gershenwald, J. E., Fong, Y., Fahey, T. J., Calvano, S. E., Chizzonite, R., Killian, P. L., Lowry, S. F. & Moldawer, L. L. (1990). Interleukin-1 receptor blockade attenuates the host inflammatory response. *Proc. Natl. Acad. Sci.*, **87**, 4966–70.

Giulian, D. & Lachman, L. B. (1985). Interleukin-1 stimulation of astroglial proliferation after brain injury. *Science*, **228**, 497–9.

Goodman, J. C., Robertson, C. S., Grossman, R. G. & Narayan, R. K. (1990). Elevation of tumour necrosis in head injury. *J. Neuroimmunol.*, **30**, 213–17.

Griffin, W. S. T., Stanley, L. C., Ling, C., White, L., MacLeod, V., Perrot, L. J.,

White, C. L. & Araoz, C. (1989). Brain interleukin-1 and S-100 immunoreactivity are elevated in Down's Syndrome and Alzheimer's disease. *Proc. Natl. Acad. Sci. USA*, **86**, 7611–22.

Groner, J. I., Brown, M. F., Stallings, V. A., Ziegler, M. M. & O'Neill, J. A. (1989). Resting energy expenditure in children following major operative procedures. *J. Pediatr. Surg.*, **24**, 825–7.

Hack, C. E., deGroot, E. R., Felt-Bersma, R. J., Nuijens, J. H., Strack van Schijndel, R. J., Erenberg-Belmer, A. J., Thijs, L. G. & Aarden, L. A. (1989). Increased plasma levels of interleukin-6 in sepsis. *Blood*, **74**, 1704–10.

Hadfield, J. (1990). Patterns of metabolic response after head injury. MSc Thesis, Manchester University, UK.

Haour, F. G., Ban, E. M., Milon, G. M., Baran, D. & Fillion, G. M. (1990). Brain interleukin-1 receptors: characterisation and modulation after lipopolysaccharide injection. *Prog. Neuro. Endocrin. Immunol.*, **3**, 196–204.

Helle, M., Brakenhoff, J. P. J., DeGroot, E. R. & Aarden, L. A. (1988). Interleukin 6 involved in interleukin-1 induced activities. *Eur. J. Immunol.*, **18**, 957–9.

Hesse, D. G., Tracey, K. J., Fong, Y., Manogue, K. R., Pallindino, M. A., Cerami, A., Shires, G. T. & Lowry, S. F. (1988). Cytokine appearance in human endotoxaemia and primate bacteremia. *Surg. Gynecol. Obstet.*, **166**, 147–53.

Higgins, G. A. & Olschowka, J. A. (1991). Induction of interleukin-1$\beta$ mRNA in adult rat brain. *Mol. Brain Res.*, **9**, 143–8.

Hinshaw, L. B., Tekamp-Olsen, P., Chang, A. C. K., Lee, P. A., Taylor, F. B. Jr, Murray, C. K., Peer, G. T., Emergon, T. E. Jr, Poassey, R. B. & Juo, G. C. (1990). Survival of primates in $LD_{100}$ septic shock following therapy with antibody to tumor necrosis factor (TNF-alpha). *Circ. Shock*, **30**, 279–92.

Holt, S., Wheal, H. & York, D. A. (1987). Hypothalamic control of BAT in Zucker lean and obese rats; effects of electrical stimulation of the VMH and other hypothalamic nuclei. *Brain Res.*, **403**, 227–33.

Horan, M. A., Gibbons, L., Hopkins, S. J., Cooper, A. L., Stijbos, P. J. L. M., Rothwell, N. J. & Little, R. A. (1989). Changes in interleukin-6 during experimentally-induced fever in humans. *Cytokine*, **1**, 138A.

Iwai, M., Hell, N. S. & Shimazu, T. (1987). Effects of VMH stimulation on blood flow of BAT in rats. *Pflügers Archiv.*, **410**, 44–7.

Jahoor, F., Desai, M., Herndon, D. N. & Wolfe, R. R. (1988). Dynamics of the protein metabolic response to burn injury. *Metabolism*, **37**, 330–7.

Jepson, M. M., Millward, D. J., Rothwell, N. J. & Stock, M. J. (1988). Involvement of the sympathetic nervous system in endotoxin-induced fever in the rat. *Am. J. Physiol.*, **255**, E617–23.

Johnson, M. D., Kameo-Pratt, J. M., Whetsell, W. O. & Pepinsky, R. B. (1989). Lipocortin-1 immunoreactivity in the normal human central nervous system and in lesions with astrocytosis. *Am. J. Clin. Pathol.*, **92**, 424–9.

Katsuura, G., Gottenschall, P. G. & Arimura, A. (1988). Identification of a high affinity receptor for interleukin-1 beta in rat brain. *Biochem. Biophys. Res. Commun.*, **50**, 61–7.

Kent, S., Bluthe, R. M., Dantzer, R., Hardwick, A. J., Kelley, K. W., Rothwell, N. J. & Varnie, J. L. (1992). Different receptor mechanisms mediate the pyrogenic and behavioural effects of interleukin-1. *Proc. Nat. Acad. Sci. USA*, **89**, 9117–20.

Kluger, M. J. (1989). Body temperature changes during inflammation: their mediation and nutritional significance. *Proc. Nutr. Soc.*, **48**, 337–45.

Kluger, M. J. (1990). Fever: role of pyrogens and cryogens. *Physiol. Rev.*, **71**, 93–127.
Koenig, J. T. (1991). Presence of cytokines in the hypothalamic–pituitary axis. *Prof. Neuro. Endocrinimmunol.*, **4**, 143–53.
Kupper, T. S., Deitch, E. A., Baker, C. C. & Wong, W. (1986). The human burn wound as a primary source of interleukin-1 activity. *Surgery*, **100**, 409–15.
Kuriyama, K., Mori, T. & Nakashima, T. (1990). Activities of interferon α and interleukin-1β on the glucose responsive necrosis of the ventromedial hypothalamus. *Brain Res.*, **24**, 803–10.
Lean, M. E. J. & James, W. P. T. (1986). Brown adipose tissue in man. In *Brown Adipose Tissue*, ed. P. Trayhurn & D. G. Nichols, pp. 339–65. London: Arnold.
LeMay, L. G., Otterness, G. I., Vander, A. J. & Kluger, M. J. (1990*a*). *In vivo* evidence that the rise in plasma IL-6 following injection of fever-inducing doses of LPS is mediated by IL-1β. *Cytokine*, **2**, 199–204.
LeMay, L. G., Vander, A. J. & Kluger, M. J. (1990*b*). Role of interleukin-6 in fever in rats. *Am. J. Physiol.*, **258**, R798–803.
Licinio, J., Wong, M. L. & Gold, P. W. (1991). Localisation of interleukin-1 receptor antagonist mRNA in rat brain. *Endocrinology*, **129**, 562–4.
Lipton, J. M. (1990). Modulation of host defence response by αMSH. *Yale J. Biol. Med.*, **63**, 173–82.
Little, R. A. (1988). Metabolic rate and thermoregulation after injury. In *Recent Advances in Critical Care Medicine*, vol. 3, ed. I. Ledingham, pp. 159–72.
Little, R. A. & Stoner, H. B. (1981). Body temperature after accidental injury. *Br. J. Surg.*, 68, 221–4.
Long, C. L. (1977). Energy balance and carbohydrate metabolism in infection and sepsis. *Am. J. Clin. Nutr.*, **30**, 1301–10.
Long, N. C., Kunkel, S. L., Vander, A. J. & Kluger, M. J. (1989). Antiserum against TNF enhances LPS fever in the rat. *Am. J. Physiol.*, **258**, R332–7.
Long, N. C., Otterness, I., Kunkel, S. L., Vander, A. J. & Kluger, M. J. (1990). Roles of interleukin 1β and tumor necrosis factor in lipopolysaccharide fever in rats. *Am. J. Physiol.*, **259**, R724–8.
Marano, M. A., Fong, Y., Modawer, L. L., Wei, H., Calvano, S. E., Tracey, K. J., Barie, P. S., Manogue, K., Cerami, A., Shires, G. T. & Lowry, S. (1990). Serum cachectin/tumour necrosis factor in critically ill patients with burns correlates with infection and mortality. *Surg. Gynecol. Obstet.*, **170**, 23–8.
Matsuda, T., Clark, N., Hariyani, G. D., Bryant, R. S., Hanumasass, M. L. & Kagan, R. J. (1987). The effect of burn wound size on resting energy expenditure. *J. Trauma*, **27**, 115–18.
McClain, C., Cohen, D., Ott, L., Dinarello, C. A. & Young, B. (1987). Ventricular fluid interleukin-1 activity in patients with head injury. *J. Lab. Clin. Med.*, **110**, 48–54.
McClain, C., Cohen, D., Phillips, R., Miller, B., Talwalker, R. & Young, B. (1990). Increased plasma interleukin-6 levels in head injury. In *The Physiological and Pathological Effects of Cytokines*, pp. 61–7. New York: Wiley-Liss.
Meldrum, B. (1990). Pathophysiology of cerebral ischaemia and trauma in relation to possible therapeutic approaches. In *Current and Future Trends in Anticonvulsant Anxiety and Stroke Therapy*, pp. 275–90. New York: Wiley-Liss.
Merrill, J. E. & Chen, I. S. (1991). HIV-1, macrophages, glial cells, and

cytokines in AIDS nervous system disease. *Fed. Am. Soc. Exp. Biol. J.*, **5**, 2391–7.

Michie, H. R., Manoque, K. R., Spriggs, D. E., Revhang, A., O'Dwyer, S., Dinarello, C. A., Cerani, A., Wolff, S. M. & Wilmore, D. W. (1988). Detection of circulating tumor necrosis factor after endotoxin administration. *N. Eng. J. Med.*, **318**, 1481–6.

Milton, A. S. (1982). Prostaglandin in fever and the mode of action of antipyretics. In *Pyretics and Antipyretics*, ed. A. S. Milton, pp. 257–97. Heidelberg: Springer-Verlag.

Minami, M., Kuraishi, Y. Yamaguchi, T., Nakai, S., Hirai, Y. & Sato, M. (1990). Convulsants induce interleukin-1$\beta$ messenger RNA in rat brain. *Biochem. Biophys. Res. Commun.*, **171**, 832–7.

Minami, M., Kuraishi, Y., Yamaguchi, T., Nakai, S., Hirai, Y. & Satoh, M. (1991). Immobilisation stress induced interleukin-1 mRNA in the rat hypothalamus. *Neurosci. Lett.*, **123**, 254–6.

Minami, M., Kuraishi, Y., Yabuuchi, K., Yamazaki, A. & Sato, M. (1992). Induction of interleukin-1$\beta$ mRNA in rat brain after transient fore brain ischaemia. *J. Neurochem.*, **58**, 389–2.

Moldawer, L. L., Gelin, J., Schersten, T. & Lundholm, K. G. (1987). Circulating interleukin-1 and tumor necrosis factor during inflammation. *Am. J. Physiol.*, **253**, R922–8.

Moore, R., Najarian, M. P. & Konvolinka, C. W. (1989). Measured energy expenditure in severe head trauma. *J. Trauma*, **29**, 1633–6.

Nicholls, D. G. & Locke, R. (1984). Thermogenic mechanisms in brown fat. *Physiol. Rev.*, **64**, 1–64.

Nijsten, N. W. N., deGroot, E. R., ten Duis, H. R., Klasen, H. R., Hack, C. E. & Aarden, L. A. (1987). Serum levels of interleukin-6 during acute phase responses. *Lancet*, **ii**, 921.

Opp, M. & Krueger, J. M. (1991). Interleukin-1 receptor antagonist blocks interleukin-1 induced sleep and fever. *Am. J. Physiol.*, **260**, R453–7.

O'Shaughnessy, C. T., Rothwell, N. J. & Shrewsbury-Gee, J. (1990). Sympathetically mediated hpermetabolic response to cerebral ischaemia in the rat. *Can. J. Phys. Pharm.*, **63**, 1334–7.

Ott, L., Young, B. & McClain, C. (1987). The metabolic response to brain injury. *J. Parenter. Enteral Nutr.*, **11**, 488–93.

Perkins, M. N., Rothwell, N. J., Stock, M. J. & Stone, T. W. (1981). Activation of brown adipose tissue thermogenesis by the ventromedial hypothalamus. *Nature*, **89**, 401–2.

Pullicino, E. A., Carli, F., Poole, S., Rafferty, B., Malik, B. & Elia, M. (1990). The relationship between circulating concentrations of interleukin-6 (IL-6) and tumour necrosis factor and the acute phase response to elective surgery and accidental injury. *Lymphokine Res.*, **9**, 231–8.

Rady, M. Y., Little, R. A., Edwards, J. D., Kirdman, E. & Faithful, S. (1991). The effect of nociceptive stimulation on the changes in hemodynamics and oxygen transport induced by hermorrhage in anaesthetized pigs. *J. Trauma*, **31**, 617–22.

Redfern, W. S., Little, R. A., Stoner, H. B. & Marshall, H. W. (1984). Effect of limb ischaemia on blood pressure and the blood pressure–heart rate reflex in the rat. *Q. J. Exp. Physiol.*, **69**, 763–79.

Relton, J. K. & Rothwell, N. J. (1993). Interleukin-1 receptor antagonist inhibits neuronal damage induced by cerebral ischaemia or NMDA-receptor activation in the rat. *Brain Res. Bull.*, **29**, 243–6.

Relton, J. K., Strijbos, P. J., Cooper, A. L. & Rothwell, N. J. (1993). Inhibition of ischaemic and excitotoxic brain damage in the rat by dietary supplementation with n-3 fatty acids. *Brain Res. Bull.*, **32**, 223–6.

Relton, J. K., Strijbos, P. J., O'Shaughnessey, C. T., Carey, F., Forder, R. A., Tilders, F. J. & Rothwell, N. J. (1991). Lipocortin-1 is an endogenous inhibitor of ischaemic damage in the rat brain. *J. Exp. Med.*, **174**, 305–10.

Revhaug, A., Mitchie, H. R., Mansin, J. M. K., Watters, J. M., Dinarello, C. A., Wolff, S. M. & Wilmore, D. W. (1988). Inhibition of cyclo-oxygenase attenuates the metabolic response to endotoxin in humans. *Arch. Surg.*, **123**, 162–70.

Rothwell, N. J. (1989*a*). CRF is involved in the pyrogenic and thermogenic effects of interleukin 1$\beta$ in the rat. *Am. J. Physiol.*, **256**, E111–5.

Rothwell, N. J. (1989*b*). Central control of thermogenesis. *Proc. Nutr. Soc.*, 48, 241–50.

Rothwell, N. J. (1990*a*). Thermogenesis in obesity and cachexia. In *Endocrinology and Metabolism–Hormones and Nutrition in Obesity and Cachexia*, ed. M. Muller, pp. 77–85. Heidelberg: Springer.

Rothwell, N. J. (1990*b*). Central effects of CRF on metabolism and energy balance. *Neurosci. Biobehav. Rev.*, **14**, 263–71.

Rothwell, N. J. (1990*c*). Central activation of thermogenesis by prostaglandins, dependence on CRF. *Horm. Metabol. Res.*, **22**, 616–18.

Rothwell, N. J. (1990*d*). Mechanisms of the pyrogenic effects of cytokines. *Eur. Cytokine Network*, **1**, 211–13.

Rothwell, N. J. (1991*a*). The endocrine significance of cytokines. *J. Endoc.*, **128**, 171–3.

Rothwell, N. J. (1991*b*). Functions and mechanisms of interleukin-1 in the brain. *Trends Pharm. Sci.*, **12**, 430–6.

Rothwell, N. J. (1992). Metabolic responses to interleukin-1. In *Interleukin-*1 *in the Brain*, ed. N. J. Rothwell & R. Dantzer, pp. 115–34. London: Pergamon Press.

Rothwell, N. J., Busbridge, N. J., Humpray, H. & Hissey, P. (1990). Central actions of interleukin-1$\beta$ on fever and thermogenesis. *Prog. Leukocyte Biol.*, **108**, 307.

Rothwell, N. J., Busbridge, N. J., LeFeuvre, R. A., Hardwick, A. J., Gauldie, J. & Hopkins, S. J. (1992). Interleukin-6 is a centrally acting endogenous pyrogen in the rat. *Can. J. Physiol. Pharmacol.*, **69**, 1465–9.

Rothwell, N. J., Little, R. A. & Rose, J. G. (1991). Brown adipose tissue activity and oxygen consumption after scald injury in the rat. *Circ. Shock*, **33**, 33–6.

Rothwell, N. J. & Relton, J. K. (1993). Involvement of cytokines in acute neurodegeneration in the CNS. *Neurosci. Behav. Rev.*, **17**, 217–27.

Rothwell, N. J., Stock, M. J. & Thexton, A. J. (1983). Decerebration activates thermogenesis in the rat. *J. Physiol.*, **342**, 15–22.

Scarpace, P. J., Bender, B. S. & Borst, S. E. (1991). *Escherichia coli* peritonitis activates thermogenesis in brown adipose tissue: relationship to fever. *Can. J. Phys. Pharm.*, **69**, 761–6.

Schmidt, K. D. & Chan, C. W. (1990). Thermoregulation and fever in normal persons and in those with spinal cord injuries. *Mayo Clin. Proc.*, **67**, 469–75.

Schobitz, B., Voorhuis, D. A. M. & deKloet, E. R. (1992). Localization of interleukin-6 mRNA and interleukin-6 mRNA in rat brain. *Neurosci. Lett.*, **136**, 189–92.

Shalaby, M. R., Waage, A., Aarden, L. & Espevik, T. (1989). Endotoxin tumor necrosis factor α and interleukin-1 induce interleukin-6 production *in vivo*. *Clin. Immunol. Immunopathol.*, **53**, 488–98.

Shenkin, A., Fraser, W. D., Series, J., Winstanley, F. P., McCartney, A. C., Burns, H. J. & Van Damme, J. (1989). The serum interleukin-6 response to elective surgery. *Lymphokine Res.*, **8**, 123–7.

Shibata, M., Benzi, R. H., Seydoux, J. & Girardier, L. (1987). Hyperthermia induced by proptic knife-cut: evidence for tonic inhibition of NST in anaesthetised rat. *Brain Res.*, **436**, 272–82.

Silva, A. T., Bayston, K. F. & Cohen, J. (1990). Prophylactic and therapeutic effects of a monoclonal antibody to TNF-alpha in experimental gram-negative shock. *J. Infect. Dis.*, **162**, 421–7.

Stoner, H. B. (1961). Critical analysis of trauma and shock model. *Fred. Proc.*, **20**, 38–50.

Strijbos, P. J. L. M., Hardwick, A. J., Relton, J. K., Carey, F. & Rothwell, N. J. (1993). Inhibition of the central actions of cytokines on fever and thermogenesis by lipocortin-1 involves CRF. *Am. J. Physiol.*, **256**, E289–97.

Strijbos, P. J. L. M., Tilders, F. J. H., Carey, F., Forder, R. & Rothwell, N. J. (1991). Localisation of immunoreactive lipocortin-1 in the brain and the pituitary gland of the rat: effects of adrenalectomy, dexamethane and colchicine treatment. *Brain Res.*, **553**, 249–60.

Stylianos, S., Wakabayashi, G., Gelfand, J. A. & Harris, B. H. (1991). Experimental hemorrhage and blunt trauma do not increase circulating tumor necrosis factor. *J. Trauma*, **31**, 1063–7.

Szabo, K. (1979). Clinical experiences with beta adrenergic blockade therapy on burned patients. *Scand. J. Plast. Reconst.*, **13**, 211–15.

Szekely, A. U. & Scolcsanyi, J. (1979). Endotoxin fever in capsaicin treated rats. *Acat. Physiol. Acta. Sci. Hung.*, **53**, 469–77.

Threlfall, C. J., Little, R. A. & Frayn, K. N. (1980). The post-scald metabolic response in the growing rat: evidence for a transient phase of muscle protein breakdown. *Burns*, **7**, 25–32.

Waage, A., Brandtzaeg, P., Halstensen, A., Kierulf, P. & Espevik, T. (1989). The complex pattern of cytokines in serum from patients with meningococcal septic shock. Association between interleukin-1, interleukin-6 and fatal outcome. *J. Exp. Med.*, **169**, 333–8.

Waage, A., Halstensen, A. & Espevik, T. (1987). Association between tumour necrosis factor in serum and fatal outcome in patients with meningococcal disease. *Lancet*, **i**, 355–7.

Wallace, B. H., Caldwell, F. T. & Cone, J. B. (1992). Ibuprofen lowers body temperature and metabolic rate of humans with burn injury. *J. Trauma*, **32**, 154–7.

Watters, J. M., Bessey, P. Q., Dinarello, C. A., Wolf, S. M. & Willmore, D. W. (1986). Both inflammatory and endocrine mediators stimulate host responses to sepsis. *Arch. Surg.*, **121**, 179–90.

Whicher, J. & Ingham, E. (1990). Cytokine measurements in body fluids. *Eur. Cytokine Net.*, **1**, 239–43.

Wilmore, D. W. (1976). Hormonal responses and their effect on metabolism. *Surg. Clin. N. Am.*, **56**, 999–1008.

Wilmore, D. W., Long, J. M., Mason, A. D. & Pruitt, B. (1974). Catecholamines: mediators of the hypermetabolic response to thermal injury. *Ann. Surg.*, **180**, 653–99.

Wilmore, D. W., Mason, A. D., Johnson, D. W. & Pruitt, B. A. (1975). Effect of ambient temperature on heat production and heat loss in burn patients. *J.Appl. Physiol.*, **38**, 593–7.

Winthrop, A. L., Wesson, D. E., Pencharz, P. B., Jacobs, D. G., Heim, T. & Filler, R. M. (1987). Injury severity, whole body protein turnover and energy expenditure in pediatric trauma. *J. Pediatr. Surg.*, **22**, 534–7.

Wolfe, R. R. & Durkot, M. J. (1982). Evaluation of the role of the sympathetic nervous system in the response of substrate kinetics and oxidation to burn injury. *Circ. Shock*, **9**, 396–406.

Wolfe, R. R., Herndon, D. N., Jahoor, F., Miyoshi, H. & Wolfe, M. (1987). Effect of severe burn injury on substrate cycling by glucose and fatty acids. *N. Eng. J. Med.*, **317**, 403–8.

Wolff, S. M., Rubinstein, M., Mulholland, J. H. & Alling, D. W. (1965). Comparison of hematologic and febrile responses to endotoxin in man. *Blood*, **26**, 190–201.

Wood, D. D., Ihrie, E. J., Dinarello, C. A. & Cohen, P. L. (1983). Isolation of an interleukin-1 like factor from human joint effusions. *Arthritis Rheum.*, **26**, 975–83.

# 12

# Central control of pain

ROBERT W. CLARKE

**Injury and pain**

In sensory physiology there is a general rule that perceived sensation is proportional to the intensity of the stimulus applied. This is true for the perception of pain as it is measured in controlled studies on human volunteers, in which increasing the strength of a stimulus towards intensities that threaten tissue damage gives rise to pain of escalating intensity (see Meyer & Campbell, 1981). In the field, however, the experience of pain is rather more difficult to predict. There are many recorded instances of quite severe injuries sustained in moments of emotional stress, which were initially unaccompanied by pain, and others, of pathological states, where acute pain was felt in the absence of noxious stimuli (see Melzack & Wall, 1988). These are extreme examples of how injury and pain may become dissociated, but they serve to illustrate that the transmission of impulses related to pain in the central nervous system (CNS) is subject to powerful modulatory influences.

The function of pain is primarily one of protection. Stimuli that cause pain activate an array of responses, including reflex withdrawal and the 'fight or flight' reaction, that have evolved to minimize tissue damage. If these strategies are not fully successful and an injury is sustained, pain acts as an urgent reminder that damage has occurred and encourages behaviours that protect the site of the lesion. In order to best serve its protective role, the nociceptive system must be adaptable to the context within which the pain message is to be generated. This chapter explores our current understanding of the nature of the central mechanisms which influence nociceptive transmission, concentrating on how traumatic stimuli themselves may activate these mechanisms. Before discussing the modulation of nociception, it is first necessary to introduce the basic elements of the nociceptive system and to look at ways in which pain may be measured.

**The nociceptive system**

Stimuli that threaten or actually cause tissue damage are detected by nociceptors located around the external surfaces of the body, within deep tissues such as muscle, and in the walls of hollow organs. Their response characteristics vary according to their location. Nociceptors in the skin may respond to mechanical distortion, temperatures above 45 °C, or irritant chemicals (for a review, see Perl, 1984), whereas those in the walls of viscera respond most readily to distension or smooth-muscle spasm (for a review, see Gebhart & Ness, 1991), i.e. tissues are equipped with nociceptors that have evolved to detect threats appropriate to their location. The afferent axons that carry nociceptor information to the CNS are at the slowly conducting end of the axonal spectrum, being small myelinated (A$\delta$ or group III) or non-myelinated (C or group IV) fibres. For cutaneous nociceptors, small myelinated axons are associated with high-threshold mechanoheat receptors, whereas receptors with non-myelinated fibres may respond to any combination of mechanical, thermal or chemical noxious stimuli, and are usually referred to as 'polymodal nociceptors' (see Perl, 1984). The combination of microstimulation with microneurography in awake volunteers has confirmed that cutaneous pain in the human arises from the activation of receptors with slowly conducting axons (Ochoa & Torebjörk, 1989; Torebjörk & Ochoa, 1990).

Afferent axons from nociceptors terminate centrally in the dorsal grey matter of the spinal cord or, if they arise from receptors in and around the face, the equivalent parts of the trigeminal nuclear complex of the brainstem. It has been shown that the terminals of nociceptive afferents from the skin are found predominantly in the outermost layers of the grey matter (i.e. laminae I and II of Rexed) (Light & Perl, 1979; Sugiura *et al.*, 1986, 1989), although small myelinated nociceptive fibres do penetrate to laminae V and X (Light & Perl, 1979). It should be noted that the terminations of axons from deep tissues are not identical with those from skin (Mense & Prabhakar, 1986; Sugiura *et al.*, 1989). The consequences of nociceptor activation are: (i) if appropriate, reflex withdrawal from the site of the stimulus; (ii) activation of the sympathetic nervous system to make the organism ready for escape or combat; and (iii) the sensation of pain with its attendant emotional reactions. Withdrawal reflexes are coordinated entirely at the segmental level, i.e. in the spinal cord or brainstem (Sherrington, 1910; Kidokoro *et al.*, 1968), although they may be modified by inputs from other parts of the central nervous system (see below)

The autonomic changes and sensory experiences that result from noxious stimuli are dependent upon spinal or trigeminal neurones, with axons that project rostrally into the brain. When classifying spinal and trigeminal neurones of animals on the basis of their responses to peripheral input, two types of cell have been described, which may be involved directly in the perception of pain. Nociceptor-specific neurones are driven only by stimuli that approach or exceed intensities that would cause pain if applied to humans, whereas multireceptive (sometimes called 'wide dynamic range') cells respond to innocuous inputs, but show greater responses when activated by noxious stimuli (see Price & Dubner, 1977; Willis & Coggeshall, 1991). Neurones in those parts of the spinal cord with inputs from the viscera also show convergent responses to both superficial and visceral nociceptors (for example, Tattersall *et al.*, 1986; Gebhart & Ness, 91). Cells that can encode noxious stimuli have been found predominantly in laminae I, II, V and X of the spinal grey matter, i.e. in areas receiving direct input from nociceptor afferents (although not all nociceptive inputs to dorsal-horn cells are monosynaptic; see Willis & Coggeshall, 1991).

Sympathetic responses to noxious stimuli result from the activation of brainstem cell groups via routes which have not yet been fully elucidated. It is possible that they may arise from noxious inflow to the ventral parts of the midbrain periaqueductal grey (PAG), which is thought to be a co-ordinating centre for defence reactions (see Bandler & De Paulis, 1991; Lovick, 1992). The sensory and emotional experiences of pain appear to be dependent on pathways ascending to the thalamus through the anterolateral quadrant of the spinal cord. The spinothalamic tract is particularly important in this respect for primates, including humans (White & Sweet, 1969), although a number of other ascending systems, such as the spinocervical and spinomesencephalic tracts, may carry information relevant to nociception (see Willis & Coggeshall, 1991). The precise distributions of spinothalamic tract neurones varies from species to species, but they are found in some common areas in most species studied, in particular laminae I, IV and V of the spinal dorsal horn.

## Measuring pain

In experiments on awake human subjects, it is possible to gauge the intensity of perceived pain by the use of carefully designed interrogatory techniques (see Reading, 1989). In studies on animals, it is necessary to observe reactions to noxious stimuli, such as withdrawal reflexes or the responses of central neurones, in what are thought to be relevant areas of the CNS, e.g. the dorsal horn of the spinal cord. The advantages of studying reflex responses or other behavioural responses to noxious stimuli (such as vocalization) are that the investigator has some knowledge of the behavioural significance of the response under investigation and the reaction is the result of the coordinated activation of functionally related populations of neurones. The disadvantage is that in every case these responses involve the activation of motor neurones and, as there is no doubt that the excitability of motor neurones and that of dorsal horn cells may be differentially controlled (see below), it is necessary to be cautious when interpreting results obtained from such studies in the context of nociception. Recordings of the responses of single central neurones gives the investigator very detailed information on the response characteristics of cells which might be involved in nociception, particularly if an intracellular penetration is achieved (for example, Cervero *et al.*, 1979; Woolf & King, 1987). It is also possible to identify the projection targets of individual cells, by antidromic activation techniques (see Brown, 1981), so that recordings can be made from spinal dorsal horn cells, which send axons to the brain and may therefore contribute to the flow of nociceptive information reaching the level of consciousness. The disadvantage of this approach is that it relies on sampling from neuronal populations, a factor that may bias the observations. It has been noted before, that even very large sample numbers represent only a trivial fraction of the total number of cells involved in sensory processing (Iggo *et al.*, 1985). Furthermore, one cannot be certain of the behavioural significance of the response of any particular cell (although see Dubner *et al.*, 1989). Recently it has become fashionable to study the expression of immediate–early-onset genes, such as c-*fos*, which are activated in spinal neurones after the application of noxious stimuli (Hunt *et al.*, 1987; Herdegen *et al.*, 1991). Although this is undoubtedly a useful technique for mapping patterns of neuronal activation following particular types of stimuli, these genes are induced by many stimuli other than those of a noxious nature. One should not be depressed by the imperfections of the techniques currently available for the study of pain; it is enough to remember that no technique alone will provide all the answers.

## Modulation of nociceptive processing

The CNS possesses mechanisms that may promote or reduce the transmission related to pain. Of these, inhibitory phenomena have been studied most extensively, particularly in relation to the transmission of nociceptive signals in the spinal cord. Spinal response to noxious stimuli may be modified by intrinsic segmental mechanisms or by pathways descending from the brain.

## Segmental inhibitory mechanisms

### *Presynaptic inhibition*

Transmission from primary afferent fibres entering the spinal cord or trigeminal nuclear complex may be reduced by depolarization of the axon terminal membrane, which reduces the voltage step induced by the arrival of an action potential (see Schmidt, 1971), or possibly by a hyperpolarizing action that blocks invasion of fine terminal branches by incoming action potentials (for example, North, 1989). Primary afferent depolarization (PAD) may be evoked by activation of afferent fibres themselves, particularly large axons from low threshold cutaneous and muscle afferents (Jänig *et al.*, 1969), or by some descending pathways (see Lundberg, 1982). Input from large myelinated cutaneous fibres induces PAD in fibres of similar type and also at the terminals of C-fibres (Woolf & Fitzgerald, 1982; Hentall & Fields, 1984), indicating that concurrent activation of large- and small-diameter afferents would result in inhibition of responses to the latter. This probably explains why gentle rubbing around a mild injury helps to relieve pain, but the effect is transient, as the duration of PAD evoked by a single A-fibre volley is no more than a few hundreds of milliseconds (Schmidt, 1971). In the original version of the gate control theory of pain (Melzack & Wall, 1965) it was hypothesized that, whereas input from large afferent fibres inhibits nociceptive transmission, the corresponding effects of small-diameter afferents would be facilitatory at the presynaptic level. However, the effects on primary afferent terminals of activation of small-diameter afferents are not straightforward. Selective electrical stimulation of non-myelinated fibres in the cat was shown to cause a positive dorsal root potential (DRP), which was taken as a sign of presynaptic facilitation (Mendell & Wall, 1964), but it was later found that activation of thermal nociceptors by heat pulses elicited the more normal negative DRP indicative of PAD (Burke *et al.*, 1971). Whatever presynaptic effects small afferents might have, there is clear evidence that activation of small fibres can potentiate transmission from large myelinated fibres to motor neurones in withdrawal reflex pathways (Behrends *et al.*, 1983; Clarke *et al.*, 1989*a*). It is not known whether such facilitation can be seen in dorsal-horn neurones.

### *Segmental inhibition by endogenous opioid peptides*

The endogenous opioid peptides are neurotransmitters with actions similar to those of the powerful analgesic drug morphine (see Duggan & North, 1984). There are three families of opioid peptides, each the product of a separate gene (for a review, see Akil *et al.*, 1984): the enkephalins, derived from the proenkephalin precursor peptide, of which the best known fragments are the pentapeptides leucine- and methionine-enkephalin; the dynorphins, cleavage products of the prodynorphin precursor; and $\beta$-endorphin, derived from the pituitary peptide proopiomelanocortin (POMC). Immunocytochemical studies in a variety of species, including humans, have demonstrated the presence of enkephalins (Hökfelt *et al.*, 1977; Glazer & Basbaum, 1981; LaMotte & De Lanerolle, 1981) and dynorphins (Cruz & Basbaum, 1985) but not $\beta$-endorphin, in neurones and terminals of the spinal cord. Opioid peptides have been found in greatest numbers in the outer laminae of the dorsal grey matter, although they are also present in more ventral areas, particularly lamina V, where enkephalin-immunoreactive terminals were found in apposition to the dendrites and somata of identified spinothalamic tract neurones (Ruda, 1982).

It is widely accepted that there are three classes of opioid receptors, namely $\mu$, $\delta$ and $\kappa$ (for a review, see Kosterlitz, 1985). The archetypal opioid agonist morphine is selective for $\mu$ receptors, as are most of the clinically useful opioid analgesics.

Amongst the endogenous opioid peptides, the enkephalins show some selectivity for $\delta$ receptors; the dynomorphins are agonists at the $\kappa$-site and $\beta$-endorphin binds with equal affinity to $\mu$ and $\delta$ receptors (see Kosterlitz, 1985). Note that none of the endogenous peptides is specific for any particular receptor type and that all of the peptides may act at any of the known receptor subtypes. All three binding sites are found in the spinal cord (Gouardarès *et al.*, 1985). The densest aggregations of opioid binding sites are found in laminae I and II (Atweh & Kuhar, 1977), paralleling the distribution of the opioid peptides.

### *Spinal actions of exogenous opioids*

Morphine and opioid peptides (or their stabilized analogues) are analgesic when applied directly to the spinal cord of animals or humans (see Yaksh & Noueihed, 1985). In spinalized animal preparations, opioids reduce spinal reflexes (Irwin *et al.*, 1951; Martin *et al.*, 1976; Clarke & Ford, 1987;

Parsons & Headley, 1989), and inhibit the responses of multireceptive neurones in the dorsal horn (Jurna & Grossman, 1976; Le Bars *et al.*, 1976; Duggan *et al.*, 1977*a*; Satoh *et al.*, 1979). This action is claimed to be selective for responses to inputs from nociceptors, so that opioids act to filter out responses to noxious inputs while not affecting those to innocuous stimuli. This effect is not mediated by a direct action on multireceptive cells. When opioids (peptides or alkaloids) are applied to the spinal cord by microelectrophoresis, the selective inhibition of nociceptor drive to multireceptive neurones is seen only when they are delivered into lamina II, i.e. dorsally to the site of recording (Duggan *et al.*, 1977a). This may be a function of $\mu$-receptor agonists, as $\kappa$-opioids directly inhibit identified spinocervical-tract neurones in the cat (Fleetwood-Walker *et al.*, 1988).

An interesting observation is that while some cells in lamina II are depressed by opioids (for example, Yoshimura & North, 1983; Jeftinija, 1988), others appear to be excited by these compounds (Fitzgerald & Woolf, 1980; Sastry & Goh, 1983; Magnusson & Dickenson, 1991). There are a number of reports of superficial dorsal horn neurones being excited by drugs or transmitters that suppress the activity of cells deeper in the dorsal horn (for example, Todd & Millar, 1983). These neurones could be an important inhibitory link in controlling the flow of nociceptive information.

### *Tonic spinal actions of endogenous opioids*

On the basis of the information presented above, it would be logical to expect that the endogenous opioids in the spinal cord would operate as part of a physiological antinociceptive mechanism. If this were so, one would expect pure opioid receptor antagonists such as naloxone to have pronociceptive actions in conditions where the endogenous opioid system was active (see Duggan & Johnson, 1983). There is some evidence to this effect. Spinal reflexes in many species (including humans) are facilitated by naloxone or other opioid antagonists (for example, Goldfarb & Hu, 1976; Clarke *et al.*, 1992*a*). The facilitation of reflexes by opioid antagonists is quite non-selective, as there are increases in the responses of somatic motor neurones to inputs from low- and high-threshold afferent fibres (Goldfarb & Hu, 1976; Catley *et al.*, 1983; Duggan *et al.*, 1984; Clarke *et al.*, 1991*a*, 1992*b*; Hartell & Headley, 1991*a*). Opioid peptides thus appear to exert a 'blanket' of tonic inhibition over afferent pathways to motor neurones, which may contribute to setting the threshold for withdrawal reflexes (Clarke *et al.*, 1991*a*, 1992*a*). It is important to note that the effects of naloxone are most easily seen in spinalized preparations. It appears that the presence of descending inhibition in non-spinalized animals masks the facilitatory effects of opioid receptor blockade (Clarke *et al.*, 1988; see also Bell *et al.*, 1985).

With respect to spinal dorsal-horn neurones, early findings suggested that administration of opioid antagonists resulted in a selective increase in the responses of multireceptive neurones to noxious stimuli (Calvillo *et al.*, 1975), but others were unable to confirm this observation (Duggan *et al.*, 1977*b*). There is now little doubt that naloxone does influence the activity of neurones in the spinal grey matter, but the effects seen are usually rather small. Neurones in ventral grey matter appear to be influenced more profoundly than those in the dorsal parts (see Duggan & North, 1984; Ford *et al.*, 1991). Some cells in lamina II are actually inhibited by naloxone (Fitzgerald & Woolf, 1980; Mokha, 1992). One way to increase the actions of endogenous opioids is to prevent their destruction by enzymes, which is, under normal circumstances, a fairly rapid process. Dickenson *et al.*, (1988) showed that direct spinal application of the enkephalinase inhibitor kelatorphan reduced C-fibre-evoked responses in rat dorsal-horn neurones, an effect that was blocked more easily by $\delta$-opioid receptor antagonists than by naloxone, which favours $\mu$ receptors. One piece of evidence further suggests that opioid receptor blockade might increase the *rostral* flow of nociceptive signals. In the cat, naloxone augmented C-fibre-evoked volleys ascending in the anterolateral quadrant of cat spinal cord, without increasing volleys resulting from A-fibre input (Duggan *et al.*, 1985). It is true to say that the role of tonically released opioids in pain perception (if there is one) has yet to be uncovered. It may be that the approach taken by Dickenson and his colleagues (see above, also Dickenson, 1986) will help to answer the question more clearly.

**Brain control of nociceptive processing**

There are several descending pathways from the brain that may modulate the transmission through the spinal cord of signals related to pain. The majority of direct pathways from the brain to the spinal dorsal horn emanate from the brainstem (see Holstege & Kuypers, 1982), in which the sites of particular interest as the sources of antinociceptive pathways are the catecholaminergic nuclei of the pons, the midline raphe and immediately surrounding reticular tissue of the rostral ventromedial medulla (RVM), and the lateral reticular tissue of the medulla. There is good evidence that some of these brainstem areas are relays for the output of more rostral structures such as the midbrain periaqueductal grey and the anterior pretectal nucleus (APtN), which in turn receive inputs from higher parts of the brain such as the hypothalamus (for example, Semenenko & Lumb, 1992).

## Antinociception from stimulation of the brain

### *The periaqueductal grey matter and rostral ventromedial medulla*

Reynolds (1969) made the dramatic claim that electrical stimulation of the PAG of the rat produced a state of analgesia in which it was possible to perform minor surgery without the aid of anaesthetics. It has since been shown that animal responses to noxious stimuli, using either withdrawal reflexes or the response of dorsal-horn cells as markers of nociception, are reduced during stimulation of many different areas of the brain (for an overview, see Willis, 1988). Most attention has focused on the PAG and the RVM, including the nucleus raphe magnus (NRM) and the various surrounding reticular nuclei (see Basbaum & Fields, 1984; Willis, 1988; Fields *et al.*, 1991).

Since the original report of Reynolds, many workers have shown that electrical stimulation of PAG or the immediately surrounding tissues suppresses withdrawal reflexes, and the responses to noxious stimuli of spinal or trigeminal neurones in the rat, cat and monkey (Mayer & Liebeskind, 1974; Oliveras *et al.*, 1974; Hayes *et al.*, 1979; Carstens *et al.*, 1980; Gebhart *et al.*, 1984; Carstens & Campbell, 1992; see Willis, 1988; Morgan, 1991). The same range of effects can be obtained from stimulation within the RVM (Mayer *et al.*, 1971; Hayes *et al.*, 1979; Zorman *et al.*, 1981; see Willis, 1988). There have been various claims and counter-claims as to whether the effects on spinal transmission evoked by electrical stimulation of these brain areas results in selective inhibition of nociceptive transmission through the cord. While it is generally accepted that neurones that encode *only* non-noxious stimuli are not usually inhibited by stimulation of the brain, it appears that all responses of multireceptive cells (i.e. to noxious and innocuous stimuli) are inhibited from the midbrain or brainstem sites (see Willis, 1988). Importantly, electrical stimulation of the PAG or more rostrally located periventricular grey (PVG) in humans can produce relief in some intractable pain states (Richardson & Akil, 1977; see Barbaro, 1988).

There is good reason to believe that the antinociceptive actions of the

PAG and RVM are linked (see Basbaum & Fields, 1984; Willis, 1988). There are few direct projections to the spinal cord from the PAG, but there are many connections from the PAG and the immediately adjacent lateral reticular tissue, to the RVM (see Holstege, 1991). The major outputs from the various parts of the RVM are to the trigeminal nuclear complex and the spinal grey matter, in particular laminae I, II and V, i.e. all those parts of the dorsal horn thought to be crucial to nociceptive transmission (Basbaum *et al.*, 1978; see also Basbaum & Fields, 1984; Fields *et al.*, 1991). Note that the major spinal projections from the caudal parts of the brainstem reticular formation are to the spinal ventral horn (see Holstege & Kuypers, 1987). Electrical stimulation within the PAG, or microinjection of excitatory amino acids into the PAG, excites many neurones in the RVM (see Fields *et al.*, 1991), and the antinociceptive effects of PAG stimulation are reduced after inactivation of the RVM (for example, Gebhart *et al.*, 1983). Furthermore, both PAG and RVM contain endogenous opioid peptides in neuronal cell bodies and terminals (Hunt & Lovick, 1982; see Reichling *et al.*, 1988; Bowker *et al.*, 1988), and microinjection of opioids into either region is claimed to reduce spinal nociceptive responses (see Yaksh, 1979; Gebhart *et al.*, 1984). This body of evidence indicates that the PAG exerts inhibitory influences over spinal transmission by means of relays in the RVM (see Basbaum & Fields, 1984; Besson & Chaouch, 1987; Willis, 1988, for more complete reviews).

Thus far, the PAG and RVM have been discussed as though they were functionally monolithic structures, which most certainly they are not. A reduction of responses to noxious stimuli is just one element in a spectrum of effects that result from stimulation in the PAG. Activation of neurones in the ventral PAG, in the region of the dorsal raphe nucleus, results in hypoalgesia in combination with reduced arterial blood pressure and 'freezing' behaviour, whereas stimulation of the lateral PAG causes antinociception with *increased* blood pressure and active escape behaviours, sometimes described as 'aversive' (DePaulis & Bandler, 1991; Lovick, 1992). Even the 'analgesic' effects that emanate from these different regions of the PAG are pharmacologically distinct. The antinociceptive actions of lateral PAG are reduced by the opioid antagonist naloxone, but that from the ventral regions is not (see Morgan, 1991). The PAG appears to be the coordinating centre for a range of defensive reactions, which may be activated according to circumstance (see Fanselow, 1991; Lovick & Lumb, 1991), and this is probably an important factor when one considers which stimuli might naturally activate endogenous antinociceptive systems.

There are other functional divisions within the midbrain–brainstem–spinal cord inhibitory network. Stimulation within PAG reduces the slope of the stimulus–response curve for multireceptive dorsal-horn neurones and spinal withdrawal reflexes, but activation of the midbrain lateral reticular formation or of the NRM raises the threshold for activation of the same responses (Carstens *et al.*, 1980; Gebhart *et al.*, 1983; Carstens & Campbell, 1992). There is also evidence that the output of the RVM may be facilitatory as well as inhibitory to nociception. Recordings made within the RVM have identified two classes of neurones that show activity related to the tail-flick reflex in the rat: 'on-cells', which discharge immediately prior to a tail flick evoked by noxious heat; and 'off-cells', which are inhibited at the same time (Fields & Heinricher, 1985; see also Fields *et al.*, 1991). Cells showing these sorts of response pattern are also found in the PAG (Heinricher *et al.*, 1987). There is a considerable body of evidence to suggest that RVM off-cells are inhibitory to spinal cord function (i.e. they have an antinociceptive function) whereas RVM on-cells are pronociceptive (see below, also Heinricher *et al.*, 1989). Opioids given systemically, or by microinjection into the RVM or PAG, cause inhibition of on-cell activity and increased firing of off-cells over the same time-course as inhibition of the tail flick (Fields & Heinricher, 1985; Fields *et al.*, 1991; Morgan *et al.*, 1992). It seems that RVM may be able to 'turn up' or 'turn down' spinal pain signals according to circumstances (see Fields, 1992).

***Brainstem adrenergic nuclei***

All of the catecholamines in the spinal cord are derived from cell bodies in the brainstem (Carlsson *et al.*, 1964). The major sources of adrenergic terminals in the cord are the A5 region of the ventrolateral medulla and the dorsolateral pontine tegmentum, including the areas variously known as A6 and A7 or locus coeruleus, or Kolliker–Fuse nucleus, depending on species (see Westlund *et al.*, 1983; Clark & Proudfit, 1991*a*; see also Clark *et al.*, 1991). I will refer to these areas under the collective name of the coerulear complex. Adrenergic terminals are found throughout the spinal grey matter, but they are particularly dense in laminae I, II, IX, X and the intermediolateral horn (see Proudfit, 1988). Electrical stimulation within A5 or the coerulear complex results in suppression of spinal withdrawal reflexes and dorsal-horn multireceptive neurones (Hodge *et al.*, 1981; Zhao & Duggan, 1988; Yeomans *et al.*, 1992; see Proudfit, 1988). The coerulear complex projects to and receives inputs from the RVM (Yeomans & Proudfit, 1990; Clark & Proudfit, 1991*b*), providing an anatomical substrate for interplay between the RVM and the dorsolateral adrenergic neurone groups.

### *The anterior pretectal nucleus*

Electrical stimulation within the anterior pretectal nucleus of the rat results in powerful depression of the tail-flick reflex and of the responses of multireceptive neurones in the spinal dorsal horn (Prado & Roberts, 1984; Rees & Roberts, 1987). APtN-induced inhibition of dorsal-horn cells is claimed to be selective for responses to noxious stimuli (Rees & Roberts, 1987). Like the PAG, this area has few direct connections to the spinal cord, and evidence has been obtained to suggest that the inhibitory outflow from the APtN is partly dependent on a relay through the lateral parts of the rostral medulla (Segal & Sandberg, 1977; Terenzi *et al.*, 1991). At present, there does not appear to be a great deal of overlap between the antinociceptive networks descending from the PAG and the APtN.

### *Tonic descending inhibition*

Blocking transmission through spinal tracts by cutting the spinal cord increases the excitability of spinal reflex pathways (for example, Sherrington & Sowton, 1915; Irwin *et al.*, 1951; Holmqvist & Lundberg, 1961). The same manoeuvre also increases the responsiveness of multireceptive dorsal-horn neurones to noxious stimuli (Hillman & Wall, 1969; Brown, 1970; Handwerker *et al.*, 1975; Duggan *et al.*, 1980; see Duggan & Morton, 1988, for review). These results show that transmission of information through and across the spinal cord is inhibited tonically by pathways emanating from the brain. In the cat, tonic descending inhibition may arise from neurones in or near the lateral nuclei (Hall *et al.*, 1982), or possibly from structures in the rostral medulla (Foong & Duggan, 1986). It is unclear whether tonic inhibition is present in conscious animals, or whether it is an artefact of surgical preparations (see Duggan & Morton, 1988).

### *Transmitters involved in brain control of spinal nociceptive circuits*

There are three main neurotransmitters that have been studied extensively for a role in descending control of spinal nociceptive function: endogenous opioid peptides, noradrenaline, and serotonin. Opioid peptides were first implicated from the observations of Akil *et al.* (1976), who claimed that the antinociceptive effects of NRM stimulation could be reduced by the opioid antagonist naloxone. It has proved difficult to substantiate the idea that descending inhibitory effects might be mediated by endogenous opioids (Aimone *et al.*, 1987; see Duggan, 1985; Willis, 1988; Fields *et al.*, 1991); this is no doubt due to the amazing complexity of descending inhibitory pathways (see below). One report has indicated that stimulation in and around the PAG may result in simultaneous release of opioids, noradrenaline and serotonin (Carstens *et al.*, 1990).

There is more convincing evidence of a role for noradrenaline in descending inhibition. This monoamine selectively inhibits the responses to noxious stimuli of dorsal-horn multireceptive neurones (Headley *et al.*, 1978), an action which is mediated through $\alpha_2$-adrenoceptors (Fleetwood-Walker *et al.*, 1985). That $\alpha_2$-receptors are responsible for adrenergic inhibition in the spinal cord, is one of the few really well-established facts relating to the mediation of descending inhibition. Selective $\alpha_2$-agonists such as dexmedetomidine are analgesic in humans (Jaakola *et al.*, 1991). The latency of the tail-flick reflex in the rat is reduced after intrathecal administration of the $\alpha_2$-antagonist yohimbine (Sagen & Proudfit, 1984; Barbaro *et al.*, 1985) and hindlimb-withdrawal reflexes in the rabbit are enhanced by the selective $\alpha_2$-blocker idazoxan (Clarke *et al.*, 1988; Harris & Clarke, 1992). While these studies indicate that noradrenaline is in some part responsible for tonic descending inhibition, there is no evidence that dorsal-horn neurones are rendered more excitable by administration of $\alpha$-receptor antagonists in the cat (Duggan, 1985; Duggan & Morton, 1988). With regards to stimulus-evoked inhibition of spinal nociceptive processes, yohimbine reduces inhibition from the APtN (Rees *et al.*, 1987) and also that from electrical stimulation within the rostral medulla. It was reported that RVM-induced inhibition was only completely abolished by co-administration of yohimbine with methysergide, an antagonist at serotonin 5-$HT_1$ and 5-$HT_2$ receptors (Barbaro *et al.*, 1985). The inhibition which results from stimulation within the coerulear complex is blocked by $\alpha_2$-adrenoceptor antagonists in the rat (Jones & Gebhart, 1986; Yeomans *et al.*, 1992), but not apparently in the cat (Hodge *et al.*, 1983; Zhao & Duggan, 1988; although see Skoog & Noga, 1991).

Serotonin is particularly interesting, because it is present in many neurones of the midline raphe nuclei throughout the brainstem, of which many project to the spinal cord (Bowker *et al.*, 1982). Unfortunately, the study of serotonergic mechanisms has been dogged by the appallingly complex pharmacology of this transmitter and the lack of selective agents for investigating the roles of different 5-HT receptors (see Frazer *et al.*, 1990). The antagonist that has been commonly used to investigate the physiological roles of 5-HT is methysergide, which does not select between 5-$HT_1$ and 5-$HT_2$ receptors, and which may also have agonist properties at some sites. The effects of serotonin on multireceptive dorsal horn cells are similar to those of noradrenaline (Headley *et al.*, 1978), but the receptor subtypes responsible for this inhibitory action have not been adequately identified. Several reports suggest that serotonin antagonists may reduce tonic inhibition of spinal dorsal-horn neurones in the rat (Rivot *et al.*, 1987) and possibly in the cat (Griersmith & Duggan, 1980). Serotonin receptor blockers have also been shown to reduce the antinociceptive effects of PAG stimulation in the cat (Carstens *et al.*, 1981) and RVM activation in the rat (for example, Barbaro *et al.*, 1985, El-Yassir & Fleetwood-Walker, 1990). Recent studies have indicated that a selective 5-$HT_3$-receptor antagonist reduces tonic inhibition of withdrawal reflexes in the rabbit (Harris *et al.*, 1992) and that intrathecal injection of a 5-$HT_3$, agonist in the rat has powerful antinociceptive effects which may be mediated through the release of the inhibitory amino acid GABA (Alhaider *et al.*, 1991).

There is no doubt that other transmitters are involved in descending control of spinal functions, for instance acetylcholine (for example, see Zhuo & Gebhart, 1991*a*) and neuropeptide Y (Duggan *et al.*, 1991), but the roles of these agents have not been widely investigated. The reader should be aware by now that descending inhibition of spinal nociceptive transmission is a rather complex phenomenon involving multiple descending pathways and more than one neurotransmitter. The situation is further complicated by the fact that different receptors for the same transmitter can have mutually antagonistic actions. For instance, while $\alpha_2$-adrenoceptors usually mediate inhibitory effects on spinal transmission (for example, Fleetwood-Walker *et al.*, 1985), $\alpha_1$-receptors are usually excitatory (for example, Lai *et al.*, 1989; see Harris & Clarke, 1992). Indeed, a particular feature of monoamine actions in the cord seems to be that, while they are inhibitory to dorsal-horn neurones, their predominant effect on motor neurones is excitation (for example, Connell & Wallis, 1988; Connell *et al.*, 1989; see Harris & Clarke, 1992). This has major implications in the study of the pharmacology of pain transmission while using motor responses as indicators of nociception. Although the situation appears to be a hopeless mess at present, there is light on the horizon in the form of highly selective agents for each of the many types of monoamine receptor. A clear picture of monoamine involvement in control of nociceptive transmission will emerge as more highly selective drugs come into use (see Harris & Clarke, 1992).

The evidence presented above suggests that there are at least two, and probably more, independently controllable 'systems' that have amongst their actions the effect of reducing the flow of nociceptive information from the spinal cord and the trigeminal nuclear complex. Of these, the network that has received the most attention is the PAG–RVM–spinal cord system, while the APtN–lateral brainstem–spinal cord pathway has been less extensively studied. Both mechanisms seem to call on catecholaminergic neurones to exert some of their effects, but exactly how this is achieved has yet to be established (see Mokha *et al.*, 1986).

**Activation of endogenous antinociceptive mechanisms**

The identification of the means of activating endogenous pain-control mechanisms to provide adequate pain relief without the need for the chronic use of drugs or invasive surgery, is the 'magic bullet' of pain research. Some techniques, such as transcutaneous electrical nerve stimulation (TENS) and acupuncture are already in common use, but are not effective in all patients or against all types of pain. Our understanding of the mechanisms that underlie TENS and acupuncture is somewhat incomplete. Both of these phenomena rely on the activation of peripheral afferent fibres, in the case of TENS by electrical stimulation through the skin, while acupuncture is effected by needles inserted at various locations (usually muscular) around the body, as defined by traditional acupuncture charts (see Sjölund & Eriksson, 1979; MacDonald, 1989; Woolf, 1989). In each case, the most effective sites at which to stimulate are usually close to the source of the pain which the manoeuvre is intended to reduce (see Melzack, 1989). Both TENS and electroacupuncture have been shown to increase the levels of endogenous opioids in human cerebrospinal fluid (see Han *et al.*, 1991) and it is generally assumed that these peptides are responsible for at least some of the analgesic effect of stimulus-evoked analgesia (for example, see Mayer *et al.*, 1977). However, it is not always possible to reverse acupuncture analgesia in humans with opioid antagonists (Chapman *et al.*, 1983). As will become clear below, this result does not mean necessarily that opioids are not involved.

***Inhibitory effects of noxious stimuli in animal experiments***

There have been many studies that have shown that activation of nociceptor afferents causes naloxone-reversible inhibitions of spinally mediated events. Repetitive activation of A$\delta$ and C-fibres of hindlimb nerves resulted in long-lasting (10–30 mins), naloxone-reversible inhibition of spinal withdrawal reflexes in cats (Sjölund & Eriksson, 1979; Chung *et al.*, 1983) and in spinalized rabbits (Catley *et al.*, 1984; Clarke *et al.*, 1989*b*). In these studies, inhibition was not seen after repetitive stimulation of low-threshold afferent fibres, although Woolf *et al.* (1980) found that iterative stimulation of large myelinated axons could increase the latency of the tail-flick reflex in the spinalized rat. Even in this instance, maximum inhibition was seen only after recruitment of A$\delta$ afferents by the conditioning stimulus. These findings indicate that spinal opioidergic neurones can be activated by inputs from nociceptor afferent fibres. Taylor *et al.* (1990) confirmed this by showing that the sural-gastrocnemius withdrawal reflex of the rabbit was depressed, in a naloxone-reversible fashion, after noxious, but not innocuous, 'natural' stimulation of the toes. Noxious mechanical stimuli were most effective in eliciting this inhibition, which could not be obtained from anywhere other than the toes in the ipsilateral hindlimb (see Catley *et al.*, 1984). The changes in spinal reflexes that follow noxious stimuli may have evolved to enhance reflex protection of injured sites (Clarke *et al.*, 1992*b*).

The inhibitory effects described above were observed in spinalized animals and must have been due to mechanisms intrinsic to the spinal cord. Noxious stimuli also activate inhibitory mechanisms emanating from the brain. Of these, probably the most extensively investigated is the phenomenon of diffuse noxious inhibitory controls (DNIC) (Le Bars *et al.*, 1979). The responses of spinal dorsal horn and trigeminal sensory multireceptive neurones are depressed by the application of intense noxious stimuli applied anywhere on the body surface outside the neurone's excitatory receptive field. Thus, cells which responded to stimulation of the skin of the hindlimb were inhibited by the application of noxious stimuli to the snout, and vice versa (Le Bars *et al.*, 1979; Dickenson *et al.*, 1980; for a review, see Le Bars & Villanueva, 1988). The inhibition that resulted from DNIC-type stimuli outlasted the stimulus by 2 to 10 min and was partially reversed by naloxone, indicating that it was to some extent dependent on the release of endogenous opioids. Curiously, DNIC is also antagonized by morphine; presumably this is because morphine reduces the noxious sensory inflow that is necessary to trigger the effect (Villanueva & Le Bars, 1986). This has led to the suggestion that DNIC may be a vital component of normal nociception in providing a contrast signal to emphasize the location of the most recent or severe noxious stimulus (Le Bars & Villanueva, 1988). The existence of DNIC also provides a good physiological basis for the many different methods of counter-irritation analgesia, such as acupuncture (Bing *et al.*, 1990). Heterotopic inhibition of nociceptive responses by noxious stimuli has been reported for spinal dorsal-horn neurones in the cat (Morton *et al.*, 1988) and monkey (Chung *et al.*, 1984), and for nociceptive reflexes in the human (Debroucker *et al.*, 1990) and rabbit (Taylor *et al.*, 1991). In the rat, DNIC depends on a supraspinal loop, as spinalization reduces the effect almost to nothing (but see Cadden *et al.*, 1983). Recent work suggests that the brainstem nucleus reticularis lateralis is an important relay in DNIC (Bing *et al.*, 1991; Villanueva *et al.*, 1991).

It has been suggested above that the heel-withdrawl reflex in the spinalized rabbit was suppressed after noxious stimulation of the foot, and that this effect was completely reversed by naloxone. If the same stimuli are applied in decerebrated *non-spinalized* rabbits, the inhibition of reflexes so produced is greater in magnitude than in spinalized preparations, and can be reversed only by co-administration of naloxone with the selective $\alpha_2$-adrenoceptor antagonist idazoxan (Clarke *et al.*, 1989*b*). Naloxone alone reduces the inhibition slightly, whereas idazoxan alone has no effect. Inhibition of reflexes in one hindlimb may be obtained from high-intensity stimulation of nerves in any of the four limbs (Taylor *et al.*, 1991). The depression of reflex responses so produced lasts for 15 to 33 min or more depending on the limb stimulated, with the most profound inhibition being evoked from the same limb as the reflex under study. This stimulus-evoked inhibition would appear to be mediated by the release in parallel of spinal opioid peptides and noradrenaline. Both have been found in superfusates of cat spinal cord after intense stimulation of the sciatic nerves (Tyce & Yaksh, 1981; Yaksh & Elde, 1981). An important lesson from this work is that the failure of a single antagonist to influence a physiological event is not enough to rule out a role for the receptors to which that antagonist binds: there may well be more than one system in play (see Clarke *et al.*, 1988, 1989*b*; Taylor *et al.*, 1991). As yet, it is not known which of the brainstem catecholaminergic nuclei is responsible for the adrenergic component of stimulus-evoked inhibition in the rabbit.

In the cat, surgical trauma has been shown to result in very prolonged inhibition of trigeminal neuronal and reflex responses to stimulation of tooth pulp (Clarke & Matthews, 1990). This phenomenon appears to be a function of the total amount of surgical preparation carried out on the animal, but some procedures, notably the use of pointed stereotaxic ear bars for head fixation, were particularly effective in generating the inhibition. It has recently been found that spinal dorsal-horn neurones in the rat are more sensitive to anaesthetics if the animal has been subjected to extensive surgical trauma (Hartell & Headley, 1991*b*), and human pain responsiveness is reduced away from the site of surgical incisions (Lund *et al*., 1990). This is probably the least understood of the inhibitory mechanisms activated by noxious stimuli, but is of some importance in view of the large amount of data collected from surgically prepared animals (and humans).

### *Stress-induced analgesia*

The work outlined above shows quite clearly that noxious stimuli themselves activate central antinociceptive mechanisms, i.e. that 'pain inhibits pain' (see Melzack, 1975). 'Stress', or anxiogenic circumstances, appears to be the other important trigger for activation of these mechanisms. The earliest studies on 'stress-induced' analgesia showed that inescapable foot-shock rendered rats less responsive to painful stimuli (Madden *et al*., 1977). On some occasions this effect was reversed by naloxone and on others it was not, depending, among other things, upon the site receiving the shock (Watkins *et al*., 1982; see Watkins & Mayer, 1982). Recent work has demonstrated that antinociceptive mechanisms are brought into play when an animal is exposed to stimuli that suggest that an attack from a predator is imminent or actually happening. Thus, handling a rat by the scruff of the neck, which is the prime site for a predator's bite, results in naloxone-reversible suppression of responses to noxious stimuli (Fanselow & Sigmundi, 1986; see also Fleischmann & Urca, 1988). This may be the major drive to the activation of the body's antinociceptive systems. The PAG receives inputs from the amygdala (Hopkins & Holstege, 1978) and the hypothalamic defence areas (Lovick & Lumb, 1991; Semenenko & Lumb, 1992; see also Fanselow, 1991). These sorts of connections would provide the routes by which antinociceptive mechanisms would be activated during anxiety or fear states, as apparently happens in human subjects (Al Absi & Rokke, 1991). One should remember that 'analgesia' systems are unlikely to be activated in isolation in the normal course of events, and that they are part of a coordinated series of physiological adaptations to threatening situations.

## Hyperalgesia after injury

Noxious stimuli also have pronociceptive actions, i.e. in some circumstances, pain begets pain. The most common experience of this process is that injured tissue becomes tender to the touch, i.e. pain may be elicited by stimuli that would not normally cause it ('allodynia') and the pain resulting from noxious stimuli is exaggerated ('hyperalgesia'). The two terms do not necessarily imply that different mechanisms are responsible for these phenomena (see Meyer *et al.*, 1992). There is no doubt that peripheral mechanisms play an important role in increased sensitivity to pain after an injury. A complex mixture of algogenic substances are released or are generated in inflamed tissue, which cause nociceptors to become more sensitive (for reviews, see Handwerker & Reeh, 1991; Treede *et al.*, 1992). Increased sensitivity is seen at the site of the injury (primary hyperalgesia) and also around the site of the lesion (secondary hyperalgesia). The distances over which secondary hyperalgesia is experienced are too great for a purely peripheral explanation to be adequate, and there is now good evidence that at least some of this effect is mediated within the spinal cord (for a more a complete introduction to these ideas, see Woolf, 1991).

Woolf (1983) showed that withdrawal reflexes in rat hindlimb flexor muscles were massively potentiated for many minutes after a thermal injury to the skin of the same limb. The effect was seen when the injury was applied away from the site from which reflexes were evoked, or if the reflexes were elicited by electrical stimulation of a cutaneous nerve, showing that the increased excitability of the reflex pathway was not the result of changes in the periphery. After the injury, it was possible to evoke reflexes by stimuli that previously were too weak to elicit withdrawal (a correlate of allodynia) and the responses to noxious pinch were greatly enhanced (analogous to hyperalgesia). This was the first evidence of sustained increases in the excitability of central circuits after a noxious stimulus. Further work from the same author and his colleagues demonstrated that withdrawal reflexes were also enhanced after the application of brief trains of electrical stimuli of the non-myelinated axons of peripheral nerves, and that activation of afferents from deep tissue, particularly muscle and joints, caused more prolonged enhancement of transmission (up to 3 h after the stimulus) than did stimulation of C-fibres in cutaneous nerves (Woolf & Wall, 1986). This finding is in good agreement with human experience of pain resulting from damage to deep tissues, although it should be noted that stimulation of afferents from muscles was not found to be especially effective in enhancing flexion reflexes in the rabbit (Clarke *et al.*, 1991*b*).

Studies on species other than the rat have confirmed that transmission through withdrawal reflex pathways is facilitated after intense electrical stimulation of small afferent nerve fibres or the application of noxious stimuli (Mense & Skeppar, 1991; Clarke *et al.*, 1991*b*, 1992*b*). The behavioural significance of the increased excitability of withdrawal reflexes, particularly a decrease in threshold for evoking these responses, is likely to be to afford increased reflex protection of damaged tissue. Further evidence from animal studies indicates that these phenomena relate to more than just the motor responses to painful stimuli. The receptive fields of spinal dorsal-horn neurones in the rat expand towards or actually embrace sites where intense thermal, chemical or mechanical noxious stimuli are applied close to the original receptive field (McMahon & Wall, 1984; Laird & Cervero, 1989; Woolf & King, 1990; see also Hu *et al.*, 1992). A similar phenomenon has been observed in cat dorsal-horn cells with input from deep muscular receptors, after injection of irritant chemicals into the same muscles (Hoheisel & Mense, 1989). In the same species, spinal neurones, which normally respond to 'painful' manipulation of the knee joint, became sensitive to movements in the normal range after induction of inflammation of the joint by injection of carageenin (Schaible *et al.*, 1987). In primates, the area from which multireceptive spinothalamic tract cells could be excited expanded after a thermal injury made *outside* their 'normal' receptive fields (Simone *et al.*, 1991), and the neurones showed markedly increased sensitivity to mechanical stimuli, particularly those of an innocuous nature (Kenshalo *et al.*, 1982). Injury-induced changes in the receptive fields of monkey spinothalamic-tract cells followed a similar time-course to the spread of secondary hyperalgesia in humans after a similar thermal stimulus (Simone *et al.*, 1989), which is consistent with the view that there is a central component to human hyperalgesia. More conclusive evidence for this process was obtained in a recent study in human volunteers. In normal subjects, microstimulation of afferent axons from low-threshold mechanoreceptors never induced the sensation of pain, regardless of the frequency with which stimuli were applied (Wiesenfeld-Hallin *et al.*, 1984). However, if the C-fibre stimulant-cum-neurotoxin capsaicin was injected into the receptive field for low-threshold mechanoreceptors, stimulation of the afferent axons from these receptors resulted in the sensation of pain (Torebjörk *et al.*, 1992). As this sensation was the result of axonal stimulation it *must* have resulted from a change in the central processing of the input from those afferents. The alterations in dorsal-horn processing that have been seen in animals (see above) would provide an adequate substrate for such a change in the processing of inputs from low-threshold mechanoreceptors. It is important to note that these reactions are not global events, as tissue damage at one site does not lead to an increase in sensitivity over the whole body (for example, Lund *et al.*, 1990).

**Transmitters involved in hyperalgesia and allodynia**

Excitatory amino acids are almost certainly involved in the prolonged increases in the excitability of withdrawal reflexes which follow noxious stimuli in the rat: this effect is blocked by the *N*-methyl-D-aspartic acid (NMDA)-receptor-channel blocker MK-801 (Woolf & Thompson, 1991). There may also be a role for some peptide transmitters such as the tachykinins, substance P and neurokinin A (Woolf & Wiesenfeld-Hallin, 1986; Xu & Wiesenfeld-Hallin, 1992). Both peptides are released in response to noxious stimuli in the spinal cord of the cat, but, while substance P persists for only a few minutes after a stimulus and its spread is restricted to lamina II (Duggan & Hendry, 1986), neurokinin A, once released, spreads throughout the spinal grey matter and persists for more than an hour (Duggan *et al.*, 1990). The time-course of release (and presumably, therefore, action) of this peptide may well be responsible for some of the protracted changes that occur in spinal processing after tissue damage. To support the view that central hyperalgesia–allodynia results from cooperative actions of excitatory amino acids with tachykinins, a recent study has shown that combined iontophoretic application of substance P with NMDA results in prolonged sensitization of spino-thalamic-tract cells in the monkey (Dougherty & Willis, 1991).

That neuropeptides are important in adaptive changes to injury is beyond doubt, but the exact nature of the roles they play has yet to be fully established. The most convincing case has been made for substance P (see above), which is released after noxious stimuli, and which, when applied to dorsal-horn neurones *in vitro*, reproduces the long-lasting excitatory post-synaptic potentials, which are similar to those seen after repetitive stimulation of C-fibre dorsal-root afferents (Urban & Randic, 1984). There is also a marked reduction in tissue levels of substance P in the spinal segments affected by severe thermal injury in the rat (De Ceballos *et al.*, 1990). There is enhanced induction of the c-*fos* gene (Leah *et al.*, 1992) and long-term changes in many peptides, or the RNA that encodes for peptides, after chronic tissue or nerve damage (see Dubner, 1991).

The data outlined above indicate that tissue-damaging stimuli result in a barrage of impulses in small-diameter afferent fibres and the subsequent release of excitatory amino acids and tachykinins in the spinal cord. The effect of such a barrage is to sensitize spinal neurones to inputs from or near the site at which the stimulus was applied, decreasing the threshold for evoking all pain reactions from the site of injury, and enhancing protective behaviour. These events almost certainly underlie the prolonged pain that accompanies injuries, and may also contribute to the pain syndromes resulting from traumatic deafferentation (see Tasker & Dostrovsky, 1989). Longer-term alterations in neuropeptides may also have a role in the physiological and pathophysiological sequelae of injury. Knowing that the pronociceptive changes described above are triggered by input from nociceptive afferents, it follows that reduction or blockade of nociceptive inputs to the central nervous system during the application of traumatic stimuli should reduce the intensity of any subsequent pain. This appears to be the case, as pretreatment of surgical cases with either opioid analgesics or local anaesthetics results in significantly decreased postoperative pain or demands for analgesic therapy (Jebeles *et al.*, 1991; Kiss & Kilian, 1992; McQuay *et al.*, 1992; Tverskoy *et al.*, 1992).

**Other pronociceptive mechanisms**

A number of recent reports indicate that the brain possesses mechanisms that can facilitate transmission through spinal nociceptive networks (see Fields, 1992). The on-cells of the RVM were mentioned above. It has been hypothesised that on-cells all fire in unison and that this discharge facilitates responses to nociceptor input all over the body (Fields & Heinricher, 1985). This conclusion is supported by the finding of Ramirez & Vanegas (1989) that tooth-pulp stimulation advances the tail-flick reflex in the rat. Also in the rat, low intensity electrical stimulation of the nucleus reticularis paragigantocellularis (NRPG) of the brainstem enhances the tail-withdrawal flick reflex evoked by noxious heat and the responses of dorsal-horn neurones to similar stimuli (Zhuo & Gebhart, 1991*b*). The behavioural significance of such putative descending pronociceptive systems has not yet been established.

***Descending facilitation of motor neurones***

It was noted above that there are a number of descending pathways which are excitatory to motor neurones. Some of these come from areas close to those, such as the coerulear complex, associated with inhibition of sensory responses to noxious stimuli (Fung & Barnes, 1981). These projections and their effects on spinal reflex pathways have the potential to cause a great deal of confusion in the study of motor responses as models of pain transmission (see above).

## Conclusions

From the preceding discussion, it is clear that noxious stimuli themselves activate central mechanisms, which may be pro- or antinociceptive. It has been suggested that the antinociceptive systems may act as a form of negative feedback on the transmission of nociceptive information (see Basbaum & Fields, 1984; Cervero & Wolstencroft, 1984; Le Bars *et al.*, 1992). However, there is little evidence that the inhibitory systems activated by noxious stimuli are actually directed against the spinal or trigeminal neurones from which the original signal was generated. Rather, it seems that an injury generates for itself a 'bright spot' in the nociceptive system, enhancing the responses of neurones immediately concerned with transmitting that signal. The contrast of the signal is improved by the simultaneous, generalized inhibition of nociceptive responses in the rest of the body. The brightness of this spot (the intensity of the pain message) may be reduced by interference from other nociceptive bright spots (counterirritation) or attentional or emotional factors such as fear and anxiety (see Fanselow, 1991; Al Absi & Rokke, 1991).

## Acknowledgements

My thanks to Mary Heinricher and Mike Morgan for opening my eyes and to Susan for her patience. All work from my own laboratory was supported by the AFRC.

## References

Aimone, L. D., Jones, S. L. & Gebhart, G. F. (1987). Stimulation produced descending inhibition from the periaqueductal gray and nucleus raphe magnus of the rat: mediation by spinal monoamines but not opioids. *Pain*, **31**, 123–35.

Akil, H., Mayer, J. D. & Liebeskind, J. C. (1976). Antagonism of stimulation-produced analgesia by naloxone, a narcotic antagonist. *Science*, **191**, 961–2.

Akil, H., Watson, J., Young, E., Lewis, M. E., Khachaturian, H. & Walker, J. M. (1984). Endogenous opioids: biology and function. *Annu. Rev. Neurosci.*, **7**, 223–56.

Al Absi, M. & Rokke, P. D. (1991). Can anxiety help us tolerate pain? *Pain*, **46**, 43–52.

Alhaider, A. A., Lei, S. Z. & Wilcox, G. L. (1991). Spinal 5-$HT_3$ receptor-mediated antinociception – possible release of GABA. *J. Neurosci.*, **11**, 1881–8.

Atweh, S. F. & Kuhar, M. J. (1977). Autoradiographic localisation of opiate receptors in rat brain. I. Spinal cord and lower medulla. *Brain Res.*, **124**, 53–67.

Bandler, R. & De Paulis, A. (1991). Midbrain periaqueductal gray control of defensive behaviour in cat and rat. In *The Midbrain Periaqueductal Gray Matter*, ed. A. De Paulis & R. Bandler, pp. 175–98. New York: Plenum.

Barbaro, N. M. (1988). Studies of PAG/PVG stimulation for pain relief in humans. *Prog. Brain Res.*, **77**, 165–73.

Barbaro, N. M., Hammond, D. L. & Fields, H. L. (1985). Effects of intrathecally administered methysergide and yohimbine on microstimulation produced antinociception in the rat. *Brain Res.*, **343**, 223–9.

Basbaum, A. I., Clanton, C. H. & Fields, H. L. (1978). Three bulbospinal pathways from the rostral medulla of the cat: an autoradiographic study of pain modulating systems. *J. Comp. Neurol.*, **178**, 209–24.

Basbaum, A. I. & Fields, H. L. (1984). Endogenous pain control systems: brainstem spinal pathways and endorphin circuitry. *Annu. Rev. Neurosci.*, **7**, 309–38.

Behrends, T., Schomberg, E. D. & Steffens, H. (1983). Facilitatory interactions between cutaneous afferents from low threshold mechanoreceptors and nociceptors in segmental reflex pathways to α-motoneurons. *Brain Res.*, **260**, 131–4.

Bell, J. A., Sharpe, L. G. & Pickworth, W. B. (1985). Electrophysiologically recorded C-fiber reflexes in intact and spinal cats: absence of naloxone facilitation in intact cats. *Neuropharmacology*, **24**, 555–9.

Besson, J.-M. & Chaouch, A. (1987). Peripheral and spinal mechanisms of nociception. *Physiol. Rev.*, **67**, 67–186.

Bing, Z., Villanueva, L. & Le Bars, D. (1990). Acupuncture and diffuse noxious inhibitory controls – naloxone-reversible depression of activities of trigeminal convergent neurons. *Neuroscience*, **37**, 809–18.

Bing, Z., Villanueva, L. & Le Bars, D. (1991). Acupuncture-evoked responses of subnucleus reticularis dorsalis neurons in the rat medulla. *Neuroscience*, **44**, 693–703.

Bowker, R. M., Abbott, L. C. & Dilts, R. P. (1988). Peptidergic neurons in the nucleus raphe magnus and the nucleus gigantocellularis: their distributions, interrelationships, and projections to the spinal cord. *Prog. Brain Res.*, **77**, 95–127.

Bowker, R. M., Westlund, K. N., Sullivan, M. C. & Coulter, J. D. (1982). Organisation of descending serotonergic connections to the spinal cord. *Prog. Brain Res.*, **57**, 239–65.

Brown, A. G. (1970). Effects of descending impulses on transmission through the spinocervical tract. *J. Physiol.*,**219**, 103–25.

Brown, A. G. (1981). *Organization of the Spinal Cord.* Berlin: Springer.

Burke, R. E., Rudomin, P., Vyklicky, L. & Zajac, F. E. III (1971). Primary afferent depolarisation and flexion reflexes produced by radiant heat stimulation of the skin. *J. Physiol.*, **213**, 185–214.

Cadden, S. W., Villanueva, L., Chitour, D. & Le Bars, D. (1983). Depression of activities of dorsal horn convergent neurones by propriospinal mechanisms triggered by noxious inputs: comparison with diffuse noxious inhibitory controls (DNIC). *Brain Res.*, **275**, 1–11.

Calvillo, O., Henry, J. L. & Neuman, R. S. (1975). Effects of morphine and naloxone on dorsal horn neurons in the cat. *Can. J. Physiol. Pharmacol.*, **52**, 1207–11.

Carlsson, A., Falck, B., Fuxe, K. & Hillharp, N. Å. (1964). Cellular location of monoamines in the spinal cord. *Acta Physiol. Scand.*, **60**, 112–19.
Carstens, E. & Campbell, I. G. (1992). Responses of motor units during the hind limb flexion withdrawal reflex evoked by noxious skin heating – phasic and prolonged suppression by midbrain stimulation and comparison with simultaneously recorded dorsal horn units. *Pain*, **48**, 215–26.
Carstens, E., Culhane, E. S. & Banisadr, R. (1990). Partial involvement of monoamines and opiates in the inhibition of rat spinal nociceptive neurons evoked by stimulation in midbrain periaqueductal gray or lateral reticular formation. *Brain Res.*, **522**, 7–13.
Carstens, E., Fraunhoffer, M. & Zimmerman, M. (1981). Serotonergic mediation of descending inhibition from midbrain periaqueductal gray, but not reticular formation, of spinal nociceptive transmission in the rat. *Pain*, **10**, 149–67.
Carstens, E., Klumpp, D. & Zimmerman, M. (1980). Differential inhibitory effects of medial and lateral midbrain on spinal neuronal discharges to noxious skin heating in the cat. *J. Neurophysiol.*, **43**, 332–42.
Catley, D. M., Clarke, R. W. & Pascoe, J. E. (1983). Naloxone enhancement of spinal reflexes in the rabbit. *J. Physiol.*, **339**, 61–73.
Catley, D. M., Clarke, R. W. & Pascoe, J. E. (1984). Post-tetanic depression of spinal reflexes in the rabbit and the possible involvement of opioid peptides. *J. Physiol.*, **352**, 483–93.
Cervero, F., Molony, V. & Iggo, A. (1979). An electrophysiological study of neurons in the substantia gelatinosa Rolandi in the cat's spinal cord. *Q. J. Exp. Physiol.*, **64**, 297–314.
Cervero, F. & Wolstencroft, J. (1984). A positive feedback loop between spinal cord nociceptive pathways and antinociceptive areas of the cat's brain stem. *Pain*, **20**, 125–38.
Chapman, C. R., Benedetti, C., Colpitts, Y. H. & Gerlach, R. (1983). Naloxone fails to reverse pain thresholds elevated by acupuncture: acupuncture analgesia reconsidered. *Pain*, **16**, 13–31.
Chung, J. M., Fang, Z. R., Cargill, C. L. & Willis, W. D. (1983). Prolonged, naloxone-reversible inhibition of the flexion reflex in the cat. *Pain*, **15**, 35–53.
Chung, J. M., Fang, Z. R., Hori, Y., Lee, K. H. & Willis, W. D. (1984). Prolonged inhibition of primate spinothalamic tract cells by peripheral nerve stimulation. *Pain*, **19**, 259–75.
Clark, F. M. & Proudfit, H. K. (1991*a*). The projection of noradrenergic neurons in the A7 catecholamine cell group to the spinal cord in the rat demonstrated by anterograde tracing combined with immunocytochemistry. *Brain Res.*, **547**, 279–88.
Clark, F. M. & Proudfit, H. K. (1991*b*). Projections of neurons in the ventromedial medulla to pontine catecholamine cell groups involved in the modulation of nociception. *Brain Res.*, **540**, 105–15.
Clark, F. M., Yeomans, D. C. & Proudfit, H. K. (1991). The noradrenergic innervation of the spinal cord – differences between two substrains of Sprague-Dawley rats determined using retrograde tracers combined with immunocytochemistry. *Neurosci. Lett.*, **125**, 155–8.
Clarke, R. W. & Ford, T. W. (1987). The contributions of $\mu$-, $\delta$- and $\kappa$-opioid receptors to the actions of endogenous opioids on spinal reflexes in the rabbit. *Br. J. Pharmacol.*, **91**, 579–89.
Clarke, R. W., Ford, T. W. & Taylor, J. S. (1988). Adrenergic and opioidergic modulation of a spinal reflex in the rabbit. *J. Physiol.*, **404**, 407–17.

Clarke, R. W., Ford, T. W. & Taylor, J. S. (1989*a*). Reflex actions of selective stimulation of sural nerve C fibres in the rabbit. *Q. J. Exp. Physiol.*, **74**, 681–90.
Clarke, R. W., Ford, T. W. & Taylor, J. S. (1989*b*). Activation by high intensity peripheral nerve stimulation of adrenergic and opioidergic inhibition of a spinal reflex in the decerebrated rabbit. *Brain Res.*, **505**, 1–6.
Clarke, R. W., Galloway, F. J., Harris, J. S. & Ford, T. W. (1992*a*). Opioidergic inhibition of flexor and extensor reflexes in the rabbit. *J. Physiol.*, **449**, 493–501.
Clarke, R. W., Harris, J., Ford, T. W. & Taylor, J. S. (1991*a*). Opioidergic inhibition of reflexes evoked by selective stimulation of sural nerve C-fibres in the rabbit. *Exp. Physiol.*, **76**, 987–90.
Clarke, R. W., Harris, J., Taylor, J. S. & Ford, T. W. (1992*b*). Prolonged potentiation of transmission through a withdrawal reflex pathway after noxious stimulation of the heel in the rabbit. *Pain*, **49**, 65–70.
Clarke, R. W., Isherwood, S. G. & Harris, J. (1991*b*). Excitability changes in hindlimb flexor reflexes after intense afferent barrage in the decerebrated and spinalized rabbit. *J. Physiol.*, **438**, 197P.
Clarke, R. W. & Matthews, B. (1990). The thresholds of the jaw-opening reflex and trigeminal brainstem neurons to tooth-pulp stimulation in acutely and chronically prepared cats. *Neuroscience*, **36**, 105–14.
Connell, L. A. & Wallis, D. I. (1988). Response to 5-hydroxytryptamine evoked in the hemisected spinal cord of the neonate rat. *Br. J. Pharmacol.*, **94**, 1101–14.
Connell, L. A., Majid, A. & Wallis, D. I. (1989). Involvement of $\alpha_1$-adrenoceptors in the depolarizing but not the hyperpolarizing responses of motorneurones in the neonate rat to noradrenaline. *Neuropharmacology*, **28**, 1399–404.
Cruz, L. & Basbaum, A. I. (1985). Multiple opioid peptides and the modulation of pain: immunohistochemical analysis of dynorphin and enkephalin in trigeminal nucleus caudalis and the spinal cord of the cat. *J. Comp. Neurol.*, **240**, 331–48.
Debroucker, T., Cesaro, P., Willer, J.-C. & Le Bars, D. (1990). Diffuse noxious inhibitory controls in man – involvement of the spinoreticular tract. *Brain*, **113**, 1223–34.
De Ceballos, M. L., Jenner, P. & Marsden, C. D. (1990). Increased [met]enkephalin and decreased substance P in spinal cord following thermal injury to one limb. *Neuroscience*, **36**, 731–6.
De Paulis, A. & Bandler, R. (eds.) (1991). *The Midbrain Periaqueductal Gray Matter*. New York: Plenum Press.
Dickenson, A. H. (1986). A new approach to pain relief? *Nature*, **320**, 681–2.
Dickenson, A. H., Le Bars, D. & Besson, J.-M. (1980). Diffuse noxious inhibitory controls (DNIC). Effects on trigeminal nucleus caudalis of the rat. *Brain Res.*, **200**, 293–305.
Dickenson, A. H., Sullivan, A. F. & Roques, B. P. (1988). Evidence that endogenous enkephalins and a $\delta$ opioid receptor agonist have a common site of action in spinal antinociception. *Eur. J. Pharmacol.*, **148**, 437–9.
Dougherty, P. M. & Willis, W. D. (1991). Enhancement of spinothalamic neuron responses to chemical and mechanical stimuli following combined micro-iontophoretic application of *N*-methyl-D-aspartic acid and substance-P. *Pain*, **47**, 85–93.
Dubner, R. (1991). Neuronal plasticity and pain following peripheral tissue

inflammation or nerve injury. In *Proceedings of the VIth World Congress on Pain*, ed. M. R. Bond, J. E. Charlton & C. J. Woolf, pp. 263–76. Amsterdam: Elsevier.

Dubner, R., Kenshalo, D. R. Jr, Maixner, W., Bushnell, M. C. & Oliveras, J.-L. (1989). The correlation of monkey medullary dorsal horn neuronal activity and the perceived intensity of noxious heat stimuli. *J. Neurophysiol.*, **62**, 450–7.

Duggan, A. W. (1985). Pharmacology of descending control systems. *Philosoph. Trans. R. Soc. London B*, **308**, 375–81.

Duggan, A. W., Griersmith, B. T. & North, R. A. (1980). Morphine and supraspinal inhibition of spinal neurones: evidence that morphine decreases tonic descending inhibition in the anesthetized cat. *Br. J. Pharmacol.*, **69**, 461–6.

Duggan, A. W., Hall, J. G., Foong, F. W. & Zhao, Z. Q. (1985). A differential effect of naloxone on transmission of impulses in primary afferents to ventral roots and ascending spinal tracts. *Brain Res.*, **344**, 316–21.

Duggan, A. W., Hall, J. G. & Headley, P. M. (1977*a*). Enkephalins and dorsal horn neurones in the cat: effects on responses to noxious and innocuous stimulation. *Br. J. Pharmacol.*, **61**, 399–408.

Duggan, A. W., Hall, J. G., Headley, P. M. & Griersmith, B. T. (1977*b*). The effect of naloxone on the excitation of dorsal horn neurones of the cat by noxious and non-noxious cutaneous stimulation. *Brain Res.*, **138**, 185–9.

Duggan, A. W. & Hendry, I. A. (1986). Laminar localization of the sites of release of immunoreactive substance P in the dorsal horn with antibody-coated microelectrodes. *Neurosci. Lett.*, **68**, 134–40.

Duggan, A. W., Hope, P. J., Jarrott, B., Schaible, H. G. & Fleetwood-Walker, S. M. (1990). Release, spread and persistence of immunoreactive neurokinin A in the dorsal horn of the cat following noxious stimulation: studies with antibody microprobes. *Neuroscience*, **35**, 195–202.

Duggan, A. W., Hope, P. J. & Lang, C. W. (1991). Microinjection of neuropeptide-Y into the superficial dorsal horn reduces stimulus-evoked release of immunoreactive substance P in the anaesthetized cat. *Neuroscience*, **44**, 733–40.

Duggan, A. W. & Johnson, S. M. (1983). Narcotic antagonists: problems in interpretation of their effects in laboratory and clinical research. In *Advances in Pain Research and Therapy*, ed. J. J. Bonica, V. Lindblom & A. Iggo, pp. 309–21. New York: Raven.

Duggan, A. W. & Morton, C. R. (1988). Tonic descending inhibition and spinal nociceptive transmission. *Prog. Brain Res.*, **77**, 193–211.

Duggan, A. W., Morton, C. R., Johnson, S. M. & Zhao, Z. Q. (1984). Opioid antagonists and spinal reflexes in the cat. *Brain Res.*, **297**, 33–40.

Duggan, A. W. & North, R. A. (1984). Electrophysiology of opioids. *Pharmacol. Rev.*, **35**, 219–81.

El-Yassir, N. & Fleetwood-Walker, S. M. (1990). A 5-$HT_1$-type receptor mediates the antinociceptive effect of nucleus raphe magnus stimulation in the rat. *Brain Res.*, **523**, 92–9.

Fanselow, M. S. (1991). The midbrain periaqueductal gray as a coordinator of action in response to fear and anxiety. In *The Midbrain Periaqueductal Gray Matter*, ed. A. De Paulis & R. Bandler, pp. 151–73. New York: Plenum.

Fanselow, M. S. & Sigmundi, R. A. (1986). Species-specific danger signals, endogenous opioid analgesia, and defensive behaviour. *J. Exp. Psychol.*, **12**, 301–9.

Fields, H. L. (1992). Is there a facilitating component to central pain modulation? *Am. Pain Soc. J.*, **1**, 139–41.
Fields, H. L. & Heinricher, M. M. (1985). Anatomy and physiology of a nociceptive modulatory system. *Philosoph. Trans. R. Soc. B*, **308**, 143–56.
Fields, H. L., Heinricher, M. M. & Mason, P. (1991). Neurotransmitters in nociceptive modulatory circuits. *Annu. Rev. Neurosci.*, **14**, 219–45.
Fitzgerald, M. & Woolf, C. J. (1980). The stereospecific effect of naloxone on rat dorsal horn neurones: inhibition in superficial laminae and excitation in deeper laminae. *Pain*, **9**, 293–306.
Fleetwood-Walker, S. M., Hope, P. J., Mitchell, R., El-Yassir, N. & Molony, V. (1988). The influence of opioid receptor subtypes on the processing of nociceptive inputs in the dorsal horn of the cat. *Brain Res.*, **451**, 213–26.
Fleetwood-Walker, S. M., Mitchell, R., Hope, P. J., Molony, V. & Iggo, A. (1985). An $\alpha_2$-receptor mediates the selective inhibition by noradrenaline of nociceptive responses of identified dorsal horn neurones. *Brain Res.*, **334**, 243–54.
Fleischmann, A. & Urca, G. (1988). Different endogenous analgesia systems are activated by noxious stimulation of different body regions. *Brain Res.*, **455**, 49–57.
Foong, F. W. & Duggan, A. W. (1986). Brain-stem areas tonically inhibiting dorsal horn neurones: studies with microinjection of the GABA analogue piperidine-4-sulphonic acid. *Pain*, **27**, 361–71.
Ford, T. W., Harris, J. & Taylor, J. S. (1991). The effects of naloxone on spinal neurones with excitatory input from the sural nerve in the decerebrated and spinalized rabbit. *J. Physiol.*, **435**, 61P.
Frazer, A., Maayani, S. & Wolfe, B. B. (1990). Subtypes of receptors for serotonin. *Annu. Rev. Pharmacol. Toxicol.*, **30**, 307–48.
Fung, S. J. & Barnes, C. D. (1981). Evidence of facilitatory coeruleospinal action in lumbar motoneurons of cats. *Brain Res.*, **216**, 299–311.
Gebhart, G. F. & Ness, T. J. (1991). Mechanisms of visceral pain. In *Proceedings of the VIth World Congress on Pain*, ed. M. R. Bond, J. E. Charlton & C. J. Woolf, pp. 351–64. Amsterdam: Elsevier.
Gebhart, G. F., Sandkühler, J., Thalhammer, J. G. & Zimmerman, M. (1983). Inhibition of spinal nociceptive information by stimulation of the midbrain in the cat is blocked by lidocaine microinjected into nucleus raphe magnus and the medullary reticular formation. *J. Neurophysiol.*, **50**, 1446–57.
Gebhart, G. F., Sandkühler, J., Thalhammer, J. G. & Zimmerman, M. (1984). Inhibition of spinal cord antinociceptive information by electrical stimulation and morphine microinjection at identical sites in the midbrain of the cat. *J. Neurophysiol.*, **51**, 75–89.
Glazer, E. J. & Basbaum, A. I. (1981). Immunohistochemical localization of leucine-enkephalin in the spinal cord of the cat: enkephalin-containing marginal neurons and pain modulation. *J. Comp. Neurol.*, **196**, 19–30.
Goldfarb, J. & Hu, J. W. (1976). Enhancement of reflexes by naloxone in acute spinal cats. *Neuropharmacology*, **15**, 785–92.
Gouardarès, C., Cros, J. & Quirion, R. (1985). Autoradiographic localization of mu, delta and kappa opioid receptor binding sites in rat and guinea pig spinal cord. *Neuropeptides*, **6**, 331–42.
Griersmith, B. T. & Duggan, A. W. (1980). Prolonged depression of spinal transmission of nociceptive information by 5HT administered in substantia gelatinosa: antagonism by methysergide. *Brain Res.*, **187**, 231–6.
Hall, J. G., Duggan, A. W., Morton, C. R. & Johnson, S. M. (1982). The

location of brain stem neurones tonically inhibiting dorsal horn neurones in the cat. *Brain Res.*, **244**, 215–22.

Han, J. S., Chen, X. H., Sun, S. L., Xu, X. J., Yuan, Y., Yan, S. C., Hao, J. X. & Terenius, L. (1991). Effect of low- and high-frequency TENS on met-enkephalin-arg-phe and dynorphin A immunoreactivity in human lumbar CSF. *Pain*, **295**–8.

Handwerker, H. O., Iggo, A. & Zimmerman, M. (1975). Segmental and supraspinal actions on dorsal horn neurons responding to noxious and non-noxious skin stimuli. *Pain*, **1**, 147–65.

Handwerker, H. O. & Reeh, P. W. (1991). Pain and inflammation. In *Proceedings of the VIth World Congress on Pain*, eds M. R. Bond, J. E. Charlton & C. J. Woolf, pp. 59–70. Amsterdam: Elsevier.

Harris, J. & Clarke, R. W. (1992). An analysis of adrenergic influences on the sural-gastrocnemius reflex of the decerebrated rabbit. *Exp. Brain Res.*, **92**, 310–17.

Harris, J., White, D. P. & Clarke, R. W. (1992). The roles of 5-HT in modulating a spinal reflex in the decerebrated rabbit. *Neurosci. Lett.*, **42** (Suppl.), S14.

Hartell, N. A. & Headley, P. M. (1991*a*). The effect of naloxone on spinal reflexes to electrical and mechanical stimuli in the anaesthetized, spinalized rat. *J. Physiol.*, **442**, 513–26.

Hartell, N. A. & Headley, P. M. (1991*b*). Preparative surgery enhances the direct spinal actions of three injectable anaesthetics in the anaesthetized rat. *Pain*, **46**, 75–80.

Hayes, R. L., Price, D. D., Ruda, M. A. & Dubner, R. (1979). Suppression of nociceptive responses in the primate by electrical stimulation of the brain or by morphine administration: behavioural and electrophysiological comparisons. *Brain Res.*, **167**, 417–21.

Headley, P. M., Duggan, A. W. & Griersmith, B. T. (1978). Selective reduction by noradrenaline and 5-hydroxytryptamine of nociceptive responses of cat dorsal horn neurones. *Brain Res.*, **145**, 185–9.

Heinricher, M. M., Barbaro, N. M. & Fields, H. L. (1989). Putative nociceptive modulating neurons in the rostral ventromedial medulla of the rat: firing of on- and off-cells related to nociceptive responsiveness. *Somatosens. Motor Res.*, **6**, 427–39.

Heinricher, M. M., Cheng, Z. & Fields, H. L. (1987). Evidence for two classes of nociceptive modulating neurons in the periaqueductal gray. *J. Neurosci.*, **7**, 271–8.

Hentall, I. & Fields, H. L. (1984). Actions of opiates, substance P and serotonin on the excitability of primary afferent terminals and observations of interneuronal activity in the neonatal rat's dorsal horn *in vitro*. *Neuroscience*, **9**, 521–8.

Herdegen, T., Kovary, K., Leah, J. & Bravo, R. (1991). Specific temporal and spatial distribution of JUN, FOS, and KROX-24 proteins in spinal neurons following noxious transsynaptic stimulation. *J. Comp. Neurol.*, **313**, 178–91.

Hillman, P. & Wall, P. D. (1969). Inhibitory and excitatory factors influencing the receptive fields of lamina 5 spinal cord cells. *Exp. Brain Res.*, **9**, 284–306.

Hodge, C. J., Apkarian, A. V., Stevens, R. T., Vogelsong, G. D., Brown, O. & Frank, I. J. (1983). Dorsolateral pontine inhibition of dorsal horn cell responses to cutaneous stimulation: lack of dependence on catecholaminergic system in cat. *J. Neurophysiol.*, **50**, 1220–35.

Hodge, C. J., Apkarian, A. V., Stevens, R., Vogelsong, G. & Wisnicki, H. J.

(1981). Locus coeruleus modulation of dorsal horn unit responses to cutaneous stimulation. *Brain Res.*, **204**, 415–20.

Hoheisel, U. & Mense, S. (1989). Long-term changes in discharge behaviour of cat dorsal horn neurones following noxious stimulation of deep tissues. *Pain*, **36**, 239–47.

Hökfelt, T. T., Ljungdahl, A., Terenius, L., Elde, R. & Nilsson, G. (1977). Immunohistochemical analysis of peptide pathways possibly related to pain and analgesia: enkephalin and substance P. *Proc. Nat. Acad. Sci. USA*, **74**, 3081–5.

Holmqvist, B. & Lundberg, A. (1961). Differential supraspinal control of synaptic actions evoked by volleys in the flexion reflex afferents in alpha motoneurones. *Acta Physiol. Scand.* (54 Suppl.) **186**, 1–51.

Holstege, G. (1991). Descending pathways from the periaqueductal gray and adjacent areas. In *The Midbrain Periaqueductal Gray Matter*, ed. A. De Paulis & R. Bandler, pp. 239–66. New York: Plenum.

Holstege, G. & Kuypers, H. G. J. M. (1982). The anatomy of brain stem pathways to the spinal cord in the cat. A labelled amino acid tracing study. *Prog. Brain Res.*, **57**, 145–75.

Holstege, J. C. & Kuypers, H. G. J. M. (1987). Brainstem projections to spinal motoneurons: an update. *Neuroscience*, **23**, 809–21.

Hopkins, A. & Holstege, G. (1978). Amygdaloid projections to mesencephalon, pons, and medulla oblongata in the cat. *Exp. Brain Res.*, **32**, 529–47.

Hu, J. W., Sessle, B. J., Raboisson, P., Dallel, R. & Woda, A. (1992). Stimulation of craniofacial muscle afferents induces prolonged facilitatory effects in trigeminal nociceptive brain-stem neurones. *Pain*, **48**, 53–60.

Hunt, S. P. & Lovick, T. A. (1982). The distribution of serotonin, met-enkephalin and $\beta$-lipotropin-like immunoreactivity in neuronal perikarya of the cat brain stem. *Neurosci. Lett.*, **30**, 1341–5.

Hunt, S. P., Pini, A. & Evans, G. (1987). Induction of c-*fos*-like protein in spinal cord neurons following sensory stimulation. *Nature*, **328**, 632–4.

Iggo, A., Steedman, W. M. & Fleetwood-Walker, S. M. (1985). Spinal processing: anatomy and physiology of spinal nociceptive processing. *Philosoph. Trans. R. Soc. London B*, **308**, 235–52.

Irwin, S., Houde, R. W., Bennett, D. R., Hendershot, L. C. & Stevens, M. H. (1951). The effects of morphine, methadone and meperidine on some reflex responses of spinal animals to nociceptive stimulation. *J. Pharmacol. Exp. Ther.*, **101**, 132–43.

Jaakola, M.-L., Salonen, M., Lehtinen, R. & Scheinin, H. (1991). The analgesic action of dexmedetomidine – a novel $\alpha_2$-adrenoceptor agonist – in healthy volunteers. *Pain*, **46**, 281–6.

Jänig, W., Schmidt, R. F. & Zimmerman, M. (1969). Two specific feedback pathways to the central afferent terminals of phasic and tonic mechanoreceptors. *Exp. Brain Res.*, **6**, 116–29.

Jebeles, J. A., Reilly, J. S., Gutierrez, J. F., Bradley, E. L. Jr & Kissin, I. (1991). The effect of pre-incisional infiltration of tonsils with bupivacaine on the pain following tonsillectomy under general anaesthesia. *Pain*, **47**, 305–8.

Jeftinija, S. (1988). Enkephalins modulate excitatory synaptic transmission in the superficial dorsal horn by acting at $\mu$-opioid receptor sites. *Brain Res.*, **460**, 260–8.

Jones, S. L. & Gebhart, G. F. (1986). Characterisation of coeruleospinal inhibition of the nociceptive tail-flick reflex in the rat: mediation by spinal $\alpha_2$-adrenoceptors. *Brain Res.*, **364**, 315–30.

Jurna, I. & Grossman, W. (1976). The effects of morphine on the activity evoked in ventrolateral tract axons of the cat spinal cord. *Exp. Brain Res.*, **24**, 473–84.

Kenshalo, D. R., Leonard, R. B., Chung, J. M. & Willis, W. D. (1982). Facilitation of the response of primate spinothalmic tract cells to cold and to tactile stimuli by noxious heating of the skin. *Pain.* **12**, 141–52.

Kidokoro, Y., Kubota, K., Shuto, S. & Sumino, R. (1968). Reflex organization of cat masticatory muscles. *J. Neurophysiol.*, **31**, 695–708.

Kiss, I. E. & Kilian, M. (1992). Does opiate premedication influence postoperative analgesia? A prospective study. *Pain*, **48**, 157–8.

Kosterlitz, H. W. (1985). Opioid peptides and their receptors. *Proc. R. Soc. London B*, **25**, 27–40.

Lai, Y.-Y., Strahlendorf, H. K., Fung, S. J. & Barnes, C. D. (1989). The actions of two monoamines on spinal motoneurons from stimulation of the locus coeruleus in the cat. *Brain Res.*, **484**, 268–72.

Laird, J. M. A. & Cervero, F. (1989). A comparative study of the changes in receptive-field properties of multireceptive and nocireceptive rat dorsal horn neurons following noxious mechanical stimulation. *J. Neurophysiol.*, **62**, 854–63.

LaMotte, C. C. & De Lanerolle, D. (1981). Human spinal neurons: innervation by both substance P and enkephalin. *Neuroscience*, **6**, 713–23.

Leah, J. D., Sandkühler, J., Herdegen, T., Murashov, A. & Zimmerman, M. (1992). Potentiated expression of fos protein in the rat spinal cord following bilateral noxious cutaneous stimulation. *Neuroscience*, **48**, 525–32.

Le Bars, D., Dickenson, A. H. & Besson, J.-M. (1979). Diffuse noxious inhibitory controls (DNIC). I. Effects on dorsal horn convergent neurones in the rat. *Pain*, **6**, 283–304.

Le Bars, D., Guilbaud, J., Jurna, I. & Besson, J.-M. (1976). Differential effects of morphine on response of dorsal horn lamina V type cells elicited by A and C fibre stimulation in the spinal cat. *Brain Res.*, **115**, 518–24.

Le Bars, D. & Villanueva, L. (1988). Electrophysiological evidence for the activation of descending inhibitory controls by nociceptive afferent pathways. *Prog. Brain Res.*, **77**, 275–99.

Le Bars, D., Villanueva, L. & Willer, J.-C. (1992). Pain modulation: from a negative feedback loop to a positive feedback loop? *Am. Pain Soc. J.*, **1**, 155–9.

Light, A. R. & Perl, E. R. (1979). Spinal terminations of functionally identified primary afferent neurons with slowly conducting myelinated fibers. *J. Comp. Neurol.*, **183**, 133–50.

Lovick, T. A. (1992). Inhibitory modulation of the cardiovascular defence response by the ventrolateral periaqueductal grey matter in rats. *Exp. Brain Res.*, **89**, 133–9.

Lovick, T. A. & Lumb, B. M. (1991). The defence reaction and inhibition of viscerosomatic reflexes. In *Proceedings of the VIth World Congress on Pain*, ed. M. R. Bond, J. E. Charlton & C. J. Woolf, pp. 389–94. Amsterdam: Elsevier.

Lund, C., Hansen, O. B. & Kehlet, H. (1990). Effect of surgery on sensory threshold and somatosensory evoked potentials after skin stimulation. *Br. J. Anaesth.*, **65**, 173–6.

Lundberg, A. (1982). Inhibitory control from the brain stem of transmission from primary afferents to motoneurons, primary afferent terminals and ascending pathways. In *Brain Stem Control of Spinal Mechanisms*, ed. B. Sjölund & A. Björklund, pp. 179–224. Amsterdam: Elsevier.

Macdonald, A. J. (1989). Acupuncture analgesia and therapy. In *Textbook of Pain*, ed. P. D. Wall & R. M. Melzack, R. M., pp. 906–19. Edinburgh: Churchill Livingstone.
Madden, J., Akil, H., Patrick, R. L. & Barchas, J. D. (1977). Stress-induced parallel changes in central opioid levels and pain responsiveness in the rat. *Nature*, **265**, 358–60.
Magnusson, D. S. K. & Dickenson, A. H. (1991). Lamina-specific effects of morphine and naloxone in dorsal horn of rat spinal cord *in vitro*. *J. Neurophysiol.*, **66**, 1941–50.
Martin, W. R., Eades, C. G., Thompson, J. A., Huppler, R. E. & Gilbert, P. E. (1976). The effects of morphine and nalorphine-like drugs in the non-dependent and morphine-dependent chronic spinal dog. *J. Pharmacol. Exp. Ther.*, **197**, 517–32.
Mayer, D. J. & Liebeskind, J. C. (1974). Pain reduction by focal electrical stimulation of the brain: an anatomical and behavioural analysis. *Brain Res.*, **68**, 73–93.
Mayer, D. J., Price, D. D. & Rafii, A. (1977). Antagonism of acupuncture analgesia in man by the narcotic antagonist naloxone. *Brain Res.*, **121**, 368–72.
Mayer, D. J., Wolfe, T. L., Akil, H., Carder, B. & Liebeskind, J. C. (1971). Analgesia from electrical stimulation of the brain stem of the rat. *Science*, **174**, 1351–4.
McMahon, S. B. & Wall, P. D. (1984). Receptive fields of rat lamina I projection cells move to incorporate a nearby region of injury. *Pain*, **19**, 235–47.
McQuay, H. J., Carroll, D. & Moore, R. A. (1992). Postoperative orthopaedic pain – the effect of opiate pre-medication and local anaesthetic blocks. *Pain*, **33**, 291–5.
Melzack, R. M. (1975). Prolonged relief of pain by brief, intense transcutaneous somatic stimulation. *Pain*, **1**, 357–73.
Melzack, R. M. (1989). Folk medicine and sensory modulation of pain. In *Textbook of Pain*, ed. P. D. Wall & R. M. Melzack, pp. 897–905. Edinburgh: Churchill Livingstone.
Melzack, R. & Wall, P. D. (1965). Pain mechanisms: a new theory. *Science*, **150**, 971–8.
Melzack, R. M. & Wall, P. D. (1988). *The Challenge of Pain*. London: Penguin.
Mendell, L. M. & Wall, P. D. (1964). Presynaptic hyperpolarization: a role for fine afferent fibres. *J. Physiol.*, **172**, 274–94.
Mense, S. & Prabhakar, N. R. (1986). Spinal terminations of nociceptive afferent fibres from deep tissues in the cat. *Neurosci. Lett.*, **66**, 169–74.
Mense, S. & Skeppar, P. (1991). Discharge behaviour of feline gamma-motoneurones following the induction of artificial myositis. *Pain*, **46**, 201–11.
Meyer, R. A. & Campbell, J. N. (1981). Peripheral coding of pain sensation. *Johns Hopkins APL Tech. Digest*, **2**, 164–71.
Meyer, R. A., Treede, R.-D., Srinivasa, N. R. & Campbell, N. A. (1992). Peripheral versus central mechanisms for secondary hyperalgesia. Is the controversy resolved? *APS J.*, **1**, 127–31.
Mokha, S. S. (1992). Differential effect of naloxone on the responses of nociceptive neurons in the superficial versus the deeper dorsal horn of the medulla in the rat. *Pain*, **49**, 405–13.
Mokha, S. S., McMillan, J. A. & Iggo, A. (1986). Pathways mediating

descending control of spinal nociceptive transmission from the nuclei locus coeruleus (LC) and raphe magnus (NRM) in the cat. *Exp. Brain Res.*, **61**, 597–606.

Morgan, M. M. (1991). Differences in antinociception evoked from dorsal and ventral regions of the caudal periaqueductal gray matter. In *The Midbrain Periaqueductal Gray Matter*, ed. A. De Paulis & R. Bandler, pp. 139–50. New York: Plenum.

Morgan, M. M., Heinricher, M. M. & Fields, H. L. (1992). Circuitry linking opioid-sensitive nociceptive modulatory systems in periaqueductal gray and spinal cord with rostral ventromedial medulla. *Neuroscience*, **47**, 863–71.

Morton, C. R., Du, H.-J., Xiao, H., Maisch, B. & Zimmerman, M. (1988). Inhibition of nociceptive responses of dorsal horn neurones by remote noxious afferent stimulation in the cat. *Pain*, **34**, 75–83.

North, R. A. (1989). Drug receptors and the inhibition of nerve cells. *Br. J. Pharmacol.*, **98**, 13–28.

Ochoa, J. & Torebjörk, E. (1989). Sensations evoked by intraneural microstimulation of C nociceptor fibres in human skin nerves. *J. Physiol.*, **415**, 583–600.

Oliveras, J.-L., Besson, J.-M., Guilbaud, G. & Liebeskind, J. C. (1974). Behavioural and electrophysiological evidence of pain inhibition from midbrain stimulation in the cat. *Exp. Brain Res.*, **20**, 32–44.

Parsons, C. G. & Headley, P. M. (1989). Spinal antinociceptive actions of $\mu$- and $\kappa$-opioids: the importance of stimlulus intensity in determining 'selectivity' between reflexes to different modalities of noxious stimulus. *Br. J. Pharmacol.*, **98**, 523–32.

Perl, E. R. (1984). Characterization of nociceptors and their activation of neurons in the superficial layers of the dorsal horn: first steps for the sensation of pain. In *Advances in Pain Research and Therapy*, ed. L. Kruger & J. C. Liebeskind, pp. 25–31. New York: Academic Press.

Prado, W. A. & Roberts, M. H. T. (1984). An assessment of the antinociceptive and aversive effects of stimulating identified sites in the rat brain. *Brain Res.*, **340**, 219–28.

Price, D. D. & Dubner, R. (1977). Neurons that subserve the sensory-discriminative aspects of pain. *Pain*, **3**, 307–88.

Proudfit, H. K. (1988). Pharmacologic evidence for the modulation of nociception by noradrenergic neurons. *Prog. Brain Res.*, **77**, 357–70.

Ramirez, F. & Vanegas, H. (1989). Tooth pulp stimulation advances both medullary off-cell pause and tail flick. *Neurosci. Lett.*, **100**, 153–6.

Reading, A. E. (1989). Testing pain mechanisms in persons in pain. In *Textbook of Pain*, ed. P. D. Wall & R. M. Melzack, pp. 269–83. Edinburgh: Churchill Livingstone.

Rees, H., Prado, W. A., Rawlings, S. & Roberts, M. H. T. (1987). The effects of intraperitoneal administration of antagonists and development of morphine tolerance on the antinociception produced by stimulating the APtN of the rat. *Br. J. Pharmacol.*, **92**, 769–79.

Rees, H. & Roberts, M. H. T. (1987). Anterior pretectal stimulation alters the responses of spinal dorsal horn neurones to cutaneous stimulation in the rat. *J. Physiol.*, **385**, 415–36.

Reichling, D. B., Kwiat, G. C. & Basbaum, A. I. (1988). Anatomy, physiology and pharmacology of the periaqueductal gray contribution to antinociceptive controls. *Prog. Brain Res.*, **77**, 31–46.

Reynolds, D. V. (1969). Surgery in the rat during electrical analgesia induced by focal brain stimulation. *Science*, **164**, 444–5.

Richardson, D. E. & Akil, H. (1977). Pain reduction by electrical brain stimulation in man. I. Acute administration of periaqueductal and periventricular sites. II. Chronic self-administration in the periventricular gray matter. *J. Neurosurg.*, **47**, 184–94.

Rivot, J. P., Calvino, B. & Besson, J.-M. (1987). Is there a serotonergic tonic descending inhibition on the responses of dorsal horn convergent neurons to C-fiber inputs? *Brain Res.*, **403**, 142–6.

Ruda, M. A. (1982). Opiates and pain pathways: demonstration of enkephalin synapses on dorsal horn projection neurons. *Science*, **215**, 1523–5.

Sagen, J. & Proudfit, H. (1984). Effect of intrathecally administered noradrenergic antagonists on nociception in the rat. *Brain Res.*, **310**, 295–301.

Sastry, B. R. & Goh, J. W. (1983). Actions of morphine and met-enkephalin-amide on nociceptor driven neurones in substantia gelatinosa and deeper dorsal horn. *Neuropharmacology*, **22**, 119–22.

Satoh, M., Kawajiri, S.-I., Ukai, Y. & Yamamoto, M. (1979). Selective and non-selective inhibition by enkephalins and noradrenaline of nociceptive response of lamina V type neurons in the spinal dorsal horn of the rabbit. *Brain Res.*, **177**, 384–7.

Schaible, H.-G., Schmidt, R. F. & Willis, W. D. (1987). Enhancement of the responses of ascending tract cells in the cat spinal cord by acute inflammation of the knee joint. *Exp. Brain Res.*, **66**, 489–99.

Schmidt, R. F. (1971). Presynaptic inhibition in the vertebrate central nervous system. *Rev. Physiol. Biochem. Pharmacol.*, **63**, 21–101.

Segal, M. & Sandberg, D. (1977). Analgesia produced by electrical stimulation of catecholamine nuclei in the rat brain. *Brain Res.*, **123**, 369–72.

Semenenko, F. M. & Lumb, B. M. (1992). Projections of anterior hypothalamic neurones to the dorsal and ventral periaqueductal grey in the rat. *Brain Res.*, **582**, 237–45.

Sherrington, C. S. (1910). Flexion reflex of the limb, crossed extension reflex and reflex stepping and standing. *J. Physiol.*, **40**, 28–121.

Sherrington, C. S. & Sowton, S. C. M. (1915). Observations on reflex responses to single break shocks. *J. Physiol.*, **49**, 331–48.

Simone, D. A., Baumann, T. K. & LaMotte, R. H. (1989). Dose-dependent pain and mechanical hyperalgesia in humans after intradermal injection of capsaicin. *Pain*, **38**, 99–107.

Simone, D. A., Sorkin, L. S., Oh, U., Chung, J. M., Owens, C., LaMotte, R. H. & Willis, W. D. (1991). Neurogenic hyperalgesia – central neural correlates in responses of spinothalamic tract neurons. *J. Neurophysiol.*, **66**, 228–46.

Sjölund, B. H. & Eriksson, M. B. E. (1979). The influence of naloxone on analgesia produced by peripheral conditioning stimulation. *Brain Res.*, **173**, 295–301.

Skoog, B. & Noga, B. R. (1991). Do noradrenergic descending tract fibres contribute to the depression of transmission from group-II muscle afferents following brainstem stimulation in the cat. *Neurosci. Lett.*, **134**, 5–8.

Sugiura, Y., Lee, C. L. & Perl, E. R. (1986). Central projections of identified, unmyelinated (C) afferent fibers innervating mammalian skin. *Science*, **234**, 358–61.

Sugiura, Y., Terui, N. & Hosoya, Y. (1989). Difference in distribution of central terminals between visceral and somatic unmyelinated (C) primary afferent fibers. *J. Neurophysiol.*, **62**, 834–40.

Tasker, R. R. & Dostrovsky, J. O. (1989). Deafferentation and central pain. In *Textbook of Pain*, ed. P. D. Wall & R. M. Melzack, pp. 154–79. Edinburgh: Churchill Livingstone.

Tattersall, J. E. H., Cervero, F. & Lumb, B. M. (1986). Viscerosomatic neurons in the lower thoracic spinal cord of the cat: excitations and inhibitions evoked by splanchnic and somatic nerve volleys and by stimulation of brain stem nuclei. *J. Neurophysiol.*, **56**, 1141.

Taylor, J. S., Neal, R. I., Harris, J., Ford, T. W. & Clarke, R. W. (1991). Prolonged inhibition of a spinal reflex after intense stimulation of distant peripheral nerves in the decerebrated rabbit. *J. Physiol.*, **437**, 71–83.

Taylor, J. S., Pettit, J. S., Harris, J., Ford, T. W. & Clarke, R. W. (1990). Noxious stimulation of the toes evokes long-lasting, naloxone-reversible suppression of the sural-gastrocnemius reflex in the rabbit. *Brain Res.*, **531**, 263–8.

Terenzi, M. G., Rees, H., Morgan, S. J. S., Foster, G. A. & Roberts, M. H. T. (1991). The antinociception evoked by anterior pretectal nucleus stimulation is partially dependent upon ventrolateral medullary neurones. *Pain*, **47**, 231–9.

Todd, A. J. & Millar, J. (1983). Receptive fields and responses of iontophoretically applied noradrenaline and 5-hydroxytryptamine of units recorded in laminae I–III of the spinal cord. *Brain Res.*, **288**, 159–68.

Torebjörk, H. E., Lundberg, L. E. R. & LaMotte, R. H. (1992). Central changes in processing of mechanoreceptive input in capsaicin-induced secondary hyperalgesia in humans. *J. Physiol*, **448**, 765–80.

Torebjörk, H. E. & Ochoa, J. L. (1990). New method to identify nociceptor units innervating glabrous skin of the human hand. *Exp. Brain Res.*, **81**, 509–14.

Treede, R. D., Meyer, R. A., Raja, S. N. & Campbell, J. N. (1992). Peripheral and central mechanisms of cutaneous hyperalgesia. *Prog. Neurobiol.*, **38**, 397–421.

Tverskoy, M., Cozacov, C., Qyache, M., Bradley, E. L. & Kissin, I. (1992). Postoperative pain after inguinal hernography with different types of anaesthesia. *Anaesth. Analg.*, **70**, 29–35.

Tyce, G. M. & Yaksh, T. L. (1981). Monoamine release from cat spinal cord by somatic stimuli: an intrinsic modulatory system. *J. Physiol.*, **314**, 513–31.

Urban, L. & Randic, M. (1984). Slow excitatory transmission in cat dorsal horn: possible mediation by peptides. *Brain Res.*, **290**, 336–41.

Villanueva, L., De Pommery, J., Menetrey, D. & Le Bars, D. (1991). Spinal afferent projections to subnucleus reticularis-dorsalis in the rat. *Neurosci. Lett.*, **134**, 98–102.

Villanueva, L. & Le Bars, D. (1986). Indirect effects of intrathecal morphine upon diffuse noxious inhibitory controls (DNICs) in the rat. *Pain*, **26**, 233–43.

Watkins, L. R., Cobelli, D. A., Faris, P., Aceto, M. D. & Mayer, D. J. (1982). Opiate vs non-opiate footshock-induced analgesia (FSIA): the body region shocked is a critical factor. *Brain Res.*, **242**, 299–308.

Watkins, L. R. & Mayer, D. J. (1982). Organization of endogenous opiate and non-opiate pain control systems. *Science*, **216**, 1185–92.

Westlund, K. N., Bowker, R. M., Ziegler, M. G. & Coulter, J. D. (1983). Noradrenergic projections to the spinal cord of the rat. *Brain Res.*, **263**, 15–31.

White, J. C. & Sweet, W. H. (1969). *Pain and the Neurosurgeon*. Springfield: Thomas.

Wiesenfeld-Hallin, Z., Hallin, R. G. & Persson, A. (1984). Do large diameter cutaneous afferents have a role in the transmissiion of nociceptive messages. *Brain Res.*, **311**, 375–9.

Willis, W. D. (1988). Anatomy and physiology of descending control of nociceptive responses of dorsal horn neurons: comprehensive review. *Prog. Brain Res.*, **77**, 1–29.

Willis, W. D. & Coggeshall, R. E. (1991). *Sensory Mechanisms of the Spinal Cord*, 2nd edn. New York: Plenum.

Woolf, C. J. (1983). Evidence for a central component of post-injury pain hypersensitivity. *Nature*, **306**, 686–88.

Woolf, C. J. (1989). Segmental and afferent fibre-induced analgesia: transcutaneous electrical nerve stimulation (TENS) and vibration. In *Textbook of Pain*, ed. P. D. Wall & R. M. Melzack, pp. 884–96. Edinburgh: Churchill Livingstone.

Woolf, C. J. (1991). Generation of acute pain – central mechanisms. *Br. Med. Bull.*, **47**, 523–33.

Woolf, C. J. & Fitzgerald, M. (1982). Do opioid peptides mediate a presynaptic control of C-fibre transmission in rat spinal cord? *Neurosci. Lett.*, **29**, 67–72.

Woolf, C. J. & King, A. E. (1987). Physiology and morphology of multireceptive neurons with C-afferent inputs in the deep dorsal horn of the rat lumbar spinal cord. *J. Neurophysiol.*, **58**, 460–79.

Woolf, C. J. & King, A. E. (1990). Dynamic alterations in the cutaneous mechanoreceptive fields of dorsal horn neurons in the rat spinal cord. *J. Neurosci.*, **10**, 2717–26.

Woolf, C. J., Mitchell, D. & Barrett, G. D. (1980). Antinociceptive effect of peripheral segmental electrical stimulation in the rat. *Pain*, **8**, 237–52.

Woolf, C. J. & Thompson, S. W. N. (1991). The induction and maintenance of central sensitization is dependent of *N*-methyl-D-aspartic acid receptor activation – implications for the treatment of post-injury pain hypersensitivity states. *Pain*, **44**, 293–9.

Woolf, C. J. & Wall, P. D. (1986). Relative effectiveness of C primary afferent fibres of different origins in evoking a prolonged facilitation of the flexor reflex in the rat. *J. Neurosci.*, **6**, 1433–42.

Woolf, C. J. & Wiesenfeld-Hallin, Z. (1986). Substance P and calcitonin gene-related peptide synergistically modulate the gain of the nociceptive flexor withdrawal reflex in the rat. *Neurosci. Lett.*, **66**, 226–30.

Xu, X. J. & Wiesenfeld-Hallin, Z. (1992). Intrathecal neurokinin-A facilitates the spinal nociceptive flexor reflex evoked by thermal and mechanical stimuli and synergistically interacts with substance-P. *Acta Physiol. Scand.*, **144**, 163–8.

Yaksh, T. L. (1979). Direct evidence that spinal serotonin and noradrenaline terminals mediate the spinal antinociceptive effects of morphine in the periaqueductal gray. *Brain Res.*, **160**, 180–5.

Yaksh, T. L. & Elde, R. P. (1981). Factors governing the release of methionine-enkephalin-like immunoreactivity from mesencephalon and spinal cord in the cat *in vivo*. *J. Neurophysiol.*, **46**, 1056–75.

Yaksh, T. L. & Noueihed, R. (1985). The physiology and pharmacology of spinal opiates. *Annu. Rev. Pharmacol. Toxicol.*, **25**, 433–62.

Yeomans, D. C., Clark, F. M., Paice, J. A. & Proudfit, H. K. (1992). Antinociception induced by electrical stimulation of spinally projecting noradrenergic neurons in the A7 catecholamine cell group of the rat. *Pain*, **48**, 449–61.

Yeomans, D. C. & Proudfit, H. K. (1990). Projections of substance P-immunoreactive neurons located in the ventromedial medulla to the A7 noradrenergic nucleus of the rat demonstrated using retrograde tracing combined with immunocytochemistry. *Brain Res.*, **532**, 329–32.

Yoshimura, M. & North, R. A. (1983). Substantia gelatinosa neurones hyperpolarized *in vivo* by enkephalin. *Nature*, **305**, 529–30.

Zhao, Z.-Q. & Duggan, A. W. (1988). Idazoxan blocks the action of noradrenaline but not spinal inhibition from electrical stimulation of the locus coeruleus and Kolliker-Fuse nucleus of the cat. *Neuroscience*, **25**, 997–1005.

Zhuo, M. & Gebhart, G. F. (1991*a*). Tonic cholinergic inhibition of spinal mechanical transmission. *Pain*, **46**, 211–22.

Zhuo, M. & Gebhart, G. F. (1991*b*). Spinal serotonin receptors mediate descending facilitation of a nociceptive reflex from the nuclei reticularis-gigantocellularis and gigantocellularis pars-alpha in the rat. *Brain Res.*, **550**, 35–48.

Zorman, G., Hentall, I. D., Adams, J. E. & Fields, H. L. (1981). Naloxone-reversible analgesia produced by microstimulation in rat medulla. *Brain Res.*, **228**, 137–48.

# 13
# The final word . . .

NANCY J. ROTHWELL

Trauma, even when restricted to a single, specific site, has effects influencing almost every homeostatic function and body system. This diverse response might be a delight to scientists, but often proves a nightmare to the clinician faced with numerous and sometimes conflicting symptoms, which in many cases have to be considered and treated independently. We hope that such diversity has been largely represented in the topics discussed in this book, although a discussion of all possible responses to trauma which might be influenced by the central nervous system (CNS) might run to several volumes.

It has been recognised for many decades that the brain directly influences or controls certain effects of trauma, such as chronic behavioural changes, pain, cardiovascular responses and disruptions in thermoregulation. The primary concern of the clinician is the acute management of the trauma patient. However, it is increasingly apparent that these associated responses directly influence outcome. Obvious examples of this are the impact on survival of body temperature, oxygen availability and cardiovascular function. Beyond the early critical phase, CNS-controlled responses clearly have profound effects on recovery time, subsequent quality of life and independence. More surprising has been the realisation that immune function and local inflammatory responses are markedly influenced by the CNS. Indeed, perhaps there is no component of the trauma patient that is not, in some way, affected by the brain.

These discoveries and the recent findings described in the various chapters unfortunately raise as many questions as they answer, but perhaps the realisation of the complexity of the problems and the interactions within the CNS is, in itself, a major step forward. The topic of CNS responses to trauma represents an excellent example of integrated research, involving numerous discplines and a parallel growth of basic research and clinical studies. Investigation into the interactions between the brain and the immune system, and in particular the role, actions and mechanisms of actions of immune mediators such as cytokines, has greatly facilitated our understanding of the responses to trauma. Future advances are likely to benefit from further dialogue and collaboration between scientists and clinicians.

Specific pathways and mechanisms that influence the body's response to traumatic insults have been identified. The important questions which must now be addressed are:

- which are the primary sites for potential intervention?
- can beneficial and detrimental responses be distinguished?
- what are the most practical means of interaction?
- can those patients most at risk be identified?
- are these interactions likely to improve long-term recovery and quality of life as well as acute survival?

The problems of diagnosis, selective, safe and efficient means of intervention, and understanding the acute and chronic mechanisms of response to trauma and their relative benefit are of obvious scientific and clinical interest, but also have important financial implications. The very rapid expansion of this field of research indicates that many of these problems may be at least partly resolved within the next decade.

# Index

Page references to charts and tables are italicized


α-MFP (α-macrofetoprotein), 48
α-MSH (α-melanocyte stimulating hormone), 50, 173–4, 175, 281
*abbreviations list*, 85–6
ACTH (adrenocorticotrophic hormone), 6, 50, 134–5, 240, 241, 242
  and neuroendocrine responses, 240, 241, 242, 245–6
ACTH–adrenal axis, 50–1, 74
acute phase
  hormones, 68–73
    defined, 33
  response, 41–2
    *see also* cytokines
  protein, *see* APP
  response, 41–2, 45–9, 53, 79, 282
  *see also* ebb phase
adipose tissue, 261–2, 283
adrenal cortex, 6
adrenal–ACTH axis, 50–1, 74
  *see also* HPA axis
adrenaline, 6, 248, 265
adrenergic nuclei, 305–6
adrenocorticotrophic hormone, *see* ACTH
affective reactions, 140–3
afferent
  axons, 296, 314
  baropreceptors, 209
  pathways, 270–4
  *see also* PAD; SNS
afferents, cardiac C-fibre, 206–8, 210, 213
AIDS (acquired immunodeficiency syndrome), 161–2
Alam and Smirk reflex, 9–10
aldosterone, 250
allodynia, 313
  transmitters and, 315–16
amygdala, lesions, 110
anaesthesia, 25
analgesia, stress-induced, 312
anaphylaxis, 108
anger, 141
angiotensins, 250
animals, 23–6, *24*
  advantages and limitations in studying, 24–6
  CNS function, study methods, 26–9
  cytokines and sickness behaviour, 156–8, *157*, *159*, 160
  experimentally induced injury, 266–8, *267*
  'freezing' response, 191–2
  infected, 153–4
  inhibitory effects of noxious stimuli, 309–12
  temperature measurement, 261
  *see also* baboons; cats; dogs; mammals, small; mice; monkeys; pigs; rabbits; rats; sheep
anterior pretectal nucleus (APtN), 306
anti-inflammatory effect, 68
anti-predatory systems, 191–2
antibiotics, 81
antibody production, 113
antinociception
  from stimulation of brain, 303–9
  mechanisms activated, 309–12
  pathways, 302
anxiety, 141
apoptosis, 34
APP (acute phase protein), 47, 48–9
  inducers, 48, 78
  synthesis, 76
APtN (anterior pretectal nucleus), 306
area postrema, 213
arousal, chronic increased, 139–40
arteries
  chemoreceptors, 208–9
  see also baroreceptors
arthritis, rheumatoid, 187
Arthus reaction, 83, 109, 110

astrocytes, 61
autocannibalism, 252–3
AVP (arginine vasopressin), 78, 173–5, 242, 246, 251, 281
axons, afferent, 296, 314

β-END (β-endorphin), 50–1, 77–8
baboons, 43
bacterial endotoxin, response to, 40–1
bacterial infections, 66, 243
baroreceptors, *212*
  afferents, 209
  and fluid loss, 242
  reflex, 205–6, 212–13, *217*
basophils, *36*, 59–60
BAT (brown adipose tissue), 261–2, 283
BBB (blood–brain barrier), 273
BCG, 112
behaviour, *see* sickness behaviour *and under* pain
biological injury, 40–5
bleeding, *see* haemorrhage
blood–brain barrier (BBB), 273
blood
  pressure, *see* hypotension
  *see also* cerebral perfusion
brown adipose tissue (BAT), 261–2, 283
burn injuries, 16, 35, 246, 247, 250
  metabolic and thermoregulatory responses, 264–5, 269–70

C-fibre afferents, 206–8, 210
C-reactive protein (CRP), 46–7
cachexia, 253, 263, 283
cancer patients, 53, 155–6
capsaicin, 60–1, 62, 314
cardiac C-fibre afferents, 206–8, 210, 213
cardiac reactions, 137–9
cardiovascular functions
  and afferent pathways, 270
  changes, 251
  homeostasis, 9–10
  *see also* blood; haemorrhage; hypotension
cardiovascular responses
  to haemorrhage, 202–15, *203*, 224–9
  to injury, 215–23
    central control, 202–31
    efferent pathways modulated, 218–22
    to injury and haemorrhage combined, 224–9
catabolic phase, *see* flow phase
catecholamines, 48, 56–7, 76–7, 248
cats, 170, 299
  cardiovascular system, 220–1
  central control of pain, 302, 303, 306, 307, 308, 311, 314, 315
CCK (cholecystokinin), 135–6
central control
  cardiovascular responses to injury, 202–31
    conclusions, 229, 231
  of pain, 295–317
central nervous system, *see* CNS
cerebral perfusion, 12–13
CGRP (calcitonin gene related peptide), 64
chemical agents, injury due to, 38
chemoreceptor reflexes, arterial, 208–9
chemoreceptors, 208–9
children, 263
  brown adipose tissue, 269
  burns, 16, 264
  cachexia, 263
  head injury, 277
  stress, 128, 137
ciliary neurotropic factor (CNTF), 48–9
circumventricular organs, 168–9
CNS (central nervous system)
  animals, 26–9
  and cardiovascular responses
    to haemorrhage, 209–15, *214*
  to 'injury', 216–18
  and haemorrhage, *214*
  and immune system, 153
  and inflammatory cells, 65
  neuroregulators, 131
  and pain, 186
  pathways, *214*, 275–82
  role, 7
  sickness behaviour controlled by, 152–7
  and trauma, 22–31
CNTF (ciliary neurotropic factor), 48–9
cold
  injury caused by, 35
  reduced response to, 7–8
colony stimulating factors (CSF), 71, 133–4
combat stress reaction (CSR), 129–30
cortex
  immunomodulation and, 111
  lesions of, 111–13
corticotropin releasing factor, *see* CRF
cortisol, 245–6
cortisone, 43
CRF, and rats, 63, 132, 171
CRF (corticotropin releasing factor), 28, 59, 63, 117, 171–2, 240–1
  and coordination of endocrine responses, 240–1
  general role, 131
  and metabolic/thermoregulatory control, 280–1
  and stress, 131–4
crime victims, 125–6, 128
  *see also* rape victims
CRP (C-reactive protein), 46–7

cryogens, and cytokines, 173–5
CSF (colony stimulating factors), 71, 133–4
CSR (combat stress reactions), 129–30
CTA (conditioned taste aversion), 153–4, 156–8
cyclooxygenase inhibitors, 172, 276–7
cytokine–endocrine response, pathways, 34–8
cytokines, 271–4
  action sites, peripheral or central, 168–71
  and acute phase, 45, 48
  behavioural effects mechanisms of, 165–73
  chemotactic proinflammatory, 55, 64–5, 83
  and cryogens, 173–5
  defined, 33, 271
  endogenous, 165–7
  and endothelium, *39*
  and humans, 161–2
  inflammatory, 55
  inhibitory, 72
  injections, 162–5, 168–71
  and local defence, 64–8
  and metabolic rate/thermoregulation, 277–80, *278*, *279*, *284*
  neural and endocrine regulation of, 49–61
  neurohormonal control of, 32–85
  conclusions, 82–5
  overview, 271
  pharmakodynamics, 162–5, *164*, *165*
  plethora of, 81, 82
  pyrogenic, 280
  released by tissue mast cells and basophils, *36*
  response to lipopolysaccharide, 41–2
  sickness behaviour induced by, 155–8, *157*, *159*, 160–5
    pharmacodynamic aspects, 162–5
  *see also* IFN (interferons); IL (interleukins); TNF (tumour necrosis factor)

defence (arousal) reaction, 11
  against injury, 61–82
  integrating visceral alerting response of, 218
  species-specific, 191–2
depression, 141
'depressor' response, 207
devitalised tissue, 80, 81
DEX (dexamethasone), 52–3, 54, 55
  acute phase, 48
dialysis, 27
diffuse noxious inhibitory controls (DNIC), 310–11
disease, defined, 190
dissociation, 142–3
DNA binding proteins, 49
DNIC (diffuse noxious inhibitory controls), 310–11
dogs
  blood pressure, 213
  'depressor' response, 207
  injury
    biological, 44
    pseudo-, 230
dorsal horn, 187, 188, 297–8, 304
  neurones, 302, 315
DSM-III, 128, 129, 136, 142

ebb phase, 5
  body temperature controlled in, 7–9
  defined, 239
  metabolic and thermoregulatory responses, 263
  and neuroendocrine response, 250–2
efferent activity, 209–13, *210–11*, *212*
  modulation of vagal, 218–19
  *see also* sympathetic efferent activity
eicosanoids, 276–7, 283
  *see also* PGs (prostaglandins)
elective surgery, 11–12, 69
  and nociceptive impulses, 11–12
electrical activity, 27, 28
electrical nerve stimulation, transcutaneous (TENS), 309
electrodermal reactions, 137–9
emotions, 241
endocrine
  regulation of cytokines, 49–61
  responses, 5–7, 240–1
  *see also* cytokine–endocrine response
endogenous antinociceptive mechanisms, activation of, 309–12
endogenous brain inhibitors, 281–2
endogenous opioids, *see* opioids, endogenous
endogenous pyrogens, 277, *278*
endothelium, cytokines produced by, *39*
endotoxins
  rats, 154
  and shock, 43–4, 81
  tolerance of, 76
energy expenditure, and temperature, 264
enzymes, *36*
epinephrine, 56
ethanol, 229
ethics, 25
exogenous opioids, *see* opioids, exogenous
experimental animals, *see* animals

fat, –see adipose tissue; BAT
fatty acids, *see* lipolysis
fever, *see* pyrexia
'fight or flight' response, 11

5-HT (5-hydroxytryptamine), 28, 227–9
flow (catabolic) phase, 5, 1
  defined, 239–40
  metabolic and thermoregulatory responses, 263
  and neuroendocrine response, 252–3
fluid loss, 7
  neuroendocrine response, 241–2
'freezing' response in animals, 191–2

GABA-ergic mechanisms, 216, 219, 221, 223, 229
gastrointestinal inflammation, 64, 83
GC (glucocorticoids), 48, 51–6, 74–6, 245–6, 252, 281
GH (growth hormone), 49–50, 241, 248
glucagon, 249, 265
glucocorticoids, *see* GC
glucose, 13, 251–1
gonadotrophins and gonadal steroids, 247
Gram-positive/-negative organisms, 80, 81, 82
granulocytes, *see* neutrophilic granulocytes
growth factor, *see* PDGF
growth hormone (GH), 49–50, 241, 248
guilt, assault-related, 130
guinea-pigs
  brain lesions, 108, 109
  metabolism/thermoregulation, *267*

haemodynamics, *see* cardiovascular
haemorrhage
  cardiovascular response, 202–15, *203*, 224–9
  cell/neurone response, 215
  combined with tissue damage, 10, 35, 224–9
  responses to, 24
  severe, 206, 208, 224, 227–8
  'simple', 202–5, *204*, *228*
heart, *see* cardiac; cardiovascular; vagal
hippocampus, 245, 275
  lesions, 110, 116
histamine, 58, 60
HIV (human immunodeficiency virus), 162
homeostasis
  cardiovascular, 9–11
  inhibition of, 9–15
    ebb phase, 14–15
    when treatment imminent, 15
homicide survivors, 127
hormones, 49–58, *75*, 245–50, *36*
  defined, 33
  secondary responses, 245–8
  *see also* ACTH; acute phase, hormones; cytokines; neurohormonal control
HPA (hypothalamic–pituitary–adrenal) axis, 130, 133
hydrocortisone, 51–2, 53–4, 265
hyperalgesia, 186, 188
  after injury, 312–15
  transmitters and, 315–16
hyperglycaemia, 250–1
hypermetabolism, 13, 263–4, 269
  children, 269
  induced, 265–6
hypersensitivity, 44, 109, 110
hypotension, 12–13, 224, 251
hypothalamic–pituitary–adrenal (HPA) axis, 130, 133
hypothalamus, 6, 115–16, 240
  and defence systems, 241
  and fluid loss, 242
  and immunomodulation, 109
  lesions of, 108–10
  and thermoregulation, 274
hypothermia, therapeutic, 16

IFN (interferons), 71
  and sickness behaviour, 155, 161
IL (interleukins), 13, 240, 271–3
  and behavioural effect mechanisms, 165–75
  central compartment of, 170
  and CNS control of sickness behaviour, 153, 155–75
  and define mechanisms against injury, 65, 68–9, 72, 74–5, 77–8, 80–4
  and flow phase, 240
  and metabolic/thermoregulatory control, 271–3, 276–83
  and neural/endocrine functions, 49–50, 52–3, 55, 57–9, 242–5, *244*
  and responses to injury, 34–9, 41, 43–5, 47–9
  and tissue damage, 242–5
illness
  defined, 190
  and pain, 195–6
IMC (intestinal mucosal mast cells), 59–60
immobility after trauma, 190–1
immune responses
  asymmetrical, 112–13
  brain lesions and, 108–13
  depression of, 252
  humoral, 66
immune system, communication with CNS, 113–15, 153
immunological injury, 44–5
immunomodulation
  brain regions involved in, 108–19
  *see also* neuroimmunomodulation
infection, 40, 66, 243
inflammation, 66–7, 83
inhibitory mechanisms and effects, 299–302, 309–12

injury
  anticipated, 11
  hyperalgesia after, 312–15
  mimicking of, *230*
  neurohormonal control of cytokines during, 32–85
    conclusions, 82–5
  and pain, 295
  phases following, 5
  treatment summarised, 14
  types, 34–5
  *see also* defence (arousal) reaction; responses to injury; tissue injury
insulin
interleukins, *see* IL
interventional studies, 29
intestinal mucosal mast cells, *see* IMC
intestinal tract, invasions of, 68
involution, 32
ischaemia, 7–8

L-NAME, *174*
labile molecule, 27
lactate, 13
lactogenic hormones, 49–50
LBP (lipopolysaccharide binding protein), 47
LEM (leukocytic endogenous mediator), 45
lesions, brain, 108–13
leukocytic endogenous mediator (LEM). 45
limbic structures, 241
  lesions, 110–13
lipocortins, 56, 281
lipolysis, 251
lipopolysaccharide, *see* LBP, LPS
liver, 45, 46, 81–2
local defence, *see* inflammation
local inflammatory response to injury, 62–4
LPS (lipopolysaccharide), 40–4, 47–8, 72
  and acute phase, 41–2, 48
  neuroendocrine response to, 42–3
  rats, 165–6, *166*, *167*
  and sickness behaviour, 165–6, *166*, *167*
lungs, 210
lymph nodes, 114
lymphocytes, *see* T lymphocytes

macrophages
  and cytokines, *37*, 58
  neural and neuropeptide regulation, 58–9
  and wound healing, 67
mammals, small
  environmental temperature and injured, 14–15
  heat production, 8–9
  *see also* guinea-pigs; mice; rats
mast cells, *36*, 55–6, 59–60
  peritoneal (PMC), 58, 59–60
mediator functions, classified, 33–4
mediators
  platelet-derived, *39*
  produced by activated monocytes–macrophages, *37*
  released by neutrophilic granulocytes, *38*
  shared, 78–9
  soluble, 32–3
metabolic rate and thermoregulation
  animals, 266–8, *267*
  basic aspects, 261–3
  benefits of changes in, 283
  central control, 260–85
  clinical relevance, 282–5
  experiments, 265–8, *267*
  and injury, 263–5
  mechanisms of responses to injury, 26, 268–70
metabolism
  responses to injury, 260–85
  and trauma, 243
  *see also* metabolic rate and thermoregulation
mice
  brain lesions, 109, 111–12
  and CRF, 171
  cytokines
    injections, 163, 165, *165*
    neural and endocrine regulation of, 49–50, 52, 53–4, 55, 56, 57
  defence mechanisms against injury, 59, 63, 72, 74
  'handedness' and immune reactivity, 118
  limb ischaemia, 7–8
  and LPS, 165
  metabolism/thermoregulation, *267*
  oxygen consumption, 7
  and prostaglandins, 172–3
  responses to injury, 34, 35–6, 41, 42, 43–4, 48
  sickness behaviour, 156, *158*, 168, 170
  temperature for survival, 15
MMPI (Minnesota Multiphasic Personality Inventory), 195–6
monkeys, 43, 303, 314, 315
monoamine actions, 308–9
monocytes, *37*, 54
motor neurones, descending
  facilitation of, 316–17
  MPD (multiple personality disorder), 142
muscular reactions, 137–9

naloxone, 40, 50, 51, 225–6, 301–2, 304, 312
natural killer (NK) cells, 109
neck suction, *217*
necrobiosis, 12
nerve growth factor (NGF), 58

neural and endocrine regulation of cytokines, 49–61
neural and endocrine regulations of cytokines, 49–61
neural and neuropeptide regulation of cytokines, 58–9
neurobiological results of trauma, 123–44
  conclusions, 143–4
neurochemical pathways, destruction of, 28
neurochemical responses to trauma, 130–6, 239–53
neuroendocrine responses
  to injury, *46*
    adaptive and maladaptive features, 250–3
    pathways to initiate, 240–5
  to LPS, 42–3
  to physical trauma, 239–53
neuroendocrine system, role, 74–9
neurogenic inflammation, 62–3
neurohormonal control of cytokines, 32–85
  conclusions, 82–5
neuroimmunomodulation, brain structures involved in, 114, 115–18
neuromodulators, 188
neurones
  classes, 305
  dorsal horn, 302, 315
  sympathoexcitatory, 222
neuropeptides, 130–1
  regulation of cytokines, 58–61
  systems, 28
neurotransmitters, 300
  defined, 33
  response to haemorrhage and injury, 224–9
neutrophilic granulocytes, 60–1
  mediators released by, *38*
NF-IL-6, 49
NGF (nerve growth factor), 58
nitric oxide, 173, 174, 276
NK (natural killer) cells, 109
nociception
  brain control of, 302–3
  distinguished from pain, 184
  impulses, 6
    afferent, 8, 10, 11–12, 270
  modulation of, 188–9, 298–9
  system, 296–7
  *see also* pronociception; antinociception *and under* spinal cord
nociceptors, 185–6
  cutaneous, 296
noradrenaline, 9, 248, 307
NRM (nucleus raphe magnus), 220
NRPG (nucleus reticularis paragigantocellularis), 316
nutrition, 262, 284–5
'observational' studies, 29
opioids
  endogenous, 225–7
    segmental inhibition by, 300
    tonic spinal actions, 301–2
  exogenous, spinal actions, 300–1
  *see also* naxolone
OVLT (organum vasculosum of lamina terminalis), 168–9, 273
oxygen
  mice, 7
  rats, 8
  tension, 208
  transport, 12

PAD (primary afferent depolarization), 299
PAF (platelet activating factor), 71
PAG (periaqueductal grey matter), *214*, 215, 219, 303–5
  caudal ventrolateral, *214*, 215
  and central control of pain, 303–5
  and defence reactions, 297
  rats, 218
pain
  acute, 184, 190
  background to, 183–4
  behaviour, 189–96
  central control of, 295–317
  chronic, 184, 188, 190, 194, 195, 196
  concept of, 183–5
  coping with, 193–5
  function, 295
  measuring, 297–8
  mechanisms, 185–6
  neuroendocrine response, 241–2
  physiological and pathological, 189
psychological and behavioural aspects, 183–97
  sensitization types, 186–8
  *see also* antinociception; nociception; pronociception
panic disorder, 135, 136
parabrachial nuclei, 214–15
paragigantocellularis lateralis (PGL), 219–20
parasites, 40, 61
paraventricular nucleus (PVN), 274
PBL (peripheral blood leukocytes), 56–7
PDGF (platelet-derived growth factor), 71
peptides, 50
  calcitonin gene related (CGRP), 64
  propiomelanocortin-derived, 50
  *see also* neuropeptides
periaqueductal grey matter, *see* PAG
peripheral effector mechanisms, 268–70
peritoneal mast cells, *see* PMC

PGL (paragigantocellularis lateralis), 219–20
PGs (prostaglandins), 172–3
phagocytes, 66
physical agents, injury due to, 34–8
physiological habituation, impaired, 140
pigs
  biological injury, 42
  haemorrhage, *225*
pituitary, 6, 240, 241, 245–8
  *see also* HPA axis
platelets, 61
  mediators derived from, *39*
PMC (peritoneal mast cells), 58, 59–60
post-mortem delay, 27
post-traumatic stress disorder, *see* PTSD
pressor response, 'injury-induced, 216
primary afferent depolarization (PAD), 299
prolactin, 49–50, 74, 248
pronociception, 316–17
proopiomelanocortin-derived peptides, 50
propranolol, 56–7
prostaglandins, 172–3
proteins, 46–9
  catabolism, 252–3
psychological results of trauma, 123–44
  conclusions, 143–4
  *see also* PTSD
psychological traumas, most commonly reported, 142
psychophysiological reactions to trauma, 136–40
PTSD (post-traumatic stress disorder), 123–30, 124–30, 135, 137–40
  chronicity of, 125–6
  defined, 123
  duration of symptoms, 124–6
  prevalence, 126–9
  subtypes, 129–30
pulmonary inflammation, rats, 63–4
push–pull perfusion, 27
PVN (paraventricular nucleus), 274
pyrexia (fever), 16, 152, 260, 261, 264
  induced, 265
pyrogens, 13, 265–6
  animals, 268
  endogenous, 277, *278*
  *see also* cytokines; endotoxins

rabbits
  biological injury, 42, 44
  and endotoxins, 170
  haemorrhage, 204–5
  pain, central control of, 308, 310, 311
  pyrexia, 16
radiation, 34
rape victims, 124, 125, 126–7, 128, 139
  trauma syndrome, 140–1
raphe pathways, response to injury, 222–3, *223*
  *see also* NRM
rats
  and AVP, 174–5
  and CRF, 63, 132, 171
  cytokines
    injections, 162–5, *164*, 168–70, *169*
    neural and endocrine regulation of, 50–1, 54, 59, 60–1
  defence mechanisms against injury, 62–4, 70–2, 74
  haemorrhage, 204, *204*
  inflammation, 270
  lesions of brain, 109, 110, 117
  limb ischaemia, 8, 11
  and LPS, 165–6, *166*, *167*
  metabolism and thermoregulation, 26, 266, 267, *267*, 272, 273, 274–6, 278, 285
  neurones, 221–2
  oxygen consumption, 7, 8
  PAG, 218
  pain, central control of, 302, 303, 305–8, 310–16
  and prolactin, 71
  and prostaglandins, 172–3
  responses to injury, 35, 41, 42–3, 44, 45, 48, 49
  scalded, 13, 266
  sickness behaviour, 154, 156–8, *157*, 160, *160*
  temperature for survival, 14–15, 16
  thyroid, 247
  trauma, 277
receptors, 205–6
  agonists and antagonists, 226–7
  opioid, 226
reflex responses, reduced, 10
reflexes, and response to haemorrhage, 205–9
reminders, reactions to, 137–9
renin–angiotensin–aldosterone, hormones, 250
research problems, 22–3
responses to injury, 3–17, 34
  cardiovascular, 202–31. 215–23
  as continuum, 5
  duration, 11–12
  interpretations and questions, 14–17
  local and general, 24
  metabolic, and thermoregulatory, 260–85
  neuroendocrine, **46**, 239–53
  normalising period, 13
  simulated, 30
  survival value, 14
responses to trauma, CNS control, 22–31
reticular formations, lesions, 110

reticular formations, lesions, 110
rheumatoid arthiritis, 187
rodents, 277–8, *278*, 279, 282, 284–5; *see also* guinea-pigs; mice; rats
rostral lesions, 110
RVLM, *see under* ventrolateral medulla

scoring systems, 23
sensitization
central, 187
peripheral, 186–7
sensory nerves, 62
sepsis, and systemic defence, 79–82
serotonin, 307–8
serum TNF, *see* TNF
sex hormones, 57–8, 77
sheep, infected, 40
shock, 37–8
causation of, 3, 5, 84
endotoxic, 43–4, 81
and systemic defence mechanisms, 79–82
sickness
defined, 152, 190
and pain, 195–6
sickness behaviour, 155–6
assessed, 153–4
cancer patients, 155–6
CNS control of, 152–76
induced, 155–65
by cytokines, 155–8, *157*, *159*, 160–5
*see also under* mice; rats
6-hydroxydopamine, 15
SMI (skeletal muscle injury), *225*
SNS (somatic afferent nerve stimulation), *255*
soluble mediators, 32–3
somatostatin, 60
SP, 60–4
*see also* substance P
species-specific defence behaviours, 191–2
spinal cord, 296–300
actions of opioids, 300–2
events mediated by, 309–10
injured, 270
nociceptive circuits, 306–9
*see also* pain, central control of
spleen, 109, 111, 113, 114
startle reactions, 137
stress, 32, 117–18
analgesia induced by, 312
CSR (combat stress reaction), 129–30
neuroendocrine response to, 79
as response, 193
*see also* psychological results of trauma; PTSD
subcortical structures, lesions of, 111–13
substance P, 58, 59, 60, 187, 188
suicide, 134
sympathetic efferent activity, 219–22
control of, 211–13, *212*
sympathetic–adrenomedullary system, 6–7, 241
and trauma, 248–50
*see also* adrenaline; noradrenaline
systemic defence mechanisms, 68–73

T lymphocytes, 53, 59
cytokines derived from, *70*
and healing, 67
taste aversion, conditioned (CTA), 153–4, 156–8
telencephalon, 241
*see also* amygdala; hippocampus
temperature, *see* metabolic rate and thermoregulation; thermogenesis; thermoregulation
TENS (transcutaneous electrical nerve stimulation), 309
TGF (transforming growth factor), 67–8
thermogenesis, 261, 274–5
non-shivering, 268–9
responses, 8
thermoneutrality, 9, 16
thermoregulation
basic aspects, 261–3
'ebb' phase, 7–9
effector mechanisms, 26
heat production, 8–9
in humans and rats, 16
responses to injury, 260–85
and thermogenesis, brain sites involved in, 274–5
*see also* metabolic rate
thyroid, 77
hormones, 241, 246–7
tissue injury
experimental methods, 23–6, *24*
and neuroendocrine responses, 242–5
tissue injury combined with haemorrhage, 10, 35, 224–9
cardiovascular response to, 224–9
tissue mast cells, *see* mast cells
TNF (tumour necrosis factor), 45, 48, 52, 53, 69, 72, 247, 272–3, 43–4
and interleukins, 243–5
response, *73*
and sickness behaviour, 156, 167
tonic descending inhibition, 306
tonic spinal actions, 300–1
transmitters
and brain control of spinal nociceptive circuits, 306–9
and hyperalgesia/allodynia, 315–16
TSH (thyroid stimulating hormone, 241, 246–7

tumour necrosis factor, *see* TNF

ultraviolet radiation, 34

vagal afferent activity
  control, 209–11, *210–11*
  modulation, 218–19, *220*
vasopressin, 6–7, 28, 246
  arginine (AVP), 78, 173–5, 242, 246, 251, 281
ventrolateral medulla, 211–13, *212*
  RVLM (rostral ventrolateral medulla), 211–12, *212*, 222, 303–5
  and central control of pain, 303–5
virus infection, 66
visceral alerting response, 217–18

war experience, 127–8, 137–9, 141, 142
  CSR (combat stress reaction), 129–30
Wiggers model, 12, 17
wounds
  demands made by, 13
  macrophages and healing, 67

X-irradiation, 34

yohimbine, 136, 307